SPORTS PSYCHIATRY

Strategies for Life Balance
and Peak Performance

22 APR 2012

JOHN

ALL THAT I'VE
LEARNED IN THIRTY
YEARS AS A MILITARY
& SPORTS PSYCHIATRIST.
GRATEFUL TO BE A PART
OF THIS ORGANIZATION & TEAM
& LOOK FORWARD TO WORKING
WITH YOU & YOUR STAFF
TO GET BETTER DAY BY DAY

DAVID

SPORTS PSYCHIATRY

Strategies for Life Balance and Peak Performance

David R. McDuff, M.D.

Clinical Professor of Psychiatry
University of Maryland School of Medicine,
University of Maryland, Baltimore;
and
Adjunct Associate Professor of Psychiatry,
F. Edward Hébert School of Medicine,
Uniformed Services University of the Health Sciences,
Bethesda, Maryland

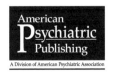

American Psychiatric Publishing
A Division of American Psychiatric Association

Washington, DC
London, England

Note: The author has worked to ensure that all information in this book is accurate at the time of publication and consistent with general psychiatric and medical standards, and that information concerning drug dosages, schedules, and routes of administration is accurate at the time of publication and consistent with standards set by the U.S. Food and Drug Administration and the general medical community. As medical research and practice continue to advance, however, therapeutic standards may change. Moreover, specific situations may require a specific therapeutic response not included in this book. For these reasons and because human and mechanical errors sometimes occur, we recommend that readers follow the advice of physicians directly involved in their care or the care of a member of their family.

Books published by American Psychiatric Publishing (APP) represent the findings, conclusions, and views of the individual authors and do not necessarily represent the policies and opinions of APP or the American Psychiatric Association.

David R. McDuff, M.D., has no competing interests to disclose during the year preceding manuscript submission.

To buy 25–99 copies of this or any other APP title at a 20% discount, please contact Customer Service at appi@psych.org or 800–368–5777. To buy 100 or more copies of the same title, please e-mail us at bulksales@psych.org for a price quote.

Copyright © 2012 American Psychiatric Association
ALL RIGHTS RESERVED

Manufactured in the United States of America on acid-free paper
16   15   14   13   12   5   4   3   2   1
First Edition

Typeset in New Baskerville and Franklin Gothic.

American Psychiatric Publishing,
a Division of American Psychiatric Association
1000 Wilson Boulevard
Arlington, VA 22209–3901
www.appi.org

Library of Congress Cataloging-in-Publication Data
McDuff, David R., 1952–
  Sports psychiatry : strategies for life balance and peak performance / by David R. McDuff. — 1st ed.
       p. ; cm.
  Includes bibliographical references and index.
  ISBN 978-1-58562-415-7 (pbk. : alk. paper)
  I. American Psychiatric Publishing. II. Title.
  [DNLM: 1. Sports—psychology. 2. Athletes—psychology. 3. Athletic Injuries—psychology. 4. Mental Disorders—therapy. 5. Physical Fitness. QT 260]
  616.890088'796—dc23

                                                        2012004141

British Library Cataloguing in Publication Data
A CIP record is available from the British Library.

This book is dedicated to
Michael Kendall Flanagan, 1951–2011
Husband, Father, Son, Friend, and Fly Fisherman

Close—but Far Away

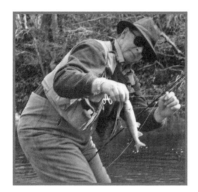 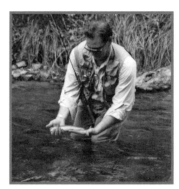

Baltimore Orioles Pitcher, Coach, Executive, and Broadcaster

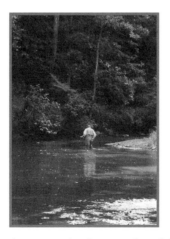

Eventually, all things merge into one, and a river runs through it. The river was cut by the world's great flood and runs over rocks from the basement of time. On some of the rocks are timeless raindrops. Under the rocks are the words, and some of the words are theirs.
I am haunted by waters.

—Norman Maclean, *A River Runs Through It and Other Stories* (1976)

Contents

Foreword ix

Preface xi

Introduction xv

1 **Scope of Practice** 1

2 **Mental Preparation** 29

3 **Stress Recognition and Control** .53

4 **Energy Regulation** 69

5 **Substance Use and Abuse** 85

    Appendix 5–1: Fact Sheets on Substance Use
    and Sports 115

6 **Injury Recovery and Pain Control** 129

7 **Common Mental Disorders** 165

8 **Teams, Medical Staff, and Sports Leadership** 195

    Appendix 8–1: Symptom Screening Form 215

9 Developmental and Cultural Competence. 219

10 Evidence Base and Future Directions 233

Index 257

Foreword

One of the important things I have learned through my journey in athletics is that performing at the highest levels requires more than just physical and intellectual talent. As team members learn more about how to handle the stress of competition and everyday life, they increase their chances of success in athletic competition. Dr. David McDuff, the team psychiatrist for the Baltimore Ravens since the franchise started in 1996, has been an important member of the staff and has helped the team win, which is always a primary focus.

Having the physical and mental talent to be a professional athlete does not mean a person has the ability necessary to compete at the highest level. When I was a player with the Cleveland Browns, owner Art Modell and head coach Sam Rutigliano used a sports psychiatrist and psychologist from the Cleveland Clinic (in the late 1970s) to create a team-based inner circle of support for Browns players with issues ranging from alcohol and drugs to family and personal problems. When the Browns moved to Baltimore in 1996, Mr. Modell required that the new sports medicine group include a sports psychiatrist with expertise in addictions and stress. Dr. McDuff was hired with the initial group from the University of Maryland School of Medicine and has been in that role ever since. When Steve Bisciotti became the owner of the Ravens in 2004, he endorsed this program of assistance for players, coaches, team and front office staff, and family members, thereby continuing a culture of player, employee, and family centered support.

Dr. McDuff provides crisis and routine services in the training room and office for stress control, substance prevention, sleep and energy improvement, injury rehabilitation, pain control, mental preparation, family support, and mental disorder treatment. He is available to the organization's staff and leadership 24 hours a day, 7 days a week. Every year he helps numerous players, coaches, team staff, front office employees, and family members address problems and concerns, improve at work and home, and become better people.

Dr. McDuff has written a timely and comprehensive book on the evolving specialty of sports psychiatry. From the perspective of a frontline psychiatrist working at all competitive levels, he provides a vital road map for mental health providers, athletic trainers, and sports medicine practitioners involved in the care of athletes (as both competitors and people). He describes a set of eight core competencies and demonstrates the expert application of these with diverse case studies from many sports. Through his descriptions of working with teams, medical staffs, and leaders, he presents a model for other sports organizations to consider and adopt. *Sports Psychiatry: Strategies for Life Balance and Peak Performance* is a book whose time has come. It has valuable lessons for anyone involved in sports—and for that matter those in other businesses and corporations—and is an important read for understanding the mental and emotional dimensions of sports competition and management.

Ozzie Newsome
National Football League Hall of Fame Tight End, Cleveland Browns;
General Manager and Executive Vice President, Baltimore Ravens

Preface

I have been consistently and passionately connected to sports for 50 years and counting. As a competitor, spectator, fan, manager, parent, coach, author, lecturer, print media contributor, mental skills trainer, and sports psychiatrist, I have come to understand the intricate behavioral routines and intense emotions of training, competition, injury, mistakes, scoring, choking, winning, and losing.

My earliest memories of sports are from attending University of Alabama football games with my father, uncle, and brother. With Paul "Bear" Bryant as head coach, the Alabama Crimson Tide football team became a national powerhouse and source of pride and inspiration for an entire state and me. From 1960 to 1969, Alabama had a 60–5–1 win-loss-tie record (.923) and won three national championships. From 1970 to 1979, the team's record was 92–15–1 (.860), and Alabama won three additional national championships.

In 1996, because of my background in sports and my expertise in addiction, military, and performance medicine, I was hired as the team psychiatrist and mental skills trainer for two professional sports teams: the Baltimore Orioles, a Major League Baseball team, and the Baltimore Ravens, a National Football League (NFL) team. Subsequently, I have worked with teams and individual athletes in other professional sports (golf and tennis) and at other levels, including collegiate, high school, and club sports. In a remarkable coincidence, I now work for Ozzie Newsome, one of Alabama's most famous football players and an NFL Hall of Fame tight end, in his current role as general manager and executive vice president of the Baltimore Ravens.

I have encountered much during my ongoing 50-year love affair with sports. However, the last 16 years as an active sports psychiatrist have provided me with a special opportunity to stand with and learn from some of the best teams, owners, general managers, athletic directors, athletes, coaches, medical staff, family members, and front office staffs. I have taken something of value from every athlete, coach, administrator, doctor, practitioner, athletic trainer, and strength and conditioning professional whose path I have crossed, and I hope to share their expertise with readers of this book. In a broader sense, I have taught and learned many of life's most fundamental lessons through the compressed time capsule of sports competition. As a parent of four athletes, I have a special commitment to the athlete's family to ensure that they say the right things, take the right steps, and stay healthy along the sports journey of their son or daughter or niece or nephew. I am motivated by a deep desire to do what I can to help athletes and coaches and those who care for them to do their best as they seek excellence and try to stay balanced and healthy in that pursuit.

I specifically want to acknowledge the influence and support of the following individuals who made this book a true narrative of my life's work.

- **My family:** Marie, DeForest, Lee, Shelley, Claire, and the Sanders family—You embraced my passions, weathered my absences, and taught me to love, to be loved, and to chill out; Charles and Carolyn—You gave me drive, creativity, conscientiousness, and a love of work; Judy, John, Carol, and Scott—You shared with me the joy and sorrow of our childhood; Oliver and Julia, Joy and Jerry, and Fred and Julie—You helped me through adversity.
- **My early friends:** Eric Blankenship, Mike Sweeting, Van Wharton, Nick Mamalis, Donna Hall, and Roy Hammock—You fueled my love of running, music, food, singing, and the arts.
- **My mentors at Spring Hill College:** Drs. MacNamara, Hemphill, Kearley, and Brandon, and Fr. Owens-Howard—You taught me a love of science and philosophy and to learn, teach, and question.
- **My medical school mentors:** Joe Sapira, Robert White, Robert Green, and Claude Brown—You gave me a love of psychiatry, neurology, and psychosomatic medicine.
- **My army mentors:** Dave Armitage, Bill Logan, Jerry Bissell, David Madison, Dan Veneziano, Tom Guyden, Bob Yaryan, Frank Abundo, Madonna Bark, Bob Sokol, Calvin Neptune, Gary Newsome, Bob Hales, Bob Ursano, Walter Reich, and Bill Boggiano—You molded my career.
- **My academic psychiatry mentors:** Walter Weintraub, George Balis, Stuart Keill, Stuart Tiegel, Jeanette Johnson, John Steinberg, Carl Soderstrom, Carlo DiClemente, and Jerry Jaffe—You encouraged my teaching, research, and writing.
- **My addiction psychiatry colleagues:** Wendy Maters, Art Cohen, Mary Klecz, Wayne Clemmons, Robert Schwartz, Tony Tommasello, Hal Crossley, Devang Gandhi, Chris Welsh, Eric Weintraub, Barbara Deluty,

Philip Hershelman, Pam Agarwahl, and Linda McCusker—You built a division and model teaching and service programs.

- **My sports psychiatry colleagues:** Don Thompson, Johannes Dalmasy, Peggy Curran Burns, Deb LeVan, Rob White, Wanda Binns, Jewell Benford, and Jessica Mohler—We all learned together.
- **My sports medicine colleagues:** Andy Tucker, Bill Goldiner, John Wilckens, Leigh Ann Curl, Bill Tessendorf, Mark Smith, Richie Bancells, Brian Ebel, Dave Walker, Tim Bishop, Jay Shiner, Alan Sokoloff, Doug Miller, and Janice Furst—You shared your knowledge, skill, energy, and compassion.
- **My sports teams' executives and staff:** Pat Gillick, Mike Flanagan, Dave Stockstill, Don Buford, Lenny Johnston, Ozzie Newsome, Dick Cass, Kevin Byrne, and Elizabeth Jackson—You are sports professionals who care about people.
- **My students, interns, residents, fellows, and the staff at Junction:** You asked the hard questions, gave me insights, inspired me, and kept me young.

Introduction

Along with music, art, religion, theater, democracy, capitalism, unemployment, violence, taxes, urban poverty, television, the Internet, texting, and military power, sports are a central part of American culture in the twenty-first century. The cultural impact of sports is at an all-time high because of rising participation rates, expanded opportunities for women, and the popularity of professional-level sports. For example, the most recent survey of the National Federation of State High School Associations (2012) showed that high school athletic participation rates increased for the twenty-second consecutive year. For academic year 2010–2011, a total of 7,667,955 participants (4,494,406 boys and 3,173,549 girls) resulted in an astounding high school athletic participation rate of more than 55%.

The numbers of teams and participants for colleges and universities have also risen. The most recent (2009–2010) participation rates report of the National Collegiate Athletic Association (NCAA; 2010) revealed that the numbers of Divisions I, II, and III championship sports teams (17,990) and participants (430,301) were at all-time highs and up substantially from the 11,025 teams (+63.2%) and 231,985 participants (+85.5%) in 1981–1982. For NCAA schools, the gender breakdown has changed substantially over the years, primarily due to the passage of Title IX of the Education Amendments of 1972. The 2008–2009 NCAA report revealed that 53% of teams (9,470 of 17,814) and 42.8% of participants (180,347 of 421,164) were women. These changes are dramatic when compared to pre–Title IX data. According to Carpenter and Acosta's (2010) 33-year longitudinal study on women in intercollegiate sports, only 16,000 females were participating in college athletics in 1968, compared with over 180,000 just 40 years later. In addition, the average number of women's teams per school has grown from 2.5 in 1970 to 8.64 in 2010.

Professional sports in the United States are extremely popular and dominated by four media market giants: football, baseball, basketball, and ice hockey (Plunkett Research 2010). The National Football League is undeniably the top professional league, with $9 billion in annual revenue, followed by Major League Baseball ($6.8 billion), the National Basketball Association ($4 billion), and the National Hockey League ($2.3 billion). For these professional teams and all others, including college, advertisers spend an astounding $27 billion per year. This marketing and branding power explains in part the substantial influence that professional athletes have on youth and adults in general and on athletes at all competitive levels.

From a psychiatric and psychological perspective, the most interesting part of sports does not involve the rates of participation, ratings, revenue, or results, but rather the pressure and stress that daily change the emotions and actions of athletes, coaches, parents, and spectators. The emotions of competition are what make sports great and difficult. From one critical athletic moment to another, athletes shift from positive emotions, thoughts, and actions that support consistent performance to negative ones that degrade it. The key emotions of sports are the same as for other important activities in life, but are often more intense. On the positive side, individuals feel fun, joy, pride, ecstasy, excitement, accomplishment, mastery, calm, and confidence, and on the negative side, they feel anxiety, doubt, fear, pain, sadness, disappointment, embarrassment, frustration, and anger. Each of these emotions must be controlled, and the energy that creates them needs to be channeled into consistent play. The fears of training and competition—fears of mistakes, failure, injury, collapse, disappointment, criticism, embarrassment, and success (with the added pressure that success brings)—are especially important.

Fortunately, psychiatrists and other mental health clinicians interested in sports practice already have the necessary general skills to help competitive athletes to deal with adversity, stress, competitive pressure, loss and trauma, injury and pain, transitions, family conflict, tough choices, mistakes, media scrutiny, money management, and even success. These practitioners, however, are typically lacking sports-specific knowledge and skills. Beneficial knowledge includes sports culture, team structure and function, elite competition, injuries, performance-enhancing substances, urine drug testing, and family stress patterns. Useful skills include core competencies such as mental preparation, sleep and energy management, substance prevention, injury recovery, pain management, developmental and gender competency, and organizational consultation.

Because of the broad impact and popularity of sports, I have written this book with several audiences in mind. First, the book is useful for mental health professionals (i.e., social workers, licensed professional counselors, marriage and family counselors, psychiatrists, psychologists, and advanced practice psychiatric nurses) who work with or may want to work with athletes or teams. Second, the book is intended for primary care physicians and other general practitioners, sports medicine fellows and physicians, sports chiropractors and dietitians, certified athletic trainers, and strength and conditioning professionals who have periodic or regular contact with athletes and teams and who want to strengthen their emotional and behavioral intervention skill set. Third, the book is for athletes, who can obtain a formula for success in sports and life, as well as review and learn from the case examples. Fourth, the book can be used by owners, athletic directors, coaches, managers, front office staff, and line administrators who work in sports, to gain a broad perspective of the common struggles of athletes and teams and the resources that are available to assist them. Finally, parents and family members can read the book to help them better support their athletes' dreams of success and to help ensure a lasting joy of training and competition.

Throughout the book, I have included stories of success and failure and presented problems and solutions from many sports at all competitive levels. Unless otherwise noted, every story is a composite of many similar cases, and the details have been substantially altered to ensure confidentiality. Because the stories are universal and common, readers might think they recognize specific individuals. I have mixed the stories with clinical experience and the evidence base of sports psychiatry with the intent to inform, teach, encourage, and inspire. Indeed, I have written this book as a guide for athletes, teams, administrators, coaches, and providers to push for peak performance and success; however, the book emphasizes the type of success that preserves human dignity, moral perspective, and quality of life while also promoting unity, sound judgment, personal growth, pride, and a lasting sense of accomplishment.

References

Carpenter LJ, Acosta RV: Women in Intercollegiate Sport: A Longitudinal National Study Thirty Three Year Update 1977–2010. 2010. Available at: http://www.acostacarpenter.org. Accessed September 23, 2011.

National Collegiate Athletic Association: Student-Athlete Participation 1981–82–2009–10: NCAA Sports Sponsorship and Participation Rates Report. Indianapolis, IN, National Collegiate Athletic Association, 2010. Available at: http://www.ncaapublications.com/productdownloads/pr2011.pdf. Accessed September 23, 2011.

National Federation of State High School Associations: 2010–11 High School Athletics Participation Survey. Available at: http://www.nfhs.org/content.aspx?id=3282. Accessed February 2, 2012.

Plunkett Research: Sports Statistics: Sports Industry Overview. Houston, TX, Plunkett Research, 2010. Available at: http://plunkettresearch.com/Industries/Sports/SportsStatistics/tabid/273/Default.aspx. Accessed September 23, 2011.

Chapter 1

Scope of Practice

Many psychiatrists and other mental health professionals have broad and specialized skills that are useful to individuals of all ages who are involved in sports at all competitive levels—including athletes, coaches, teams, administrators, owners, sports medicine physicians, other clinicians, athletic trainers, and family members. Since the 1980s, sporadic articles and one book on the developing practice area of sports psychiatry have appeared (Begel and Burton 2000; Glick et al. 2009). In addition, in 1997 the International Society for Sports Psychiatry was founded to bring together psychiatrists with special interest and expertise in sports and to link this expertise with sports medicine, sports organizations, and the community. The earliest sports psychiatry reports focused on the diagnosis and treatment of common mental disorders in athletes, which include attention-deficit, learning, sleep, mood, anxiety, impulse control (aggression), eating, and substance use disorders, as well as the common problems of stress, risky behaviors, precompetition anxiety, choking, overtraining, fatigue, burnout, injury, and life balance. Later articles expanded into consulting with teams and organizational leaders, assisting parents, optimizing health and fitness, recovering from injury, and improving performance; however, these practitioner roles and the skills needed for them are not well defined (Gee 2010). Until recently, few descriptions of actual applied experiences or case studies have been provided. Documenting the main lessons learned from years of work in collegiate and professional sports, McDuff et al. (2005) describe various situations in which prompt assistance is effective and appreciated. This information is especially beneficial when services to athletes and the teaching to primary care sports medicine and addiction psychiatry fellows are provided where a team practices and competes.

1

In this chapter, I provide an overview of a broadened scope of practice for sports psychiatrists and mental health professionals. I briefly describe eight core clinical competencies and representative cases. The competencies have been developed from many years of providing on-site sports psychiatric services to athletes, coaches, family members, and team and front office staff at professional, collegiate, high school, and club levels of competition. The cases, which come directly from my practice and illustrate common problems and solutions along with various perspectives, are designed to be useful for clinicians, coaches, athletic trainers, and parents and other family members. The eight core competencies are 1) mental preparation; 2) stress control and life balance; 3) sleep and energy management; 4) substance use and misuse; 5) injury recovery and pain management; 6) mental disorder treatment; 7) working with teams, sports leadership, and medical staff; and 8) developmental, gender, and cultural skills. All of these competencies are important and routinely required during both the competitive season and the off-season. Figure 1–1 represents the relationships of these competencies to the athlete's talent, experience, athletic and fitness fundamentals, injury history, and coaching and family support. These core competencies are detailed in Chapters 2 through 9. In Chapter 10, I discuss the current evidence base for sports psychiatry and future directions.

Mental Preparation

Mental preparation and mental skills training become more important contributors to competitive consistency and positive results as the athletes' talent and competitive levels increase. Figure 1–2 illustrates the elements of mental preparation that are progressively more important for building self-confidence. Most teams and athletes focus almost exclusively on technical skills, tactical strategies, fitness, nutrition, and injury management, but neglect the mental and emotional aspects of practice and competition and of winning and losing.

Basic Mental Skills

The basic mental skills of breathing and relaxation, positive self-talk, focus and attention shifting, visualization and imagery, and motivation and persistence provide a pathway to competitive self-confidence. (Further discussion and case studies of each of these specific basic mental skills is provided in Chapter 2, "Mental Preparation.") The basic mental skills are useful before and during practice and competition to quiet the mind from distractions, relax the body to allow automatic fluid movement,

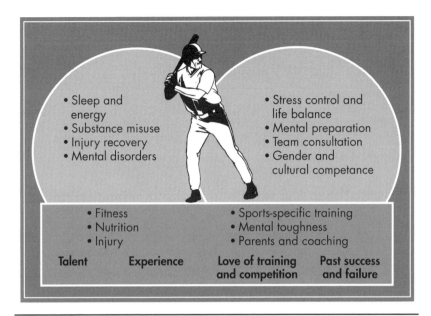

FIGURE 1–1. Sports psychiatry: core competencies (circles) enhancing athletic fundamentals (base).

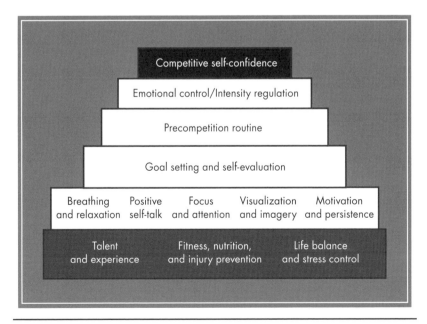

FIGURE 1–2. Pyramid of mental skills linking athletic fundamentals to competitive self-confidence.

raise energy and intensity, and finally shift attention to a state of automatic awareness and play. Relaxation is usually accomplished by breathing and stretching, although some athletes use music to detach from the other demands of the day and switch to a focus on sports. Positive self-talk is used multiple times each day, as well as during practice and competition. Short positive phrases, such as "crisp and quick" or "run light" or "play through," can be repeated and combined with visualization of successful execution or outcomes. Visualization is best done while a person is in a relaxed state with eyes closed and is sitting in a chair or on a floor or bed. Combining short periods of seeing positive play with slight motor activation allows athletes to say, see, and feel the desired athletic movement. This strategy permits the brain's auditory, visual, and kinesthetic circuits to activate in support of repetitive coordinated movement. The following case demonstrates the use of some of these basic skills.

Case Study: Precompetition Anxiety

A high school distance runner and a football player each sought assistance because of precompetition anxiety and performance inconsistency at the beginning of the season. Each athlete noted increased arousal, race/game worrying, restless sleep, and decreased appetite. On competition day, their arousal increased dramatically and included motor restlessness, muscle tightness, increased heart rate, shallow breathing, nausea and occasional vomiting, loss of appetite, and diminishing confidence. Both were seniors who had early success in their sport and felt increasing pressure to lead their teams by performing better each year.

Assessment: Each athlete was seen in the office for an initial 2-hour consultation with parental participation. Neither athlete had a history of excessive worrying or anxiety in other important life areas, including school, work, or social situations. Both were taught several basic mental skills to reduce precompetition arousal and asked to return in 2 weeks and to maintain e-mail contact between sessions.

Intervention: The athletes were educated about the need to control their activation and arousal through the following sequence: 1) quiet the mind, 2) relax the body, 3) raise and circulate energy, and 4) focus and shift attention. They were taught to quiet the mind by changing to breath cycles that strongly emphasized expiration. They were taught two exercises to practice multiple times each day: 1) three lengthening clearing breaths to reset and channel the energy of arousal and 2) a 2-minute patterned breathing exercise to produce and maintain relaxation.

The athletes were taught to use the three clearing breaths before competition. In this procedure, if arousal starts to build, the athlete stops the breath cycle and clears out all the air strongly until a small circle of tightness can be felt in the center of the abdomen just above the navel. While in a sitting or standing position, the athlete takes in air evenly through the nose until the lungs are filled fully from the bottom to the top at the level of the collar bones, and then expires the air smoothly through pursed lips to a count of 4. A second breath is taken in through the nose to a full fill, and then the air is released smoothly through pursed lips to a count of 6. After the third breath is taken in through the nose, the expiration lasts to a count of 8. Then the athlete shifts to easy breathing (nose/nose or mouth/mouth). The athlete repeats the entire "three-clear" process each time his arousal level rises.

The athletes were told to perform a 2-minute patterned breathing exercise while sitting on the floor or in a chair or while driving four to six times a day. In this exercise, the person clears out all the air; breathes in through the nose evenly to a count of 4; holds the breath to a count of 7 (while rocking to and fro with each count); and releases the breath evenly to a count of 8. Eight breath cycles are completed before shifting to easy breathing (nose/nose or mouth/mouth). This 4–7–8 pattern is best done at first with eyes closed (except when driving). The purpose of this exercise is to quiet the mind and settle the body by clearing out the excess energy and tension.

Outcome: Almost immediately, both athletes were able to reduce their worrying and physiological arousal. Many of their precompetition anxiety symptoms disappeared or diminished. Over time, they were able to control the rising energy of precompetition arousal and channel it for use during competition. In addition, both began to sleep better and were able to take in more fluids and nutrition the night before and the day of competition.

Complex Mental Skills

The more complex skills of goal setting, self-evaluation, precompetition routine, and emotional control and intensity regulation ensure that athletes and teams are ready to compete and can play with emotional control despite changes in the competitive environment (Beswick 2001; Dorfman 2000; Dorfman and Kuehl 1995; Loehr and Schwartz 2003; Porter 2003, 2004; Rotella 2004). (Further discussion and case studies of each of these specific complex mental skills is provided in Chapter 2.) The complex skills become an essential part of the process of preparing to practice and compete, with steady improvement as the main goal.

Goal Setting

Goals can be established for a short term (preseason, a tournament), intermediate term (a season), or longer period (an entire year). Goals should be written, specific, and accompanied by action steps that detail the activity, frequency, and number of repetitions. The following is an example from football for a receiver: "Improve my ability to run good routes and look the ball into my hands each time so that I increase my catches by 20% in the upcoming season." The accompanying action steps might be as follows: 1) run 20 extra routes three times each week with my position coach; 2) take 50 extra catches using the passing machine three times each week working high and low, in and out; and 3) visualize with 5% movement activation daily for 5 minutes while running sideline, crossing, and deep routes.

Self-Evaluation

Self-evaluation is also best done in written form; players should review a week or two of practice or a competition and solicit feedback from coaches or other players. A simple one-page form can be used for assessing the positives of play and how they helped, the negatives of play and how they got in the way, and the behaviors that helped to overcome the negatives (Porter 2003, p. 27). This review can then be used to create the work plan for the next week or two.

Precompetition Routine

The precompetition routine is often neglected as part of mental and emotional preparation. Typically, this routine begins many hours before competition or 30–45 minutes before practice. In addition to raising the player's heart rate and activating the kinetic chain of muscles, the routine helps to clear the athlete's mind of the clutter of the day and release the tension in the muscles so that intensity can be gradually increased and concentration sharpened. For example, a baseball or softball player could perform the following sequence: 1) relaxation breathing and visualization while getting dressed, 2) a short period (e.g., 5 minutes) of indoor cardio warm-up (e.g., using an exercise bike), 3) outdoor cardio activity (sprints) and stretching, and 4) batting practice. For each swing during batting practice, the player might practice an organized prepitch routine involving clearing breaths; adjusting the gloves and stance; and gripping, releasing, and regripping the bat. The following case demonstrates the use of some of these complex skills (Grossbard et al. 2009).

Case Study: Team Cohesion and Confidence

High school and college soccer teams sought assistance for improving game preparation, cohesion, and confidence. The high school team had established a record of competitive excellence, including several state championships, over 5 years. They were a preseason favorite to repeat as county and state champions. After winning several early season games, they tied their first two county games. In both games, they did not look ready to play and gave up early goals. The coach asked a sports psychiatrist for assistance with the pregame routine to raise and make consistent the team's intensity level.

The college team had a successful season but lost several close conference games in overtime. They made it to the National Collegiate Athletic Association (NCAA) tournament but as a low seed. They were to face an in-state rival in the first round and then, if they advanced, a high seed that had beaten them badly earlier in the season. The coach asked a sports psychiatrist for assistance with building team cohesion and confidence.

Assessment: The psychiatrist held separate meetings with the head coach and the team captains of each team. The high school team had adopted a pregame routine of quiet visualization on the bus or in the locker room before going onto the field for a short, unstructured pregame warm-up. The meetings with the psychiatrist led to the conclusion that this pregame routine was not readying the team to play and that the first 5–10 minutes of play were needed to raise the team's intensity level to that of the opponent.

The college team consisted of a talented group of experienced and first-year players who had not been able to win big games. The coach and captains were worried about a first-round upset to the in-state rival or intimidation by the higher-seeded team if their team made it to the second round. The conclusion was that the team lacked confidence in bigger games and that with the extra pressure, team communication and connection tended to fragment.

Intervention: The entire pregame routine of the high school team was revamped. Quiet individual visualization was replaced with loud, energizing music that was chosen by the team and played through a boom box. The team adopted the intent to "rock the bus" with music and movement on the way to games. The unstructured pregame routine was replaced with a fast-paced series of high-intensity small-sided drills, alternating with team stretching. Just before beginning the game, the starting team and first reserves joined together for some fast-paced seven-versus-seven play to create competitive game intensity and produce focus and rapid attention-shifting.

The college team decided to develop a team building exercise on the 4-hour bus ride to the tournament. Each team member and coach was asked to anonymously bring a single song to become the "team warm-up song." Thirty songs were played, and everyone rated each song and was asked to guess who chose the song. This process created a highly interactive process that was fun and relaxing. Three songs were eventually chosen, and the captains elected to play each of them on the ride from the hotel to the stadium. The captains and several injured experienced players began working on team communication and confidence during several facilitated team meetings and during practices and pregame warm-ups. The sports psychiatrist met with every player and asked for input about the team's strengths and areas for improvement. The statements "communicate" and "let the ball move" became unifying team concepts.

Outcome: The high school team quickly became ready to play with good team intensity for every remaining game. A focus on pressuring the ball connected the back line with the midfield and forward players. The team won all remaining county games and also won the regional and state tournaments to become state champions.

The college team players became more connected to the coaches and each other. Several team leaders called a meeting the night before the first two tournament games and symbolically passed around a piece of cloth and asked each individual to tear off a piece and wear it through the tournament. The team dominated play in the first game, winning easily, and then upset the higher-seeded team with a score of 1 to 0, with a late-game header goal and an incredible defensive effort in the last 5 minutes.

Stress Control and Life Balance

Athletic participation produces a patterned demand on athletes, coaches, and staff that results from long days, exhaustion, the pressure of competition, injury and pain, disappointment, and the requirement to balance sports with other important activities such as school, relaxation, and socializing with family and friends. The demands of sports may produce disruptions in sleep, energy, and appetite, or the increased use of substances such as alcohol, marijuana, and tobacco. In addition to the general effects of stress, four specific stress reaction patterns can interfere with performance: 1) anxiety (active thinking, worrying, arousal, tension, poor sleep); 2) depression (disappointment, sadness, isolation, loneliness, negative thinking, loss of confidence, crying spells); 3) anger (frustration, irritation, critical comments, impatience, acting out, fights); and 4) somatic symptoms (pain, gastrointestinal upset, rapid breathing and heart rate, chest pain, skin eruptions, headaches). Athletes can have one or several of these stress responses. Furthermore, athletic competition can trigger intense emotions that are normal, quick, and patterned and that tend to appear within tenths of a second in the face and core (neck, chest, and abdomen). The typical stress emotions of competition are frustration, disappointment, anxiety, and embarrassment. Each of these emotions signals its presence in the body's major organ systems (cardiovascular, musculoskeletal, gastrointestinal, respiratory, and dermatological), and each requires action to prevent performance degradation. If unmanaged, frustration changes over time to anger and resentment and shifts attention out of the present to a person or a situation; disappointment changes over time into depression and shifts attention to the past; anxiety changes into fear or panic and shifts attention to the future; and embarrassment changes into guilt or shame and also shifts attention to the past. When an outlet is not created for these signal emotions, they tend to circulate and intensify and prevent athletes from performing in the moment, such as competing point to point in tennis or shot to shot in golf.

Stress must be controlled through supportive social networks and life balance. Talking does help, and coaches, teammates, friends, family, chaplains, and mental health professionals are good resources. Life balance comes from good sleep and nutrition, an organized awakening routine to produce sufficient energy for the day, a series of short recovery breaks throughout the day, and a solid unwinding routine at night. The following are the most common stress control strategies relevant to sports: 1) triggering the body's relaxation reflex system (breathing, massage, meditation, music, stretching, etc.); 2) thinking positively and looking calm and in control; 3) developing and using a support network; 4) staying informed and avoiding rumors; 5) avoiding excessive stimulants and sedatives; 6) developing good time management skills; 7) developing positive routines and visualizing success; and 8) having fun and enjoying training, competition, and other activities. Each of these strategies is discussed in detail in Chapter 3, "Stress Recognition and Control." The following case illustrates some common stress-linked problems and solutions.

Case Study: Stress and Disappointment

A second-year college soccer player sought assistance 1 month into the season because of disappointment with her play and playing time. She played a lot in her first year and had worked hard during the preseason to move into a starting role as an attacking midfielder. She became deeply disappointed and frustrated with the head coach when her first-year roommate instead started the first six games. She began to wonder whether the coach did not like her and whether she may never become a starter again.

Assessment: The player did not have the typical history of a college soccer player in that she started playing at age 11, rather than at age 5 or 6 as did her teammates. Her primary sport had previously been basketball. Once she committed to soccer, however, she worked tirelessly to improve her game by attending camps, using an individual athletic trainer, and playing on high-level club teams. While in high school, she played for her school team and a regional travel club and participated in her state's Youth Soccer Olympic Development Program. She arrived at college with superior fitness and was ready to make an immediate impact. Her first year was filled with stress as she attempted to balance academics with soccer and to manage a minor but recurring ankle injury (her first experience with injury). In addition, she did not get along with her three suite mates; at the end of the year, she decided to move off campus with several lacrosse athletes. Throughout her first year, she had been disappointed with the consistency of her play and frustrated with the lack of recognition of her skills by the coaching staff. She did not feel that she could approach anyone on the staff to voice her concerns. Over the summer before her second year, she played regularly at home and hired soccer and fitness trainers. She returned to campus with the rest of her team 2 weeks before the fall semester, feeling confident that she would move into a starting role. She was again disappointed when her old roommate, who was not even in shape, was chosen over her.

Intervention: The sports psychiatrist helped the player to acknowledge her emotions of disappointment and frustration and to create an outlet for them by clarifying her goals for the season. This effort involved a shift of her focus from an outcome (playing time) to a process (steady improvement of several specific skills). The player approached one of the new assistant coaches and asked what areas she felt were targets for improvement. The new coach identified two important areas: the player's commitment to playing defense even though she was an attacking player and her one-versus-one skill. Between the first and second sessions with the psychiatrist, the player formally developed written goals to improve these two areas and one additional one (quality shots on goal) by establishing three specific action steps for each. The new coach was encouraging and supportive and felt that the young woman's playing time would naturally increase as her additional work paid off.

Outcome: As the next few weeks passed, the player began to feel energized by the extra work that she and one other player were doing with the new assistant coach. Her confidence began to soar, and she became more aggressive in practice, particularly in the air and on defense. Subsequently, the head coach pulled her aside after practice and told her that she would be starting the next game and that her playing time would increase because the coach had seen a side of her lately that she had not previously demonstrated. The emotions of frustration and disappointment that blocked positive play were now replaced with confidence and a stronger connection with her teammates. She was able to appreciate that her negative emotions produced negative thinking and suboptimal play.

Sleep and Energy Management

Good sleep quality is the main key to producing enough energy to supply the entire day. Because high school, college, and professional athletes often have 10- to 12-hour days of continuous work, they need high energy levels to succeed at sports and other activities (e.g., school, family, friends). Studies show that at least 4–5 but ideally 6–7 hours of uninterrupted sleep are needed to provide 80%–90% of the next day's energy requirement. Uninterrupted sleep is important because it allows the athlete to cycle through the alternating stages of deep and dream (rapid eye movement, or REM) sleep. Good sleep hygiene leads to good sleep. A 60- to 90-minute unwinding routine—consisting of listening to soft music, easy reading, family dialogue/phone calls, relaxing television, warm bath, or meditation—in a quiet, low-light area can be helpful. In addition, eating, fluid intake, exercise, intense work, video games, Internet surfing, television channel flipping (especially in a dark bedroom), and arguing should be avoided in the 2 hours before bedtime. Finally, the time for bed should be consistent and before midnight, the mattress should be correctly sized and comfortable, and the room should be the right temperature and devoid of aggravating noises.

Another main key to producing and maintaining energy is the awakening routine. In the first 3–4 hours after daylight, the body's neurohormonal system activates with a rapid rise in serum cortisol as well as body temperature. During this period, an organized awakening routine can further boost energy. Typical activities of awakening routines are 1) exercise; 2) stretching; 3) drinking something hot or cold; 4) eating breakfast; 5) going outside; 6) taking a shower; 7) using a bright light; and 8) taking in caffeine or another natural stimulant such as ginseng. Exercise can be short, consisting of as little as 5–7 minutes of cardiovascular activation (e.g., use of a treadmill or elliptical machine, jumping rope) or three 60-second full-intensity cardiovascular intervals (e.g., jumping rope, push-ups, sit-ups) separated by a few minutes' rest. This activation, if done early, can substantially raise the entire day's energy level. During sleep, the body's core temperature drops to its lowest level during a 24-hour cycle. Drinking a hot or cold beverage immediately on awakening changes the body's core temperature and delivers a signal to the brain to produce more energy. In addition, if the beverage contains a reasonable amount of caffeine (150–400 mg), then an additional boost can be obtained. Similarly, going outside where the temperature and light patterns are different, even for just a few minutes, can also boost energy production. Finally, individuals who are light sensitive and notice lower energy in winter than in summer, may benefit from morning light therapy, perhaps in the form of an alarm clock that gradually turns on a bedside light or from bright light therapy (10,000 lux) for 20–30 minutes while reading or sitting.

The final key to maintaining a steady energy level throughout the day is to eat regular meals and take breaks. Every 3–4 hours, athletes should eat a meal or snack containing a balance of carbohydrates, proteins, and fats, as well as fluids to maintain hydration. After workouts, an especially important goal is to resupply carbohydrates, because rehydration is inhibited if carbohydrate levels are too low. Breaks are also critical to energy maintenance. Even short breaks of 3–5 minutes, consisting of a change in venue (going outside, walking to another area of a building), can help. A good technique for accentuating a break is to use activation breathing (60 seconds of nasal hyperventilation—i.e., 160–180 breaths in 60 seconds with an emphasis on the exhalation), followed by patterned relaxation breathing (in through the nose for a count of four, hold for a count of seven, and out through the mouth for a count of eight, repeated eight times). Once this pattern is completed (about 3 minutes), then simple easy breathing with the eyes closed followed by simple stretching of the whole body and targeted body parts (e.g., neck and shoulders or low back) can be added.

Case Study: Active Mind and Insomnia

A rookie free-agent football player (offensive lineman) was referred to a sports psychiatrist by the athletic trainer during the second week of preseason camp because of the player's insomnia, fatigue, and difficulty concentrating in team meetings.

Assessment: Dating back to his first year of college, the player had difficulty falling asleep during high-stress periods in football and academics. He described a very active mind that would not turn off at bedtime even though his body was very tired. He often took 2–3 hours to fall asleep and would awaken early and immediately start worrying about the new day. He tended to repeatedly review his mistakes, fret over the complexity of the playbook, and worry about the talent level of other players competing for his position. He did not drink or use stimulants and had no history of anxiety, mood, or attention disorders. He had occasionally taken diphenhydramine for sleep but did not like the persistent drowsiness that he felt the next morning.

Intervention: The psychiatrist reviewed the basics of good sleep hygiene, and the player adopted an unwinding routine that included reading, relaxing, talking to family on the phone, or listening to music, and avoiding eating or drinking fluids and visually stimulating the brain by watching television or using the Internet for 2 hours before bedtime. In addition, a trial of trazodone 50 mg taken 90 minutes before bedtime was initiated.

Outcome: Over the first 5 days, the player's sleep improved moderately, so the dosage of trazodone was raised to 100 mg. This routine, along with continued reassurance that his experience was typical of first-year players moving to this level, resulted in much improved sleep and energy.

Substance Use and Misuse

Athletes use risky and addictive substances for the same reasons that persons of similar age in the community use them, as well as to boost performance and manage injuries (i.e., to improve sleep or to reduce pain, stiffness, or swelling) (Figure 1–3). The most common substances misused in collegiate and professional sports are alcohol, stimulants (caffeine, nicotine, methylphenidate, amphetamine), sedatives, and marijuana. Less common but more controversial and possibly more monitored substances are anabolic androgenic agents (i.e., steroids, growth hormone, masking agents), opiate pain medications, and cocaine. Each substance can be used for one or all three reasons shown in Figure 1–3, but drug use in sports is usually divided administratively into drugs of abuse (alcohol, marijuana, cocaine, hallucinogens, 3,4-methylenedioxymethamphetamine (MDMA; hereafter referred to as ecstasy), opiates, phencyclidine) and performance enhancers (anabolic androgenic agents, stimulants, hormones, masking agents). Some medications that are banned or disapproved, such as stimulants for attention-deficit disorder, can be taken by athletes as long as a request for a therapeutic use exemption is made by a clinician and approved by the sports authority structure. In these cases, a potentially per-

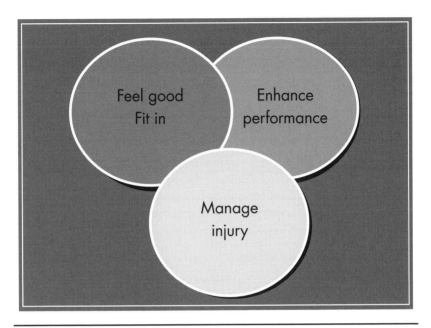

FIGURE 1–3.   Reasons athletes use substances.

formance-enhancing medication is viewed as simply restoring functioning to a normal level for athletes with a legitimate disorder.

Athletes in various sports have different patterns of substance misuse. For example, stimulant use is common among baseball players, who often use oral tobacco (35%) and sometimes concurrently use a risky mixture of caffeine, nicotine, and stronger stimulants such as amphetamines (McDuff and Baron 2005). This concurrent use is called stimulant stacking and is worrisome because of excessive cardiovascular activation (tachycardia, hypertension) and risk of heat injury. Among football players, sedative use for sleep and relaxation and opiate pain medication for injury are more common. Stimulant misuse among football players does occur and is most likely on game day when combinations of caffeine, ginseng, and/or short-acting amphetamines are typical. The most common side effects are post-game arousal and insomnia. High-dose stimulant use in any sport is likely to be accompanied by the use of a sedative-hypnotic substance, such as alcohol or benzodiazepines, and this "upper-downer" pairing can lead to escalating amounts of each substance.

Use of alcohol and marijuana is common across most sports. Players tend to use these substances to relax and unwind after practices or games and sometimes, depending on the pattern of competition, demonstrate episodic heavy use. The use of highly addictive substances, such as cocaine and heroin, or riskier substances, such as lysergic acid diethylamide (LSD), ecstasy, or phencyclidine, is uncommon. Episodic heavy alcohol use by a player is usually revealed when 1) an alcohol-related event (lateness, fight, arrest) occurs; 2) an athletic trainer smells alcohol on a player's breath early in the morning; or 3) regular urine testing for drugs of abuse includes alcohol testing. Any detection indicates heavy alcohol use the night before and can lead to a productive risk discussion with the athlete if a mental health professional is integrated into the medical staff. Marijuana use is usually detected through urine testing or through the evaluation of a problem with alcohol. The clinician discusses with the athlete the pros and cons of the use of these two substances; assesses the athlete's readiness to change, although the sports league may mandate abstinence; and helps the athlete identify and implement alternative ways to relax.

Case Study: Alcohol, Sleep, and Energy

An athletic trainer and team physician referred a second-year professional baseball player for assistance when he requested sleep medication after the all-star break. The player described both difficulties falling asleep from an active mind and regular awakenings after 3–4 hours. He was constantly tired and noted that his energy drinks and coffee were not raising his energy level as they had before.

Assessment: A review of the player's postgame patterns revealed regular drinking of four to six beers and sometimes liquor shots with teammates either at clubs or at the team hotel. He would often return to his apartment or hotel room at 3–4 A.M. and still not be tired, so he would get a snack or watch television while in bed. Eventually, he would get drowsy but would either be unable to fall asleep because of reviewing his performance or wake up far too early and not be able to fall back asleep. This pattern of insomnia and fatigue was new this season and not associated with anxiety, depression, or other drug use.

Intervention: The player already realized that his drinking and partying were likely interfering with his sleep and reducing his energy level. He was in the process of reducing his drinking nights and amounts and was open to the idea of a trial of complete abstinence. In addition, he was encouraged to stop all late-night eating, television watching, and Internet use, and to purchase a portable white noise machine for use at home and on the road. He also established a regular bedtime of 1 A.M. after night games and reduced his stimulant use from the equivalent of 750 mg of caffeine per day to 300–400 mg. Upon awakening, he started drinking a cold bottle of water and eating an energy bar before doing some simple 60-second cardiovascular intervals.

Outcome: Over a 2-week period, the player's sleep improved dramatically without medications and his energy levels soared. He began systematically reviewing his performance by completing a one-page form that identified the positives of play, the areas for improvement, and skill areas to work on with his position coach.

Case Study: Stimulant Stacking and Excessive Arousal

After becoming dizzy and overheated while warming up in the bullpen during a game on a hot day, a third-year minor league late-innings relief pitcher was examined by the team physician and noted to have sinus tachycardia, flushing, and postural blood pressure changes but a normal core temperature. The player acknowledged being a heavy sweater and to taking an extra dose of his short-acting amphetamine salts before warming up. He was treated with rest out of the sun and electrolyte replacement fluids. The physician referred the athlete to the team psychiatrist.

Assessment: The player was seen in the clubhouse by the team psychiatrist the following day and revealed that he was a regular user of pre-game caffeine (coffee and Red Bull Energy Drink), was a heavy dipper of moist snuff (using from wake-up to bedtime), and was approved to take amphetamine salts 30 mg 3 hours before the game and sometimes another 30 mg before he thought he might pitch. He had never had such an episode before and had no past history of cardiac arrhythmias or syncope. He was using on average 600–800 mg of caffeine pregame and typically would put in his mouth three or four large dips of oral tobacco in the morning before a 1 P.M. game. He liked the effect of the short-acting amphetamine salts.

Intervention: The psychiatrist reviewed with the player the pattern of his stimulant use and discussed the risks and benefits of taking such high quantities of three stimulants at the same time on a hot day. The athlete agreed to lower his use of caffeinated beverages to 1–2 cups of coffee with breakfast and to try to reduce his use of moist snuff. In addition, he agreed to change from short-acting amphetamine salts to a long-acting formulation that he would take 3–4 hours before a day or night game.

Outcome: The player's focus and concentration improved when he took the long-acting agent, and his wife noted after a few weeks that he was more social in the mornings and had become a better listener. He did not miss the caffeine, and on reviewing his past pitching, in fact reported that he was likely overstimulated, which had led to inconsistency in his pitching control. After 1 month, his long-acting agent was changed to twice daily on night games, so that he took extended-release amphetamine salts 30 mg on awakening and then 20 mg at 2 P.M. before a 7 P.M. game. This pattern further improved his sociability at home and his performance on the field. In addition, he reported that he was able to unwind more easily after games and consequently was sleeping better and waking more energized.

Injury Recovery and Pain Management

Severe injuries resulting in substantial missed time from practice or competition, as well as surgeries with long rehabilitation periods, are more common in collision sports such as rugby, boxing, mixed martial arts, football, lacrosse, ice hockey, and rodeo, than in contact sports such as basketball, soccer, and field hockey, or in noncontact sports such as golf, tennis, or baseball. Nevertheless, injury in sports is common and one of the most likely reasons for inconsistent play and diminished confidence. In collision sports, expected serious injuries include concussion; cervical spinal damage; ankle sprains; torn knee ligaments; dislocated joints in the hands, feet, and shoulders; and torn cartilage in knees or shoulders. In contact sports, the injury patterns are similar to those in collision sports but are less frequent or severe, with the exception of anterior cruciate ligaments tears (often not related to contact) in men and women in field sports. In noncontact sports, overuse injuries such as tendinitis and sprains are more common.

When an injury occurs, the person usually has intense acute pain, swelling, muscle spasm, restricted range of motion, and sleep difficulty. Most injuries are handled initially by immobilization, icing, anti-inflammatory agents, muscle relaxants, and opiate pain medications. Depending on the severity of the injury, emotions such as sadness, disappointment, apprehension, uncertainty, and frustration may arise immediately or over the first few days. The sports psychiatrist can help the athlete in several ways:

- Communicate actively with the athletic trainers and team physicians during the acute injury period as new diagnostic information is obtained and the treatment plan is clarified.
- Have brief but regular patient interactions to assess the athlete's understanding of the injury, proposed treatment, and prognosis, as well as to assess pain control and sleep.
- Monitor the emotional response to the injury.
- Monitor and manage the development of a support system.

For injuries requiring surgery and prolonged rehabilitation, the psychiatrist should continue meeting with the player during the injury, rehabilitation, and return-to-play periods. Long-term rehabilitation is painful, frustrating, discouraging, and isolating and can lead to burnout and poorer outcomes, such as weakness, residual stiffness, chronic pain, and restricted range of motion. The return-to-play phase of treatment is characterized by uncertainty and fear. Often, as the injured athlete returns to full fitness or limited practice, he or she experiences a minor setback with increased pain, swelling, and stiffness. During this time, the support and encouragement of the athletic trainers, strength and conditioning staff, chiropractors, and sports mental health clinicians are critical. As this phase is worked through and the athlete returns to full practice, the fear of reinjury often surfaces, triggering muscle chain tightness and movement tentativeness. The psychiatrist can talk the patient through the injury and healing process or ask a teammate, the athletic trainer, or team orthopedist to dispel any misconceptions.

Case Study: Ankle Surgery, Neuralgia, and Insomnia

A rookie professional football special teams player was seen by a sports psychiatrist in the training room 3 weeks after the player sustained a compound fracture of his right ankle on a kickoff. He had gone to another city after his injury to have surgery performed by a well-known foot and ankle specialist. The fracture required the insertion of several screws and a plate. By the time he returned to the team, he was complaining of severe burning foot pain, insomnia, and irritability.

Assessment: At the end of the first postsurgical week, the player began to feel that the cast was too tight. A local orthopedist in his hometown removed the cast and applied another to better accommodate the swelling that had occurred. Over the next 2 weeks, the athlete began to develop constant burning pain on the top of his right foot that did not diminish with hydrocodone and kept him awake at night. After returning to the team, he was seen by several members of the medical staff, including a consulting neurologist. The recommendation was to continue taking hydrocodone 5 mg twice during the day and again at bedtime and to begin taking pregabalin 50 mg twice daily.

Intervention: After another few days during which the athlete experienced little improvement in pain or sleep, the psychiatrist revised the medication regimen in collaboration with the head team physician. The hydrocodone dosage was changed to 7.5 mg every 3–4 hours and 15 mg at bedtime. The pregabalin dosage was increased gradually from 50 mg twice daily to 75 mg three times daily. Also, zolpidem 10 mg was added at bedtime.

Outcome: Over the first few days on this new regimen, the player's sleep improved dramatically and his irritability faded. After a week, his rating of his burning foot pain was reduced from 8 to 3–4 out of 10. His daytime dosage of hydrocodone was reduced, but his pregabalin was continued. At 6 weeks, his cast was removed and his rehabilitation shifted to improving his ankle's range of motion and strengthening his foot and lower-leg musculature, which had significantly atrophied. As he became ambulatory and more active, he took hydrocodone mainly after treatments and generally did not need it at bedtime. By week 12, his dosage of pregabalin was being tapered off, and he had stopped using zolpidem. The athlete went on to make a full recovery over the next 6 months and was able to return to full play.

Case Study: Gymnastics, Concussion, and Fear

Four weeks after missing a vault and smacking her head on the mat, sustaining a concussion, a high school senior who had just received a scholarship to a top gymnastics college was referred to a sports psychiatrist for the evaluation of fear of competing. The athlete had fallen many times before but had never sustained a concussion. She had no prior history of general or competitive anxiety or fear.

Assessment: For the first week after the fall, she experienced headaches, dizziness, light and noise sensitivity, and restless sleep, and she did not practice. Her symptoms gradually faded, and after a week she went back to light fitness training and some harness work without difficulty. In the third postfall week, at the suggestion of her coach, the gymnast tried to do the vault that she had missed. She tried several times, balking just before reaching the vault. She then tried several simpler vaults but balked at these as well. Because balance beam was her best event, she tried to do some simple routines but froze on the beam. At the time of the evaluation, she was very upset that she might not be able to compete in several large upcoming national meets and that her scholarship might be revoked.

Intervention: The athlete's anxiety and fear of practice were addressed through five primary strategies. First, she was educated about concussion and postconcussive syndrome using a brain model and Internet images. Second, she was taught relaxation and activation breathing as a way to demonstrate control over worrying, catastrophic thinking, and somatic arousal. Third, she began nightly activated visualizations (with 5% movement of the core and upper body) of successful floor, beam, uneven bars, and vault routines while sitting upright on the floor. After a week, she began doing more activated visualizations of all routines while standing. Fourth, she began to observe the faces of the most confident gymnasts in her club during practice and competition; she then practiced, at first in front of the mirror, putting their "light smiles of confidence" on her face, and then when she had gotten good at this mirror practice, she continued practicing without the mirror for short periods throughout the day and before routines at practice. Finally, she began taking propranolol 20 mg 1 hour before each practice. A graduated reentry from simpler to complex routines over 3 weeks was developed in consultation with her coach.

Outcome: Over 4 weeks, the athlete's anxiety and fear faded, and she began doing complex routines with confidence. She successfully competed in all the national meets, and although she did not do as well as she might have before the accident, she was proud that she was able to fully compete. She worked hard over the late spring and summer, and the psychiatrist last saw her in August before she headed to college. She went on to do well in her first year and developed into a strong performer for her last 3 years of college.

Common Mental Disorders

The mental disorders most frequently seen among athletes at all competitive levels are generally the same ones seen in similar populations matched for age, gender, and ethnicity in the community. The most common disorders are adjustment (stress), anxiety, mood, sleep, learning, attention-deficit, substance use, and impulse control (anger control) disorders. Some disorders are more common in certain sports than in the general population. For example, eating and compulsive exercise disorders are more common among athletes in cross country, track and field, swimming, wrestling, and gymnastics, whereas impulse control (anger) and episodic alcohol use disorders are more common among players of collision sports (e.g., football, hockey, lacrosse) or contact sports (e.g., soccer). In addition, sleep disorders are much more common among players of sports such as football, in which the athletes are extremely large, or in fatigue-producing sports such as baseball, basketball, or soccer, in which many games are played and extensive road travel through different time zones is common. Somatoform pain disorders with psychological factors are also more common in collision sports, where injury rates are high and catastrophic injuries that threaten future play are common. Fear of reinjury often contributes to the reluctance of an athlete to return to play, and the resultant stress from this fear might alter the frequency and severity of the pain in the injured area.

The treatment of mental disorders for athletes is similar to that for other groups of patients and includes individual counseling or therapy and medications. Collateral individuals, such as family members and coaches, are more often involved in the treatment of athletes than would be the case with other patients. The involvement of collateral individuals is critical to garner support, assess the level of dysfunction, and monitor changes that support peak performance.

Medication management is more challenging for athletes because of the impact that side effects can have on level of alertness, reaction time, heat regulation, weight, sexual functioning, and mental quickness. In general, lower starting dosages are used, and increases are more gradual. The combination of two medications at lower dosages is often preferred to one medication at a higher dosage. The following are examples of medication approaches for common disorders seen in athletes:

- To help with sleep, the most common medications are zolpidem or trazodone as needed. For more intractable cases of insomnia that are not caused by obstructive sleep apnea, a combination of either 1) ramelteon and zolpidem or low-dose trazodone (25–100 mg) or 2) low-dose trazodone (25–50 mg) taken 2 hours before bedtime and zolpidem at bedtime is usually helpful. If the combination strategy does not work, then low-dose quetiapine alone (25–50 mg) is used.
- For anxiety, the first options are usually low-dose benzodiazepines (5–10 mg equivalents of diazepam), low-dose selective serotonin reuptake inhibitors (SSRIs), or extended-release venlafaxine or bupropion.
- For depression, the nonsedating SSRIs (e.g., fluoxetine, citalopram) or a serotonin-norepinephrine reuptake inhibitor (SNRI) (e.g., venlafaxine, duloxetine) is used.
- For attention-deficit disorder, atomoxetine or extended-release methylphenidate is usually tried first; if those fail, then extended-release amphetamine salts are tried. In athletes who lose weight or cannot sleep with either stimulant medication, atomoxetine or bupropion is tried.

Again, in all cases, the dosage is started low and increased more slowly than for other patient groups, and the athlete's symptoms, performance, relationships, and side effects are monitored.

Case Study: Generalized Anxiety and Obsessive-Compulsive Personality

A 32-year-old married father of two children and veteran professional soccer player was referred for assistance by a teammate who was being treated for anxiety and insomnia. The player identified a long history of anxiety, obsessive thinking, compulsive sports rituals, and insomnia dating back to high school. He was most troubled by his inability to fall asleep quickly at night. Since the birth of his second child a year earlier, he would lie awake for hours listening for sounds that would indicate his son might have awakened and worrying that something bad would happen to the child. During the current soccer season, his insomnia worsened to the point that some nights he would sleep off and on, never getting more than 2–3 hours at a time. He would awaken early and fatigued and felt that his play was beginning to slip. As a veteran who had overcome several serious injuries, he was worried that he might be replaced the next season by a younger player. Before practice and as he approached the practice field, he had a number of rituals about his shoes and touching the end lines repeatedly before he could start his warm-ups. If he did not do these correctly, he would need to repeat them.

Assessment: His tendency to be a compulsive analyzer and worrier dated back to early middle school. During high school, with his dominance as a central defender on his club team, his worrying shifted over primarily to his athletic future. He attended a large Division I university and was a game starter all 4 years. Throughout college and his entire professional career, which included some time playing in Western Europe, he worried constantly and slept poorly. He had never been evaluated or treated for these difficulties and just considered himself to be an odd person. He had no history of substance misuse or mood difficulties.

Intervention: The player was started on trials of escitalopram 10 mg and trazodone 50 mg. After 10 days with little improvement, the escitalopram was raised to 20 mg and trazodone to 100 mg. After another week, with some improvement in his anxiety, worrying, and compulsive rituals but little improvement in his sleep, trazodone was discontinued and quetiapine 25 mg was added at bedtime. Almost immediately his sleep improved and his fatigue resolved. He began to get 6–8 hours of continuous sleep for the first time in his adult life. The psychiatrist saw the player on a weekly basis throughout the 6 months of the season and contacted him monthly by phone during the off-season. In addition, the psychiatrist and player spent considerable time discussing parenting and other important relationships in their meetings.

Outcome: After the player had been taking stable dosages of escitalopram 20 mg and quetiapine 25–37.5 mg at bedtime for 2 years, his presenting symptoms had resolved completely. He decided to taper off his escitalopram during the off-season, and this was done successfully. Today,

3 years later, he continues to take quetiapine nearly every night. He has not had side effects, gained weight, or developed metabolic abnormalities.

Case Study: Underachievement, Dysthymia, and Attention-Deficit Disorder

A fifth-year redshirt women's college lacrosse player was encouraged to seek assistance in midseason by an assistant coach because of the athlete's dissatisfaction with her play and general unhappiness with her life direction. She had been a starting midfielder for 4 years and a team captain for 2 years but felt that she was never able to play to her ability level. She had already received a bachelor's degree in communications and was enrolled in a master's program in business. She did not play her second year because of a torn anterior cruciate ligament that was successfully repaired with a patellar tendon graft.

Assessment: During the initial meeting with the sports psychiatrist, the player described a chronic sense of athletic and academic underachievement that dated back to early high school. Academically, she was a severe procrastinator, never studying for a test or writing a paper until the night before, and often staying up all night. Athletically, she knew she was talented but felt she never realized her potential or met the expectations of her coaches or parents, especially her father, who had been her club team coach. She became sad, tearful, and angry when discussing her father's behavior at games. He would often stand alone at the corner of the field and yell at her continuously. After the game, if he did not feel that she had played well, he would either yell at her for not competing hard enough or not speak to her. Lately, he had just stopped coming.

Intervention: It became clear over the first few weekly meetings that the player had chronic dysthymia and that during high-stress periods when projects or papers were due, she would have great difficulty sleeping and worry constantly about getting them done. More in-depth discussion of her study, research, and writing routines revealed a consistent difficulty with focus, attention shifting, distractibility, motor restlessness, and poor organization and follow-through. She was able to get focused and accomplish her work only when a time deadline approached. By completing her studying or assignments the night before, she always felt that she was not doing her best. The psychiatrist completed an in-depth assessment for attention-deficit disorder that included rating scales and collateral contact with her coaches and mother. The player was eventually diagnosed with dysthymia and adult attention-deficit disorder, combined type. Although reluctant at first, the athlete agreed to weekly therapy and trials of venlafaxine and long-acting methylphenidate.

Outcome: Over an 8-week period, the player responded well to the treatment. Her mood improved significantly, as did her sleep. Her confidence at practice and in games became solid, and she assumed a much stronger leadership role than ever before. During weeks of high academic demand, she would take two daily doses of long-acting methylphenidate (one upon awakening and a second at about 2 P.M.). She was thus able to develop a more organized approach to task completion and more comfort with seeking assistance from the faculty and library staff. With a new perspective that her chronic sense of underachievement was explained by attention deficits, she became more satisfied with her best efforts, both academically and athletically.

Working With Team Leadership, Coaches, and Medical Staff

Most team owners, general managers, athletic directors, school presidents, head coaches, and sports medicine clinicians do not have experience working with mental health professionals in training facilities, treatment rooms, and team meetings, or during practice or competitions. Only a few colleges and an even smaller number of professional sports teams employ psychiatrists, psychologists, or other mental health professionals on an ongoing basis. Many use mental health clinicians only in the case of a serious crisis, such as after a tragedy (e.g., the accidental death of a teammate), for a suicidal athlete, or after an athlete's public arrest for intoxication or assault. The exception to this trend is professional baseball. For the past 20 years, the commissioner of Major League Baseball has required each of the 30 teams to have an employee assistance program (EAP) that provides mental health and substance use screening, evaluation, brief intervention, and referral to longer-term treatment services. Some of these EAPs structure services so that the clinicians work on-site during spring training and in the clubhouse during the season. In these EAPs, a productive integration of services with team leadership and the medical staff is possible.

The ideal model for the practice of sports psychiatry or sports mental health is one that pays for the provider to be present at the practice site on a regular basis (twice a week is ideal) and to be on call continuously to respond to crises and to schedule next-day evaluations. Breaking from the EAP model of brief interventions, a well-developed sports mental health program allows for long-term treatment of athletes, team staff, and family members throughout the year, including the off-season. This practice results in a high level of continuity and consistency of care and ongoing coordination with all medical, professional development, and life skills services.

Case Study: New Head Coach's Resistance to Psychiatry

A newly hired college basketball head coach had little experience working with sports psychiatrists or mental skills trainers. He was reluctant to allow the team psychiatrist to attend practices and meet with players individually afterward in the training room. His general view was that he did not want the distractions that this activity might bring.

Assessment: The team psychiatrist scheduled a meeting with the new head coach and two assistant coaches who had been there the year before and were familiar with an on-site model for sports psychiatric service delivery. A short handout was prepared with key talking points about the rationale, the psychiatrist's role, and past successes. A lengthy dialogue ensued with active participation and support by the assistant coaches, including a testimonial by one of them about how the psychiatrist had helped him after the death of his father. It became clear that the head coach wanted his players to practice with game intensity and focus and that outside distractions would not be tolerated.

Intervention: The new coach was assured that the presence of the sports psychiatrist at practice and in the training room would not be a distraction. He agreed to a trial of this approach and a follow-up meeting. Over the ensuing weeks, the coach was able to observe multiple productive interactions between the sports psychiatrist and the players, coaches, athletic trainers, and team physicians. The head team physician, who met with the new coach routinely about injured players and who had years of experience with sports psychiatry, was able to voice his support of its value to the team.

Outcome: Over the course of the first season, the new coach fully accepted the role of a sports psychiatrist. He acknowledged at an end-of-season meeting that his lack of experience with psychiatry in past positions and his stereotypes of the profession had influenced his initial position. Over the ensuing seasons, the coach became a strong supporter of sports psychiatry and comfortably referred players, coaches, and family members for assistance.

Developmental, Gender, and Cultural Competency

To facilitate strong working alliances and effectiveness, mental health professionals must consider the developmental stage, gender, and cultural background of teams and athletes. Participation in youth sports has exploded in the United States since the 1990s, and alarming trends of early specialization to one sport, year-round training, and premature shifts to higher competitive levels have occurred. These trends have often taken the fun out of training and competition and can lead to injury, family conflict, burnout, and quitting. In some sports, club teams are unable to fill a roster because of the high quit rates of players before age 15 or 16. In addition to the athlete's developmental stage, gender differences are important to consider. For example, female athletes are more likely to note and consider the impact of starting roster decisions on their teammates and to express concern and support for those whose playing time is reduced (DiCicco and Hacker 2002). In addition, they do not respond well if a teammate is called out for a mistake or poor play in front of the group. Cultural differences are just as important as age and gender. The largest cultural groups in U.S. sports are African Americans (football, basketball), Latinos (baseball), whites (tennis, golf), and Asians (women's golf, martial arts). Each of these cultural groups has unique foods, music, languages, customs, traditions, religious views, and family structure and function. Although teams cannot expect mental health professionals to be bicultural and cannot hire only clinicians from a specific cultural group, clinicians can develop increasing cultural awareness and sensitivity though travel, readings, and in-depth conversations with individual athletes.

Case Study: Parent-Child Conflict and Achievement Pressure

A 14-year-old Asian American high school sophomore who was a highly ranked junior tennis player was referred to a sports psychiatrist for the evaluation of inconsistent play and increasing frustration with his coaches and parents over the prior 6 months. He had become nationally ranked the year before, and as a result, had changed coaches and schools. This change resulted in an increased time commitment to tennis from 2 hours a day 4 days a week to 3 hours a day 6 days a week, in addition to a longer commute. He also began to play more out-of-town tournaments on the weekends and experienced stronger competition. He was usually accompanied to tournaments by his father, and they had begun to argue more frequently before and after matches.

Assessment: The psychiatrist initially saw the father and athlete together and asked what change each of them would like to see in the player's tennis in the coming months. The father said that he wanted to see his son practice and play with more commitment and intensity and wondered whether his son really wanted to continue. The player said he wanted more breaks from tennis for time to hang out with friends and to do other things. He also expressed an interest in playing another sport in school just for fun. This discussion provoked an argument between father and son. Following a break, the psychiatrist met with the player alone. The player voiced concern about his father's intensity and involvement at matches. The athlete had begun to resent his father's constant discussion of strategy before each match and long reviews of his mistakes after each match. In addition, he felt that his father was too loud at his matches, shouting instructions in Korean and yelling at his opponent's line calls. The player found this behavior embarrassing, anxiety provoking, and distracting. The psychiatrist then met alone with the father, at the player's request, and the two discussed the father's view that his son was wasting his talent and the father's frustration that his son was now routinely being beaten by less talented players.

Intervention: The psychiatrist, father, and son decided to meet after every one or two tournaments and agreed that the player would log the positives and negatives of his play and the tactics he used to overcome the negatives after each match. The father agreed to refrain from lengthy discussions of strategy before matches to allow his son time to improve his prematch routine. At the second meeting, it became clear that the player was not enjoying his practices or competitions and that his anxiety levels in general and especially during tournaments was rising. He worked extensively with the psychiatrist to revise his prematch routine to allow him to quiet his mind, relax his body, raise his intensity, and then focus and shift his attention. He seemed initially to respond to this longer and more regimented approach, as well as to some relaxation and muscle tension–reducing strategies during matches. His performance began to improve until he went to a national tournament. Even though he had success in the early rounds, he became very upset during and after a semifinal loss when his father began shouting instructions. At a meeting following this tournament, the father acknowledged that he had broken the agreement and had upset his son. After discussion, he agreed to let his wife or his son's uncle travel to the next few tournaments because they had very different temperaments. In addition, the coach was contacted, and his perspective was that the player and his family were putting too much emphasis on the outcome of matches and not enough on enjoying competition and improving. He suggested that the player participate in another sport at school as a way to improve his fitness and have fun without so much pressure.

Outcome: After several tournaments with different travel partners and a strong commitment to play with passion and lightness, the player's confidence and play improved. Although at the early meetings he seemed to feel burned out by tennis, it became clear that the extra pressure that he was experiencing had temporarily reduced his love of the game.

Case Study: Latino Culture, Baseball Anxiety, Homesickness, and Family

A second-year Latino professional baseball position player was referred to the team's psychiatrist by the team athletic trainer and physician for the evaluation of poor concentration and declining performance with hitting and fielding. Because the player's English was not at a high level, a veteran Latino player agreed to sit in on the initial session.

Assessment: After an hour-long meeting and with the helpful involvement of the other player and collateral contacts with the former manager and current hitting coach, the psychiatrist came to understand that the player was a generally anxious young man who constantly worried about his performance while on the field and about his family in Mexico while off the field. Although he was a young adult, he still had periods of intense homesickness and longing to be with his family in his home country.

Intervention: He agreed to meet the psychiatrist once each time the team was home to work on his hitting routines and discuss his stress about his family. He was able to insert several relaxation strategies (clearing breath, grip/release/grip/release) into his hitting routines and to ventilate about his frustration over the fact that his brother was not helping his mother financially. In addition, he began taking low-dose escitalopram (5 mg), which was raised to 15 mg over the ensuing 6 weeks.

Outcome: The player's anxiety gradually diminished, and his confidence improved. He developed a very strong prepitch routine that reliably released his anxiety and tension and improved his focus. The following season, he had great success until he was injured, requiring a 6-week rehabilitation assignment. After his return, he quickly moved back to confident and consistent play using his mental skills and revised routines. Two years later, he now continues to take his medication and works to improve with the input of coaches and other players. A side benefit of the regular meetings (10 total) was that his English improved greatly and he began to socialize more with English-speaking players.

Conclusion

Sports psychiatrists and other mental health providers working from an office base or at the team's facility or practice field will be asked to assess and assist with a variety of problems or performance improvement. These clinicians need to develop a broad clinical skill set and comfort with interventions with athletes in practice settings and training rooms. In addition, comfort and skill with enlisting the support of family members and coaches in understanding players' problems and in crafting lasting solutions are critical. The eight core competencies and the case studies described in this chapter are intended as an overview of the skills that are essential for a part-time or full-time sports psychiatry or mental health practice. In the following chapters, I provide in-depth descriptions of these competencies and additional cases that demonstrate different challenges.

Key Clinical Points

- Sports psychiatric or mental health services are most effective if they are provided immediately when a need arises, are free of charge, are available on-site at a team's training facilities, and are broad in scope.

- Mental toughness and emotional control become more important for athletes at higher competitive levels.

- Proper breathing is one of the best ways to reduce precompetitive anxiety and clear out excessive muscle chain tension.

- Four stress responses—anxiety, anger, depression, and somatic symptoms—most commonly interfere with athletic performance.

- The stress of athletic performance is best managed through support networks, awakening and unwinding routines, restorative sleep, strategic breaks, quality nutrition, and life balance.

- The enemies of good sleep include eating, drinking alcohol and other fluids, exercise, Internet surfing, and television channel flipping within 2 hours of bedtime, as well as staying up too late.

- Regular or heavy in-season use of alcohol, caffeine, nicotine, marijuana, and/or medications alone or in combination slowly and subtly erodes performance over time in different ways.

- Eating, anger control, sleep, substance use, somatoform pain, and attention-deficit disorders are more likely to be encountered in sports psychiatric practice but are easier to treat if they are identified early and team support is used.

- Severe injuries produce strong emotions and chronic pain that can impede recovery, block return to play, and complicate transition out of sports.

- Age, gender, and cultural differences must be considered in sports diagnosis and treatment.

- Attitudinal and fiscal barriers to providing on-site services can be overcome with time and persistence.

References

Begel D, Burton RW (eds): Sports Psychiatry: Theory and Practice. New York, Norton, 2000

Beswick B: Focused for Soccer. Champaign, IL, Human Kinetics, 2001

DiCicco T, Hacker C: Catch Them Being Good. New York, Penguin Books, 2002

Dorfman HA: The Mental ABCs of Pitching: A Handbook for Performance Enhancement. South Bend, IN, Diamond Communications, 2000

Dorfman HA, Kuehl K: The Mental Game of Baseball: A Guide to Peak Performance. South Bend, IN, Diamond Communications, 1995

Gee CJ: Does sport psychology actually improve athletic performance? A framework to facilitate athletes' and coaches' understanding. Behav Modif 34:386–402, 2010

Glick ID, Kamm R, Morse E: The evolution of sports psychiatry, circa 2009. Sports Med 39:607–613, 2009

Grossbard JR, Smith RE, Smoll FL, et al: Competitive anxiety in young athletes: differentiating somatic anxiety, worry, and concentration disruption. Anxiety Stress Coping 22:153–166, 2009

Loehr J, Schwartz T: The Power of Full Engagement. New York, Free Press, 2003

McDuff DR, Baron D: Substance use in athletics: a sports psychiatry perspective. Clin Sports Med 4:885–897, 2005

McDuff DR, Morse E, White R: Professional and collegiate team assistance programs: services and utilization patterns. Clin Sports Med 4:943–958, 2005

Porter K: The Mental Athlete: Inner Training for Peak Performance in All Sports. Champaign, IL, Human Kinetics, 2003

Porter K: The Mental Athlete. Champaign, IL, Human Kinetics, 2004

Rotella B: The Golfer's Mind. New York, Free Press, 2004

Chapter 2

Mental Preparation

Achieving peak athletic performance with consistency requires a combination of sports-specific training, seasonally adjusted physical conditioning, injury prevention or rehabilitation, life balance, and mental preparation (Beswick 2001; Dorfman 2000; Dorfman and Kuehl 1995; Loehr 1994; Loehr and Schwartz 2003; Porter 2003, 2004; Porter and Foster 1990; Rotella 2004; Yandell 1999). The integrated use of basic and complex mental skills that can be learned through repetition produces high achievement in persons with athletic talent regardless of the competitive level or sport. To review, the basic skills are breathing and relaxation, positive self-talk, focus and attention shifting, visualization and imagery, and motivation and persistence; the complex skills are goal setting, self-evaluation, precompetition routine, and emotional control and intensity regulation (McDuff et al. 2005). Each of these mental preparation skills can link to and enhance general fitness, sound nutrition, injury recovery, life balance, and sports-specific training to produce consistent competitive self-confidence (Figure 2–1). When physical and mental training are integrated, the athlete can compete with a quiet mind, relaxed body, raised energy, and narrowed and rapidly shifting attention, producing automatic play that is described as "in the zone." In this chapter, I describe the application of five basic and five complex mental skills to individual sports (golf, tennis, track) and team sports (baseball, softball, football, soccer, ice hockey). Case studies from high school, club, intercollegiate, and professional levels are included. Recent findings from applied neuroscience and functional imaging research are introduced to validate and explain the use of these skills.

Athletes who excel at the highest levels have organized approaches for fitness, injury prevention, practice and competition, and mental prepara-

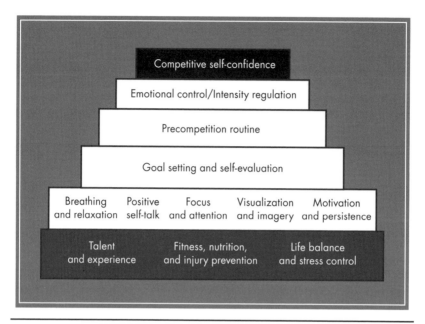

FIGURE 2–1. Pyramid of mental skills linking athletic fundamentals to competitive self-confidence.

tion. Elite players who consistently achieve peak performance despite changing competitive circumstances display quality preparation, competitive follow-through, and accurate self-evaluation. Stated more simply, they are ready to compete, get the job done, and react to results (Maher 2011). They also share a common set of emotional competencies and personality traits.

Emotional competencies are natural or learned skills that enhance an athlete's ability to compete with intensity and consistency and to become a good teammate (Aberman 2011; Anderson and Aberman 1995). The most important of these is *emotional control*—the ability to manage feelings and impulses to act while staying focused on a goal in the face of changing competitive circumstances. This competency permits individuals to play through mistakes and injuries and to bounce back when they are being outplayed. A second important competency is *self-awareness*—the ability to maintain perspective between ideal or unrealistic images of play and actual images that are based on accurate feedback from film or others. This ability prevents the development of unrealistic expectations and ensures that play occurs at the proper competitive level. A third important competency is *internal motivation,* which refers to practice or play that is based on a natural or developed love or passion for the game rather than an attempt to satisfy the expectations of others or for scholarships, fame, or social popularity. This competency prevents burnout and disappointment with playing time. A fourth competency is *empathy*—an instinctive ability to be sensitive to and supportive of others. This competency is critical to team unity and purpose. The final competency, *socialization,* refers to the ability to be an effective communicator and to bond with others while maintaining an attachment to strong competitive ideals and values. This competency is also necessary for team unity and critical for the development of a distinctive team style of play.

Group studies of Olympic champions have identified nine traits that are associated with high athletic achievement (Porter and Foster 1990). These traits, described in the following list, can be remembered using the acronym BELIEVE IT.

- **B**alances sports and other life areas. This trait refers to the ability to shift time and energy from sports to other important areas, such as family, friends, academics, hobbies, and rest. This ability follows an important principle in athletics, in which stress and recovery are described as making waves (Loehr and Schwartz 2003). Unplugging from training and competition, even if briefly, allows an athlete to return to practice and competition with renewed energy and enthusiasm. For younger athletes, this trait also refers to the ability to play and enjoy other sports or to cross-train.
- **E**ncourages and supports teammates. This trait is most necessary in team sports to ensure uniform intensity, work rate, and playing rhythm. Surprisingly, athletes who encourage competitors in other sports or on other teams seem to benefit from getting outside their own competitive arena.
- **L**ets go of mistakes and defeats easily. This trait is especially important in continuous- or repetitive-play sports, such as soccer, softball, tennis, or golf. If one or more players lose intensity or become distracted after a poor play or defeat, then the entire team's play can drop. Similarly, a bad pitch, an unforced error, or a bad shot can result in a dramatic performance decrement.
- **I**magines self and abilities in positive way. This trait means that despite winning or losing, the athlete maintains positive thoughts and feelings.
- **E**njoys training and competition. This trait means that despite a player's hard work and setbacks, his or her passion for the game and satisfaction from steady improvement dominate any negatives.
- **V**isualizes success and positive play. This trait refers to maintaining a general view that success ultimately comes from quality preparation and using visualization and positive imagery in practice and daily be-

fore competition. These mental repetitions are easy to do when in a relaxed state and provide a nice addition to the physical repetitions necessary to create the muscle memory of automatic play.

- **E**valuates performance and outcome. This trait refers to having a system for reviewing each game to identify the positives of play and areas for improvement, which are used to create actions for the next set of practices.
- **I**ntensity is maintained and regulated during practice and competition. *Intensity* is often defined as controlled and focused energy or aggression. Intensity is built slowly during the pregame routine. It requires that each player clear the mind of clutter and distractions, relax the body, and focus and rapidly shift attention while raising energy. Scoring in individual and team sports often occurs when one team's or player's intensity level rises well above that of the other team or player.
- **T**alks in positive and encouraging ways. An important goal is for teammates (as well as coaches and parents) to respond positively when they catch each other doing something well rather than groaning or shouting when mistakes are made. The best teams push players to peak play and performance through positive team talk. For individual play, a positive phrase can lock in an action and ensure that it is executed with skill and precision.

Since the late 1990s, evidence-based techniques derived from the cognitive, exercise, and neurological sciences have been introduced to bring a more valid and reliable approach to performance improvement training in sports (Carlstedt 2007; Yandell 1999; Zetou et al. 2002). These neuropsychophysiological approaches include cognitive profiling or brain typing, brain wave and heart rate variability biofeedback, and videotape self-modeling. Cognitive profiling involves testing an athlete before performance using cognitive and neuropsychological measures that assess mind-body interplay relevant to key moments in competition, such as a pass under pressure in soccer or a serve for a set point in tennis. Testing might assess, for example, sustained attention, physiological reactivity, and mistake coping. Biofeedback involves the measurement, feedback, and alteration of physiological parameters such as heart rate variability or brain wave patterns in athletes during a series of interventions over time. These interventions are designed to help a player change a current pattern to one that is more favorable to peak performance, such as decelerating heart rate before a field goal in football or a birdie putt in golf. Videotape self-modeling employs the use of edited video of repetitive, successful demonstrations (staged or actual) of one or more skills that are critical to a specific sport, such as a free-throw in basketball or making solid contact in baseball.

One evidence-based neurophysiological program developed by Carlstedt (2007) advocates a multistep approach. Each step is part of a long-term process designed to help athletes create and maintain a "seamless transition" in competition between the left and right brain hemispheres. In this approach, mental skills training is organized to help athletes improve left hemispheric activation for internal (strategic) planning for a shot or a play before shifting to right hemispheric activation for task or action completion with an external visual-perceptual focus. In addition, the training is designed to prevent the disruptive effects that negative thinking and stress can have on this left-right (internal-external) shift during critical athletic movements. The four steps of Carlstedt's program are summarized as follows:

- Step 1 requires determination of the athlete's personality profile in three areas empirically relevant to peak performance: 1) hypnotic susceptibility/subliminal attention (i.e., effortless attention—"zone trait"); 2) neuroticism/subliminal reactivity (i.e., reactivity to pressure—"zone buster"); and 3) repressive/subliminal coping (i.e., letting go of mistakes—"zone facilitator"). These three traits are strongly associated with the previously mentioned basic skills of relaxation, attention (focus), and self-talk and the complex skills of emotion and intensity regulation and self-evaluation. The ideal profile of *high* effortless attention, *low* reactivity to pressure, and *high* letting go of mistakes is strongly associated with consistent mind-body control and peak performance. In addition, these traits can serve as strong predictors of the mental skills of intervention acceptance, follow-through, and coachability.
- Step 2 involves extensive neurocognitive testing of attention, decision making, impulse control, and brain wave mapping.
- In Step 3, laboratory (timed serial subtractions) and field (repetitive perfect shot making) stress or pressure testing is conducted using heart rate variability measurement.
- Step 4 involves actual in-game monitoring of brain wave and heart rate patterns during critical athletic events using portable monitoring technology.

Basic Mental Skills

Breathing and Relaxation

Athletes, like all people, have two "hard-wired" neurological and neurohormonal systems that operate up and down the mind-brain-body axis.

These opposing stress and relaxation systems activate quickly and auto-matically during critical movements and can either enhance or degrade athletic performance. The operation and balance of these two systems during practice and competition are vital for coordinated movement and competitive self-confidence. The stress system electrically and hormon-ally activates the body's cardiovascular, neuromuscular, and visual-perceptual systems, which are critical to athletic movement and intensity. Too much stress activation, however, can lead to excessive physiological arousal, negative thoughts and emotions, and disrupted concentration, which can interfere with the rapid left (internal)–right (external) brain shift that must occur during critical athletic movements.

Stress-related thinking and breathing patterns, facial expressions, and body posture are easy to recognize. Stress breathing tends to be rapid, shallow, and noisy. In addition to use of the diaphragm to move air in and out, stress breathing involves use of accessory facial, neck, throat, and upper chest muscles. The focus of the breath cycle in stress breath-ing is on inhalation (getting air in). Stress breathing in particular and stress activation in general utilize large amounts of energy that may be-come unavailable for fitness training, practice, or competition.

Fortunately, the stress system can be opposed by the body's relaxation system. The relaxation system is designed to deactivate thinking, analyz-ing, and physiological arousal and to trigger calm and relaxation. The drop in cardiovascular intensity and the release of neuromuscular ten-sion allow for a fluid left-right brain shift and technically correct motor actions during critical athletic movements. Relaxation breathing is dis-tinctly different from stress breathing in that the former tends to be slow, quiet, and deep, and it uses mainly the diaphragm to move air. Relax-ation breathing emphasizes exhalation and tension release, and exhala-tion tends to be significantly longer than inhalation. The relaxation system can be activated by many activities, such as meditation, stretching, sunning, exercise, reading, naps, massages, socialization, walks, good nu-trition, and specialized breathing techniques.

Three specialized relaxation breathing techniques adapted from Weil (1999) can be easily learned and used to immediately quiet the mind, release tension, and reduce unnecessary emotional intensity. *Pat-terned relaxation breathing* consists of breathing in through the nose quietly and evenly for 4 counts, holding for 7 counts, and then breathing out through the mouth evenly for 8 counts—this pattern is repeated eight times and takes about 2 minutes. Breathing in through the nose warms, moistens, and filters the air, allowing the lungs to relax and fill com-pletely and evenly. Holding the breath (while counting and/or rocking) allows the mind to quiet and the body to settle. Breathing out allows for the release of mental and physical tension and strengthens the mind-body connection. In addition, the nose-mouth pathway activates a relaxing electrical circuit that facilitates tension release. A single breath cycle can be strengthened by saying, "in–2, 3, 4; hold–2, 3, 4, 5, 6, 7; out–2, 3, 4, 5, 6, 7–one…" while breathing.

The second technique is controlled *nasal hyperventilation*. This involves breathing rapidly (2–2.5 breath cycles per second with good rhythm) in and out through the nose for either three sets of 15–20 seconds each (with easy nose-mouth breathing in between) or one long cycle of 60 seconds (aiming for about 160–180 breath cycles in 60 seconds). Each episode of hyperventilation is likely to produce some mild symptoms resulting from low carbon dioxide and respiratory alkalosis (e.g., light-headedness, blurred vision, extremity tingling). These symptoms will disappear quickly, however, after two or three clearing breaths (in through the nose for a count of four and out through the mouth for eight counts or more) followed by easy nose-mouth breathing.

The third technique is the *clearing breath*. This involves starting a breath cycle by clearing all the air out through the mouth until a small knot is felt in the midline just above the navel. A smooth inhalation through the nose follows to a count of 4 until the lungs are filled to the level of the collar bone. Finally, a smooth exhalation through the mouth over 8–12 counts clears out substantial tension. The clearing breath is frequently used in competition just before a critical action, such as a penalty kick in soccer, a free throw in basketball, a serve in tennis, or a putt in golf. A triple clear, a variation of the clearing breath, consists of three lengthening breath cycles (in 4–out 4, in 4–out 6, in 4–out 8) and is used to dampen rising physiological arousal or intense worrying.

Case Study: I Get Too Amped Up Before Games

A college defensive back got so "amped up" before games that he could not take in adequate pregame nutrition or regulate his game intensity, which spiraled upward, resulting in multiple late-game penalties and mistakes.

Intervention: He was taught nasal hyperventilation and patterned breathing. Over a few weeks, he discovered that two to three repetitive sets of nasal hyperventilation every few hours starting the day before a game effectively countered his stress response, allowing him to eat and regulate his pregame and late-game intensity.

Case Study: I Feel Much More Pressure at This Level

After moving up to a higher competitive level, a professional baseball player felt anxiety, increased muscle tension, and poor command of his pitches.

Intervention: He was taught patterned breathing and clearing breathing exercises to repeat four to six times per day. In addition, he started using a clearing breath between pitches while throwing on the side, during warm-up, and in competition. He used a three-step process, in which he would occasionally walk off the mound, face away from the plate, and clear out the tension and focus on his core using a breath in through the nose and a prolonged exhalation out through the mouth. This release of tension allowed him to mechanically get on top of his pitches again and get the ball down in the zone. This improvement was possible because he was relaxed enough to rotate his shoulder, get his arm up, and finish his pitches with good wrist action and feel.

Brain Imaging Research

Meditation is a useful way to promote activation of the body's relaxation system. One of the most basic forms of meditation is concentration meditation, in which sustained attention is focused on an object, such as a small visual stimulus, or the breath. In a functional magnetic resonance imaging (fMRI) study comparing expert meditators to novices, Brefczynski-Lewis et al. (2007) found that activation of brain regions involved in sustained attention was stronger in experts. In addition, when distracter sounds were presented during meditation, expert meditators had less brain activation in regions related to analyzing and emotion, and more activation in regions related to response inhibition. The authors suggested that meditation may improve cognitive processes through negative self-talk inhibition.

Positive Self-Talk

The language areas of the brain have strong neural track connections with important emotional, attentional, and neuromuscular brain areas that are vital to critical athletic movements. According to Rotella (2004), movements in sports are most likely to be graceful and rhythmic if athletes use the unconscious (instinctive, intuitive) mind rather than the conscious (analytical, self-critical) mind. Positive self-talk during practice and competition is a good way to turn on the subconscious mind and get to automatic play. Effective positive self-talk must be simple, trigger a light and easy facial expression, relax and coordinate opposing large muscle groups, and fit within the specific rhythmical pattern of the sport. For example, during a golf swing, a tennis serve, or a baseball pitch, an athlete can say "back and thru" or "up and thru" to turn off analytical, left brain thinking, and to trigger a smooth shift to automatic, right brain action. Choosing short, simple phrases that literally command an athlete to correctly execute a critical movement without excessive thinking or analysis is desirable. In distance running, an athlete can quietly say "rise-up" when running up hills ("rise" is said during exhalation and "up" during shorter inhalation) or "recover-down" ("recover" is said during a long exhalation) on flat sections or downslopes. Saying "rise-up" with an external focus provides lift and acceleration, whereas saying "recover-down" drops the heart rate, releases muscle tension, and clears out metabolic toxins.

Positive self-talk can also be effective when preparing for an athletic action as part of a broader prepitch (baseball), preshot or prehit (golf, basketball, soccer, softball), or visualization routine (Dorfman 2000; Dorfman and Kuehl 1995). For example, in baseball or softball, a pitcher could occasionally say, between pitches or while visualizing, something like "down in the zone" or a shortened version like "DZ" or "hit my spots." A golfer could say "target line," "back of the cup," or "make it," whereas a tennis player could say "crosscourt," "down the line," or "breathe." When positive self-talk is used as part of a precompetitive or competitive routine, it is even more effective if used along with patterned breathing and visualization. When these different brain areas are activated together, the athlete is literally able to "see, say, and feel" any critical athletic movement, thereby reinforcing its execution.

Case Study: Sometimes I Just Can't Get Negative Thoughts Out of My Head

A professional golfer noted frequent nervousness and negative thinking on the tee box ("don't choke or don't hit the ball right") and competitive self-doubt ("the wheels keep falling off when I make mistakes").

Intervention: He was taught to use the patterned and clearing breathing techniques while holding his driver. At critical times in competition, he learned to walk to the edge of the tee box, face away from the target and his competitor, and take several clearing breaths while gripping the club hard during inhalation and releasing the tension during exhalation. This revised preshot routine helped turn off negative thinking by sending his attention down into his body.

Case Study: I'm Obsessed With Scoring Goals

A high school senior and club soccer player who wanted to play in college was putting too much pressure on herself by repeatedly saying that she needed to score more goals in games. This triggered negative self-talk and self-criticism and generated increased muscle tension, overthinking, and poor touch in competition.

Intervention: Instead of focusing on the desired outcome (goals, assists), she learned to shift her attention to positive play by saying repeatedly to herself "get to the ball," "make runs," or "work rate." By focusing on process rather than outcome, she shifted her talk and emotions from negative to positive and released excessive muscle tension.

Brain Imaging Research

Simple words like "no" and "yes" (and their associated negative and positive commands) are learned in childhood but continue to operate in adult life. In addition, these words and commands are associated with strong and quick emotionality and variable cognitive and motor response times. In an fMRI study, Alia-Klein et al. (2007) found that the emphatic use of "no" and "yes" vocalizations was associated with opposite brain-behavior response patterns. The "no" vocalization evoked negative emotions and slower response times, whereas the "yes" vocalization produced positive emotions and faster response times. This study supports the idea that positive and negative self-talk and supportive comments by teammates and parents can have quick and opposite influences on emotion, mental processing, and motor reaction times, possibly enhancing or diminishing critical athletic movements. The suggestion by DiCicco et al. (2002) for coaches and parents to "catch them [athletes] being good" may well have an evidence base.

Focus and Attention Shifting

According to sports psychologist Robert Nideffer (1993), playing in the zone and choking are both examples of altered states of consciousness. Altered states of consciousness are characterized by a change in sense of time, perception of the world, or ability to think and remember. For example, time distortion occurs when a person is engrossed in an enjoyable movie and surprised that 2 hours have just passed. This distortion is known as time compression.

The same thing can happen in sports during critical athletic movements. When an athlete is playing well, everything seems more natural; every pass or shot is accurate. When the athlete is not playing well, every pass or shot is off, and the body feels tense or out of balance. Whether the athlete is playing well or poorly, a specific state of consciousness (whether positive or negative) develops during attention shifting. Four distinct attention areas must be understood and mastered:

- **Broad internal focus** involves thinking, planning, or analyzing (e.g., when analyzing information from a scouting report of an opposing team). The goal is to make sense out of a lot of information. This type of focus may also involve broad attention to the body through scanning for muscle looseness and warmth, comfort, and coordination.
- **Narrow internal focus** is required when rehearsing a personal act of performance before doing it (e.g., when an athlete considers what to do if the ball is passed or hit to him or her). This level of attention is also useful when a player shifts to a narrow physical focus, such as his grip on a golf club or bat, her core tension level and breathing, or his foot position or balance.

- **Broad external focus** is used when an athlete is monitoring what is occurring around him or her. For example, a softball player uses this focus when deciding where to hit the ball or checking the position of the outfielders or base runners. A soccer player uses it when checking the position of the nearby players while dribbling into open space or the position of the goalkeeper when shooting.
- **Narrow external focus** is about reacting and performing. In soccer, if a player is dribbling down the flanks and the ball is crossed, the other players' attention narrows while positioning to receive or one-touch the ball. During putting in golf, the player's attention shifts from finding a line for the putt to executing the shot with feel and confidence.

Typically, attention rapidly shifts among these four areas. Playing in the zone happens when attention shifts effortlessly and an athlete is strongly locked in on a narrow external or internal area. Generally, when playing well, a player shifts attention less frequently and his or her focus is more external, with less time "in his or her head." Athletes often describe the experience as automatic thinking—"It just happens." In contrast, poor performance often happens when a player's focus is mostly internal and he or she is thinking and analyzing excessively.

When a player's attention is predominately external, performance seems automatic. At these times, the sense of control and predictability is enhanced. During choking, focus is usually too internal and analytical so that situations do not seem clear, and anticipation and attention shifting are difficult. For improved attention, therefore, the goal in practice and competition is to move steadily toward a narrowing, external focus. To move along a continuum toward a narrow external focus, the athlete needs to develop ways to shift from the analyzing brain to an external target. This involves identifying distractions and refocusing attention. No athlete is able to stay in the zone all or even most of the time. The goal, therefore, is to build momentum toward the development of concentration skills and the ability to quiet distractions. Sports psychologist Shane Murphy (1996) suggests using the four Rs when distracted: react, relax, reflect, and renew. These techniques should take only a few moments and can be used in virtually any situation:

- **React:** Athletes often get upset when mistakes are made. They need to allow the emotional reaction to surface and be released, but keep it controlled and in perspective.
- **Relax:** Athletes should use one of the following methods to help settle down after the mistake: positive self-talk, clearing breath, muscle relaxation, imagery, or inner focus.

- **Reflect:** Athletes need to figure out what interfered with performance, then move on. For example, if the ball came faster or higher than expected, an athlete must make an adjustment for the next play.
- **Renew:** Athletes need to refocus, with the goal of shifting from an internal, in-the-head focus to a narrow, external focus, as before the error was made.

Case Study: I Get Mentally Fatigued and Lose Focus at the End of Games

A junior club ice hockey goalie and a collegiate soccer goalie each became mentally fatigued late in their games and gave up late goals.

Intervention: Both goalies were introduced to the importance of taking attention breaks during the course of each game by using the phrase "lock and release." They were taught that while the puck or the ball was near the opposite goal, they should give their visual-perceptual system a short break (i.e., a release) by looking down blankly and sending attention narrowly to their core and by taking one or two strong clearing breaths while moving easily in front of the goal. Following this break, they should then lock back into the external action either broadly or narrowly.

Case Study: I Can't Control My Anger

A nationally ranked junior tennis player and a competitive high school golfer were both having frequent breaks in attention and drops in performance due to anger over bad shots.

Intervention: Both were instructed to develop an attention shifting routine to get over the mistake and continue playing point to point or shot to shot. The tennis player learned to turn away from the court and say "breathe," then squeeze his racket with both hands while breathing in through his nose, and then let go of the bad shot and frustration or anger while breathing out. The golfer was instructed to walk up the course, allowing a release of emotion with a strong exhalation, until she reached a certain landmark in the fairway (tree, yardage marker). At that landmark, she quit thinking about the mistake and moved on to making a good recovery shot.

Case Study: I Can't Put Up a Soft Shot; I Think I'm Too Tight

A collegiate basketball center was having difficulty making her free throws, frequently putting up hard shots ("bricks").

Intervention: She adopted a new preshot routine, using multiple clearing breaths and visual and balance shifting. She started each free throw in a good balanced position on the line with a strong internal focus, completing one full breath cycle. Her focus would then go external during inhalation to visually scan the other players in the lane. Her attention then shifted internally to her hands as she slowly expired and dribbled the ball four or five times. Finally, she looked up to the basket and took in a deep breath while locking in on a narrow visual focus (the back of the rim). She completed the shot while exhaling partially or holding her breath. This routine reduced physiological activation and released tension so she could put up a soft shot.

Brain Imaging Research

Most talented athletes learn quickly that technical repetitions are one of the main keys to performing critical athletic movements well while under pressure. Basketball players usually shoot hundreds of free throws on their own time each week, and middle infielders in baseball and softball take dozens of extra ground balls each day to improve. These repetitions allow the mind of the high-achieving athlete to remain cool and focused. A study by Milton et al. (2007) showed that during motor planning, the fMRI brain activation patterns of expert golfers were markedly different from those of novice golfers. Specifically, expert golfers had much simpler activation patterns in the visual, premotor, and motor areas, whereas the novices had additional activation of areas associated with emotions and emotional memory. Another fMRI study by Wright et al. (2010) demonstrated that in cortical areas associated with observing and understanding others' actions, the activation patterns of expert badminton players to anticipating stroke direction from a brief video clip were stronger than those of novices.

Visualization and Imagery

Mental imagery or visualization involves imagining oneself practicing a task (e.g., a golf swing or football pass) using sight and feel without any (or with limited) physical movement. This technique is now widely used by athletes and coaches at all levels in individual and team sports, such as golf, tennis, baseball, and soccer (Beswick 2001; Dorfman 2000; Dorfman and Kuehl 1995; Rotella 2004). Support for this technique comes from fMRI research in which actual and imagined motor repetitions were compared and found to show identical supplementary, premotor (action planning), and primary motor (action execution) cortical area activation patterns, but different activation patterns in feedback (frontal lobe somatosensory) and opposite-side posterior cerebellar (motor inhibition) areas (Lotze et al. 1999; Nyberg et al. 2006).

Critical movements in all sports involve activation of the brain's visual and perceptual systems and their links to cortical and subcortical (cerebellum, midbrain, and brain stem) motor control areas. As athletic movements progress, feedback from the somatosensory cortex (in front of the motor cortex) is activated, linking with specialized posterior parietal areas for visual and spatial integration to correct actions during sports with either continuous play (soccer, lacrosse, tennis) or interrupted play (golf, baseball, football). Motor repetitions in practice are a key to success in athletics so that automatic play (the seamless left-to-right brain shift mentioned in the opening section of this chapter) occurs during competition without interference from negative thinking or emotions. Early motor repetitions in childhood produce a basic muscle memory foundation that allows for more sophisticated movements to be added as experience increases.

Case Study: I Have Regular Images of Shanked Punts

A punter on a college football team was plagued throughout his career with inconsistency and recurrent negative images of shanking punts short and to the right.

Intervention: As part of a revised prepunt routine, the player was taught to break down the act of punting into small manageable steps ("snap, catch, lock, step, drop, and kick"). He set about saying these words and seeing himself repeatedly punting correctly when relaxed at home and at practice with good follow-through and long hang time. This combination of positive self-talk and visualization resulted in steady improvement in his consistency.

Case Study: If I Don't Stop Dropping Passes, I'll Be Dropped From the Team

A wide receiver on a professional football team was having problems with dropping the ball in practice and in games.

Intervention: In addition to improving his preplay relaxation and attention shifting skills, this athlete began daily visualization sessions during preseason camp. For 3–5 minutes each day, he would see himself surveying the defense, clearing out his tension, running his routes well, and looking the ball into his hands. As he worked on this revised routine more, his confidence and performance began to rise and he began making catches with consistency.

Case Study: If I Want More Playing Time, I Need to Improve My Goal Scoring

A college soccer athlete who played outside midfielder and forward had low confidence when attacking and shooting on goal. She would commonly engage in negative self-talk and imagine negative outcomes (shots struck poorly, blocked, or missed wide or high).

Intervention: She learned to use visualization of a current positive in her game (i.e., challenging for balls in the air on defense) and of goals scored in prior games and in practice as a basis to begin a daily regimen of visualizing strong, confident attacking with well-struck shots on frame. After the player used nightly visualization for a few weeks, her confidence began to rise and she attacked with greater certainty and success.

Brain Imaging and Brain Wave Research

Electroencephalographic (EEG) brain wave patterns and fMRI brain activation patterns are not the same for expert athletes as they are for less skilled athletes. In an fMRI mental imagery study of golfers with handicaps ranging from 0 to 16, Ross et al. (2003) found expected activation patterns in visual-perceptual, planning, execution, and error detection areas in all golfers, but far less activation of the cingulate gyrus or basal ganglia in experts than in novices. In addition, golfers with low handicaps had less overall activation with swing visualization than did golfers with higher handicaps, suggesting that the former had a simpler, more focused brain pattern. A preliminary study by Quencer et al. (2003) using portable EEG biofeedback also supports this finding by showing that expert golfers, compared to students, had a detectable quiet time just before hitting a shot. This quiet time may well indicate that an automatic swing has been learned, making more consistent ball striking possible. Using EEG, electromyography, and measures of muscle strength and power, Fontani et al. (2007) compared three groups of trained adult karate students learning a new skill over a month (i.e., students practicing the skill, students visualizing the skill, and control students who did not practice or visualize). The visualization group showed positive changes in muscle strength, power, and work similar to those of the action group but did not improve on reactivity. In addition, electromyographic findings documented changes in the movement-related brain macropotentials over time.

Motivation and Persistence

As athletes move from one competitive level to another, they discover that 1) more time is required and expected; 2) the competitors are more talented, athletic, and skilled; 3) fitness training and practice are more intense; and 4) the speed of play and competitive pressure are substantially greater. The athletes do not necessarily know or learn that desire, commitment, and persistence become vital to their long-term success. Each jump in competitive levels—from recreational to club, high school to college, or college to professional sports—requires an adjustment period that can last up to a full year or more. During this adjustment period, high-achieving athletes typically develop a stronger commitment to the sport and develop a formal improvement plan. Dorfman and Kuehl (1995) describe the critical sequence in high achievers as an inner desire to get better, the development of goals that allow that to happen, and unwavering dedication to future success. Many athletes also discover during these transitions that the mental and emotional aspects of sports become more important. In addition, some young athletes begin to question whether they want to commit to additional hours of training and competition and to worry about the loss of time in other important areas of their life, such as socialization, family, leisure, or academics.

Case Study: I'm Not Sure I Want to Play Soccer in College

A high school sophomore forward on a high-level club soccer team wasn't sure she wanted to continue playing on the team or play in college even though her club coach and mother were encouraging the further development of her talent. She was worried that she would not have time for studies or just having fun.

Intervention: The sports psychiatrist and player discussed the positives (teammates, socialization, competition, team success) and negatives (not enough time, practices too repetitive, player and coaching changes, injuries) of playing soccer. The psychiatrist emphasized the importance of having fun and good life balance. Together, they developed a set of simple short-term (1–3 months) and intermediate-term (6-month) goals. The athlete decided she wanted to improve her fitness in the short term and her attacking skills and leadership in the intermediate term, and then she would decide on continuing or quitting. Just knowing that she had the option to quit and permission to prioritize other life areas (friends, school) seemed to create new energy and enthusiasm, and she ultimately decided to continue playing.

Complex Mental Skills

Goal Setting

Most high-achieving athletes have a formal system to evaluate performance and improve play (Porter 2003; Porter and Foster 1990). The main intent of such evaluation systems should be steady improvement rather than perfection. These systems are created with specific preseason, in-season, and postseason goals in mind. Goal setting is a formal process that allows athletes at all levels to periodically assess strengths and weaknesses. Weaknesses then become targets for improvement. Goal setting means aiming to achieve a specific level of performance in a certain amount of time using a written action plan. Goals can be short term (30 days), intermediate (6 months), or long term (1 year). Individual goals should be chosen freely without strong external pressure; each goal, large or small, should be something internal that generates interest and excitement. The seven important steps to effective goal setting are listed and discussed below. Each goal must be accompanied by at least three specific action steps that are worked on regularly.

1. **Set goals that are specific and measurable.** Use numbers to specify exactly what to do and to enable measurement of gains.

   Examples: "Increase my soft toss hitting from occasionally to three times per week for 20 minutes." "Increase my touches on the ball from 20 to 30 per soccer game." "Increase my movement off the ball so that I get five additional open looks at the basket per practice."

2. **State each goal in positive terms.** Phrase goals to indicate what to do rather than what to avoid.

   Examples: "Increase quality shots on goal" rather than "Reduce shots off frame." "Increase the number of good at-bats or hits" rather than "Reduce the number of strikeouts."

3. **Set goals that are challenging but realistic.** Find the right balance between pushing for success rather than setting up for failure. Overly difficult goals will lower self-confidence.

   Example: "Increase my pass coverage intensity" rather than "Don't ever get beat by the wide receiver."

4. **Establish a timetable for completion.** A timetable allows for checks on progress and for devising goals that are realistic.

   Example: "Off season—Improve my touch on the ball through daily juggling and drills. Improve my foot speed by doing plyometric training 3 days a week. In season—Increase my assists by 20%. Win 50% more balls in the air."

5. **Personalize and internalize each goal.** Each goal must make sense and be adopted for positive self-improvement rather than forced by a parent or coach. Seek input from others when choosing or modifying goals.

6. **Monitor and evaluate progress.** Obtain regular feedback to determine progress. Chart results on an index card or graph. Ask others to help record results, such as good contact with the ball in baseball or softball. Progress may require that goals be modified.

7. **Link athletic goals to life goals.** Goal achievement should allow sports to be seen in a broader life context. Improvements in teamwork, discipline, commitment, and patience can lead to academic success and improved relationships.

An athlete should work on two or three goals at a time. For each goal, a time frame should be determined, the goal's purpose should be defined, and specific action steps should be developed. Figure 2–2 shows examples of intermediate- and long-term goals and action steps for a soccer player.

Self-Evaluation

Successful athletes have organized approaches for reviewing and evaluating the positives and negatives of play in practice and competition (Por-

Intermediate-term goal (6 months)	Long-term goal (12 months)
As a central defender, I want to improve my play in the air. This means anticipating well, getting into better position, challenging more strongly, and clearing the ball or directing it to my teammates. I will improve my strong challenges in the air during scrimmages and games by 50%. This improvement will allow me to break into the starting lineup.	Improve my shooting on goal by attacking the box more aggressively, isolating defenders one on one, shooting more quickly, and picking up a strong target in the back of the net. This will allow me to average three quality shots on goal and score one goal per game.
Step 1. Have a partner deliver 25 crosses for heading three times per week.	**Step 1.** Practice shooting on goal alone for 20 minutes a day three times a week.
Step 2. Have a partner toss balls for heading for 10 minutes three times per week.	**Step 2.** Dribble and practice one-on-one moves for 15 minutes three times per week.
Step 3. Head juggle 200 times per day, working up to 100 continuous juggles.	**Step 3.** Play in an indoor league over the winter.
Step 4. Strengthen core muscles with large-ball stabilization exercises three times a week.	**Step 4.** Participate in small-group tactical training twice weekly over the summer.
Step 5. Improve vertical leap with vertimax training three times a week.	**Step 5.** Improve first-step quickness through year-round plyometric training.
Step 6. Improve agility and balance with wobble board training for 15 minutes every day	**Step 6.** Improve flexibility by developing a new pregame warming and stretching routine.
Step 7. Visualize successful play in the air for 5 minutes every day.	**Step 7.** Practice turning on goal and shooting against a defender for 30 minutes a week.
Step 8. Watch several soccer matches and note the techniques of skilled defenders.	**Step 8.** Watch 30 soccer matches and/or goal scoring highlights.
	Step 9. Visualize successful shots daily for 5 minutes in the days before each game.

FIGURE 2–2. Examples of goals and action steps for soccer.

ter 2003; Porter and Foster 1990). These can include watching films, completing a postgame evaluation form, and/or discussing the game with parents, teammates, coaches, or a sports psychologist or mental skills trainer. An immediate purpose of the review is to identify technical areas for improvement and specific actions for skill development during the next few training sessions. Broader purposes are to stay positive and humble, to assume responsibility for results, to focus only on those areas that are controllable, and to commit to ongoing improvement.

Case Study: I Can't Play as Well After Being Away

A high school and club soccer player (a forward) was just returning to play after a broken arm had kept her away from training and competition for 3 months. She had lost her fitness and confidence and was demoted to a lower-level club team because of inconsistent play.

Intervention: She committed herself over a 2-month period to improve her fitness, speed of play, and touches on the ball. After each game, she completed a game review form that consisted of 1) the positives of her play (in technical, tactical, and mental areas) and how they helped her and the team, and 2) the negatives of her play and what she did to try to overcome these. In addition, the sports psychiatrist asked her to identify three areas to work on during practice the following week. Regular follow-up meetings were held every few weeks over the entire season. This systematic approach to improvement helped her to get back on track with her fitness and technical training and to regain her playing confidence.

Precompetition Routine

An athlete who is well prepared every time he or she competes sets the stage for consistent, high-level performance. Preparation increases the likelihood of success and reduces mistakes. A precompetition routine includes organized actions from awakening until a competition begins. These routines vary with the time of the competition (day or night) or its location (home or away). Developing a slightly different routine for each circumstance is useful. Routines are not rituals; they are adaptable and adjustable depending on the situation.

Precompetition routines have three stages: wake-up, arrival at the field, and final preparation. Each stage contains physical and mental components. The wake-up stage addresses nutrition and equipment. During this stage, an athlete or team needs to confirm that everything that needs to be taken to the field has been gathered and checked for wear and tear. Items might include socks, cleats, uniform, ball, gloves, and so forth. Other components of this stage include energy production, hydration, meals, meetings, cardiovascular system activation, stretching, and treatment. Mental preparation during this stage involves reviewing the opponent or finalizing strategy and style of play. Some athletes also engage in relaxation, meditation, music listening, movie watching, or journal writing.

After arriving for competition, an athlete needs to warm up and stretch before engaging in organized drills, such as throwing, kicking, hitting, passing, or shooting. All fitness and technical drills should lead to a quiet mind, relaxed body, increased energy, and narrow focus. If time permits, an athlete can do extra work on a specific skill that was identified in the postcompetition reviews.

During the final preparation stage, fine-tuning is usually all that is necessary. Each athlete makes adjustments to his or her strategy, relaxation, positive thinking, or imagery. Bull et al. (1996) divided the final phase into three distinct parts: preparation (mainly physical—occurs during warm-up), focusing (mainly visual—occurs just after warm-up), and execution (mainly positive talk—just before competition). Attention cues (physical, visual, or verbal) are used during this stage to strengthen preparation. These cues help with relaxation, concentration, and intensity regulation. No set cues are used; instead, unique groups of cues are used by each athlete. Physical cues require doing something specific and narrow (e.g., grabbing some grass, pulling up socks, staying on toes, taking a deep breath). Visual cues involve intense focus on something narrow and external in the environment (e.g., the athlete's locker, a picture, a word phrase, the writing on the ball, cleat laces, an advertisement, the net of the goal). Verbal cues are single words or word phrases that are repeated silently (e.g., "be ready," "play hard," "protect the goal," "be aggressive," "focus," "relax and go").

Case Study: I Don't Take Enough Energy Into the Game

A professional late-innings relief pitcher was having difficulty getting his energy up and his focus sharp before entering the game.

Intervention: An inning or two before it looked like he might enter the game, the player started visualizing himself dominating the hitters with location and power. He began to activate himself physically while still seated by chewing tart gum, doing brief (10-second) sets of nasal hyperventilation, and stretching and then releasing the large muscle groups of his back and shoulders several times with strong clearing breaths. He further activated himself mentally by visually locking onto a narrow external target, such as home plate or a spot on the fence, and then releasing in sync with a breath cycle. When he got up to throw, he did some additional sets of rapid breathing with progressive core tightening, followed by strong clearing breaths. Between warm-up pitches, he took one strong clearing breath, then repeated a positive statement ("dominate") while giving his visual system a break from looking at the bullpen catcher and mitt. This revised routine resulted in raised energy, sharper focus, and improved confidence.

Case Study: I Can't Score If I Can't Make Putts

A club professional golfer was having difficulty with putts and chips during tournaments. Although he had tried different putters and grips, he was still giving away too many strokes.

Intervention: His prechip/preputt routine was reviewed and revised to make sure he released excess muscle tension and narrowed his focus. To lock onto his target and line more strongly, he introduced a strong clearing breath while still standing behind the ball. On inhalation, he would tighten his grip on the club slightly, survey the green, and see the line, whereas on exhalation, he would lock onto the line and the target while releasing his grip and saying "see it" or "lock in." He repeated this routine while standing over the ball, except this time he would say "make it" on exhalation. This revised routine seemed to raise his confidence by clearing tension and doubt and replacing them with solid focus and certainty.

Brain Imaging Research

Mental skills training was introduced in individual sports such as golf, tennis, and track many years before its use in team sports. Preshot (golf), prereturn/pre-serve (tennis), and prerace (sprints, middle distance) routines have long been recognized as keys to success, with a shot-to-shot emphasis in golf, a point-to-point emphasis in tennis, and a lap-to-lap emphasis in track. As mentioned previously, in the "Focus and Attention Shifting" section, an fMRI study by Milton et al. (2007) showed that motor activation patterns during the preshot routine were much simpler in expert than in novice golfers. The authors concluded that experts in golf achieve "focused and efficient" neural networks through their preshot routines and repetitions from practice and play.

Emotional Control and Intensity Regulation

Emotional control and intensity are difficult to maintain during practice and competition for both individual and team sports. For individuals, mistakes often trigger quick emotional reactions, such as fear, frustration, anger, or disappointment, from automatic (subcortical) brain areas. These quick emotions may be followed by additional mistakes (e.g., hitting another poor shot in golf, giving up a second home run in baseball, committing a needless foul in soccer or basketball) unless the athlete adopts a planned behavioral approach to prevent these reactions. Intensity is a complex blend of determination, energy, work rate, and focus. It cannot be raised quickly but rather must be raised during pregame warm-ups or at half-time by clearing the mind of distractions (including poor play), relaxing the body, raising the energy, and narrowing and focusing attention. In team sports, members may have difficulty starting or continuing to play with a consistent intensity level. Therefore, runs in basketball, momentum shifts in football, and goals in soccer often occur when one team's intensity level rises well above that of the other.

Case Study: I Can't Let Go of Mistakes

A collegiate soccer player regularly lost her intensity during competition after an early and simple mistake on defense or in the attack. The mistake led to quick disappointment and self-doubt that turned on her analyzing left brain, dramatically slowing her speed of play and decision making.

Intervention: The athlete created images of positive play from reviewing games and practices via film and discussion. She reinforced these images of power, certainty, and confidence with strong positive phrases, such as "power up" or "take someone on." Over time, she learned to use these images and positive self-talk before and during competition to prevent drops in her intensity and to maintain a positive attitude.

Conclusion

Recent advances in brain science, especially functional brain imaging and brain wave biofeedback, provide a strong evidence base to support the integration of mental preparation into an overall approach to training and competition that has previously focused on physical, technical, and tactical areas. Newer approaches such as life balance skill development, stress control, and mental skills training can be easily introduced into the fitness facility, training room, or practice areas in collaboration with athletic trainers, nutritionists, coaches, strength and conditioning staff, and team physicians and chiropractors. This chapter describes some behavioral and emotional traits of high-achieving athletes and the use of a set of basic and complex mental skills to enhance performance. Examples from different sports illustrated the actual application of these skills to a wide range of problems with performance. As new portable imaging and biofeedback technology becomes available, more specific measures of the positive effects of mental preparation on performance can be documented during practice or competition.

Key Clinical Points

- Five basic mental skills—breathing and relaxation, positive self-talk, focus and attention shifting, visualization and imagery, and motivation and persistence—can be used to enhance individual and team performance.

- Five complex mental skills—goal setting, self-evaluation, precompetition routine development, intensity regulation, and emotional control—are critical to competitive self-confidence and consistent play.

- Five emotional competencies—control, self-awareness, internal motivation, empathy, and socialization—are necessary for intensity regulation, overcoming mistakes and disappointment, burnout prevention, and team unity and resilience.

- The following nine behavioral traits, remembered using the acronym BELIEVE IT, are associated with high-achieving athletes: **B**alances,

Encourages, **L**ets go, **I**magines, **E**njoys, **V**isualizes, **E**valuates, **I**ntensity, **T**alks positively.

- In evidence-based cognitive profiles from neuroscience, three cognitive traits—high effortless attention, low reactivity to pressure, and high letting go of mistakes—are associated with steady improvement in competitive play; these traits comprise the ideal personality profile for an athlete.

- Three practical breathing techniques that emphasize exhalation— patterned relaxation breathing, nasal hyperventilation, and the clearing breath—can be used to control arousal and anxiety, reduce muscle chain tension, and improve focus and attention shifting.

- Positive word phrases that fit within the rhythm of the sport, trigger positive emotions, and turn on positive images can be used to maintain positive play or shift play from a negative to a positive pattern.

- Brief but regular mini-breaks during competition are necessary to maintain focus and attention shifting.

- Daily visualization of positive practice and play, if paired with partial movement, activates the same brain areas as actual athletic repetition and therefore builds muscle memory.

- Sports goals should be freely chosen, specific and measurable, stated in positive terms, challenging but realistic, personalized and internalized, and monitored and evaluated.

- Precompetition routines are effective when they quiet the mind, relax the body, balance energy, control emotions, and narrow focus and shift attention.

References

Aberman R: The Performance Sweet Spots. Minneapolis, MN, Lennick Aberman Group, 2011

Alia-Klein N, Goldstein RZ, Tomasi D, et al: What is a word? No versus yes differentially engage the lateral orbitofrontal cortex. Emotion 7:649–659, 2007

Anderson J, Aberman R: Why Coaches Quit and How You Can Stay in the Game. Minneapolis, MN, Fairview Press, 1995

Beswick B: Focused for Soccer. Champaign, IL, Human Kinetics, 2001

Brefczynski-Lewis JA, Lutz A, Schaefer HS, et al: Neural correlates of attentional expertise in long-term meditation practitioners. Proc Natl Acad Sci USA 104:11483–11488, 2007

Bull J, Albinson JG, Shambrook CJ: The Mental Game Plan. Eastbourne, UK, Sports Dynamics, 1996

Carlstedt R: Integrative evidence based athlete assessment and intervention: a field-tested and validated protocol. Journal of the American Board of Sport Psychology 1:1–30, 2007

DiCicco T, Hacker C, Salzberg C: Catch Them Being Good. New York, Penguin Books, 2002

Dorfman HA: The Mental ABCs of Pitching: A Handbook for Performance Enhancement. South Bend, IN, Diamond Communications, 2000

Dorfman HA, Kuehl K: The Mental Game of Baseball: A Guide to Peak Performance. South Bend, IN, Diamond Communications, 1995

Fontani G, Migliorini S, Benocci R, et al: Effect of mental imagery on the development of skilled motor actions. Percept Mot Skills 105:803–826, 2007

Loehr JE: The New Toughness Training for Sports. New York, Plume, 1994

Loehr J, Schwartz T: The Power of Full Engagement. New York, Free Press, 2003

Lotze M, Montoya P, Erb M, et al: Activation of cortical and cerebellar motor areas during executed and imagined hand movements: an FMRI study. J Cogn Neurosci 11:491–501, 1999

Maher C: The Complete Mental Game of Baseball. New York, AuthorHouse, 2011

McDuff DR, Morse E, White R: Professional and collegiate team assistance programs: services and utilization patterns. Clin Sports Med 24:943–958, 2005

Milton J, Solodkin A, Huistik P, et al: The mind of expert motor performance is cool and focused. Neuroimage 35:804–813, 2007

Murphy S: The Achievement Zone. New York, Berkley Books, 1996

Nideffer R: Psyched to Win. Champaign, IL, Leisure Press, 1993

Nyberg L, Eriksson J, Marklund P: Learning by doing versus learning by thinking: an fMRI study of motor and mental training. Neuropsychologia 44:711–717, 2006

Porter K: The Mental Athlete-Inner Training for Peak Performance in All Sports. Champaign, IL, Human Kinetics, 2003

Porter K: The Mental Athlete. Champaign, IL, Human Kinetics, 2004

Porter K, Foster J: Visual Athetics: Visualization for Peak Sports Performance. Dubuque, IA, William C Brown, 1990

Quencer RM, Winters R, Leadbetter D: Editorials: unlocking the mental aspects of the golf swing: can functional MR imaging give us insights? Am J Neuroradiol 24:1033–1034, 2003

Ross JS, Tkach J, Ruggieri PM, et al: The mind's eye: functional MR imaging evaluation of golf motor imagery. Am J Neuroradiol 24:1036–1044, 2003

Rotella B: The Golfer's Mind. New York, Free Press, 2004

Weil A: Breathing: The Master Key to Self-Healing. Boulder, CO, Sounds True, 1999

Wright MJ, Bishop DT, Jackson RT, et al: Functional MRI reveals expert-novice differences during sport-related anticipation. Neuroreport 21:94–98, 2010

Yandell J: Visual Tennis. Champaign, IL, Human Kinetics, 1999

Zetou E, Tzetzis G, Vernadakis N, et al: Modeling in learning two volleyball skills. Percept Mot Skills 94:1131–1142, 2002

Chapter 3

Stress Recognition and Control

Athletes, especially those at higher competitive levels, perform repeatedly under a spotlight and have their personal lives examined under a microscope. They must adapt to unpredictable events and situations in short time frames while meeting the high expectations of themselves and others. They must perform and produce and look good doing it.

Athletic training and competition are demanding, often requiring year-round commitment and self-sacrifice for athletes to perform with consistency under changing competitive circumstances. The unique demands of competitive sports, such as performance expectations, long practices, infrequent days off, changing schedules, travel, family separations, lack of privacy, media attention, exhaustion, and injury, must be managed with other priorities in life, such as relationships, family, children, financial security, and future education or career planning. Therefore, at times during a playing season, the demands of life and sports may temporarily exceed an athlete's ability to cope, and day-to-day functioning and performance may suffer. Recognizing the early symptoms of stress is often the first step for preventing performance drops and maintaining general functioning.

At its most basic levels, stress is necessary for survival and personal growth and development. At low to moderate levels, stress is positive, time limited, and manageable; however, at higher levels, it is additive and disruptive to relationships, performance, and health. Stress produces strong physiological reflexes that prepare the mind and body to meet nonroutine demands. The nervous system's energy level rises, emotional intensity increases, problem-solving brain systems activate, and hormonal patterns change. Fortunately, an equally powerful counterbalancing relaxation reflex exists. This reflex slows heart rate and breathing, releases muscle tension, quiets mental excitation, and narrows attention. Living a healthy lifestyle involves balancing these two opposing systems. Fortunately, many effective stress control techniques are available to help busy people. Like many other habits or practices in life, however, these techniques must be learned through repetition and are most effective if incorporated into daily routines.

Stress is best defined as a rapid, automatic (hard-wired) reaction to high, sustained levels of routine, novel, or unexpected demands. These demands (stressors) typically cluster into physical and mental categories (Table 3–1) but vary significantly in pattern across individual athletes and sports. Awareness of the different types of stressors can lead to an action plan with specific stressor management strategies. For example, maintaining fluid intake on long road trips can prevent dehydration, and avoidance of excessive stimulant intake (i.e., caffeine, nicotine) or alcohol use (i.e., three or more drinks per occasion) can prevent insomnia or delayed adjustment to jet lag.

TABLE 3–1.   Types of physical and mental stressors

Physical stressors	Mental stressors
Environmental	**Cognitive**
Physical work	Information (too much, too little)
Heat, cold, wetness	Sensory overload or deprivation
Bright lights, darkness	Time pressure, waiting
Noise, excitement, crowds	Uncertainty, unpredictability
Travel, jet lag	Hard choices, no choices
Infection, toxic agents	Recognition of impaired performance
Physiological	**Emotional**
Sleep debt	Fear or anxiety from threats of injury, disease, pain, loss, failure
Dehydration, poor nutrition	
Poor hygiene	Grief from important losses
Illness or injury	Resentment, anger, rage
Overuse or underuse of muscles	Frustration, guilt
Fatigue	Boredom-producing inactivity
Substance use (e.g., alcohol, tobacco)	Conflicting demands (home vs. job)
	Interpersonal feelings (rejection, shame)
	Temptation causing loss of faith

High-demand states lead to four common stress reactions: anxiety, depression, anger, and somatic (physical) response (Figure 3–1). These reactions are produced by automatic circuits in subcortical brain areas and must be countered by simple but organized stress control routines and assistance from support networks. Although many individuals have one main type of stress reaction, some have a mixture of symptoms from several reactions. As shown in Figure 3–1, sleep difficulties (too much or too little), decreased energy, increased substance use (alcohol, tobacco, marijuana, pills), and altered activity level (overactive vs. social isolation) are common to all four reaction types.

Fortunately, high stress levels are usually temporary, and the common stress reactions that interfere with general functioning and athletic performance decrease over time. Many strategies can be used for managing common stressors and preventing stress reactions from lasting too long or interfering too much. To control stress, individuals can try three targeted approaches: 1) identify, organize, prioritize, and develop an action plan to reduce all current stressors; 2) identify and manage the current stress response through support network assistance, counseling, medications, and an intent to create more positive moments and short-term success; and 3) identify those background factors that have predisposed to the high stress state (such as trauma, loss, personality style, and mental disorder), and work through these with therapy, pastoral counseling, or self-help (Figure 3–2). For additional discussion on the impact of background factors on injury response and recovery and the impact of mental disorders, see Chapter 6, "Injury Recovery and Pain Control," and Chapter 7, "Common Mental Disorders.

If not recognized and controlled, high-stress lifestyles threaten an athlete's general health and well-being. Sustained stress can produce health changes, aggravate existing illnesses, or impede or complicate injury recovery. For more than 50 years, physicians have recognized that certain chronic illnesses are linked with stress. In 1950, Franz Alexander described seven classic psychosomatic disorders (essential hypertension, neurodermatitis, bronchial asthma, rheumatoid arthritis, hyperthyroidism, ulcerative colitis, and peptic ulcer). Today, the disorders have changed (heart disease, migraine headaches, irritable bowel syndrome, hyperventilation syndrome, chronic fatigue, fibromyalgia, hives, hypoglycemia, and dizziness), but the mechanisms are the same (Hackett and Cassem 1987; Strain 1978). The following 12 stress control tips and case studies are presented as strategies to quickly and simply reduce stress levels and restore optimal functioning and performance (Asmundson and Taylor 2005; Childre 1998; Loehr and Schwartz 2003; Rollnick et al. 2000; Weil 1999).

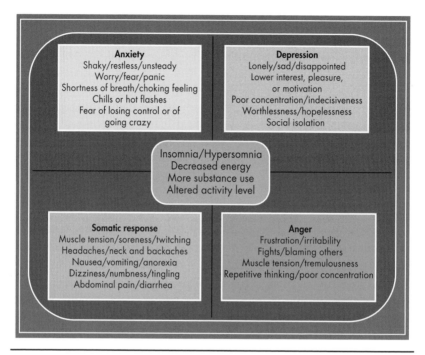

FIGURE 3–1. Symptoms of the four common stress reactions.

The list in the centrally located box indicates symptoms that are common to all four stress reactions. Use this figure to assist athletes in identifying their specific stress-response profile.

Tip 1: Know the Facts About Stress

Stress is necessary for survival and for human growth and development. It is usually a normal reaction to an abnormal situation. Reactions to stress are initially positive, but they can become unhealthy if stress is prolonged without breaks. Stress in one life area increases stress in other life areas.

Case Study: Newborn Baby and Sleep

A professional football player was having difficulty staying awake in team meetings and was struggling with film watching and playbook studying at home. He was married with two children, a 3-year-old daughter and a 6-month-old son. He identified a significant change in his sleep pattern after the birth of his son. From birth, his son was in a crib next to the wife's side of their bed. Because the player was a light sleeper, he had difficulty falling asleep and would awaken when his son needed to nurse. In addition, his daughter had become jealous and wanted to sleep in her parents' bedroom. They agreed to let her sleep between them for a few nights, but 6 months later, she was still coming into their room in the middle of the

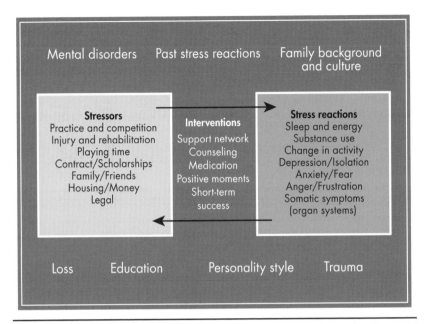

Mental disorders   Past stress reactions   Family background and culture

Stressors
Practice and competition
Injury and rehabilitation
Playing time
Contract/Scholarships
Family/Friends
Housing/Money
Legal

Interventions
Support network
Counseling
Medication
Positive moments
Short-term success

Stress reactions
Sleep and energy
Substance use
Change in activity
Depression/Isolation
Anxiety/Fear
Anger/Frustration
Somatic symptoms
(organ systems)

Loss   Education   Personality style   Trauma

FIGURE 3–2. Common sports stressors, stress reactions, background factors, and interventions.

night. She was a restless child, and her constant movement added to the athlete's sleep problems. The demands of parenting and the presence of both children in the parental bedroom were identified as major stressors. The lack of sleep was interfering with the player's energy and concentration and was negatively impacting his football performance.

Intervention: A plan was developed to transition both children out of the parents' bedroom. First, the older child was told she needed to be a big girl and start sleeping in her own bedroom. The player committed to putting her to bed nightly by reading a story and leaving on a night-light. Each time she tried to come into the parents' bedroom, her father took her back to her room and stayed with her until she fell asleep. Over a 3-night period, she adjusted to sleeping in her room and began sleeping through the night. Because the master bedroom was quite large and had a sitting area, the baby's crib was moved into the sitting area. The additional distance resulted in longer sleep intervals and fewer awakenings. The player began sleeping 5–6 hours each night, and this greatly improved his energy and learning.

Tip 2: Recognize Symptoms of Stress Early

Athletes should become aware of stressors in their life and remember that high stress levels are just as likely to occur when many small stressors are present as when one or two large stressors are present. Although most individuals have one main stress reaction pattern—anxiety, depression, anger, or somatic response—a mix of symptoms from each area is also possible. Changes in sleep and energy (too much or too little), altered activity level, and increased substance use (caffeine, nicotine, alcohol, marijuana) are common to all four stress reaction types.

Case Study: Unresolved Grief

A professional baseball player went to one of the athletic trainers complaining of restless sleep and concern about his wife's mood. The couple had been discussing having their first child for about 6 months, and gradually over this period of time, his wife had become more anxious, withdrawn, and depressed. They began fighting more when she stopped doing the routine things to maintain the condominium (i.e., shopping, cleaning, laundry, bill paying).

Intervention: The sports psychiatrist met with the player the next day in the clubhouse. The player speculated whether the discussion of having a child had triggered sadness in his wife because her mother had died of breast cancer 2 years earlier, and her father had died in the same year from an unexpected heart attack. The psychiatrist scheduled an appointment for the player's wife 2 days later. The evaluation revealed significant anxiety, unresolved grief, and current depression. The wife was treated with an antianxiety/antidepressant medication and weekly short-term grief therapy. She improved greatly over the next 3 months. Then the couple was seen once a month to explore their relationship and plans for a child. After a few meetings, they decided the time was right to try for a pregnancy, agreeing that they had good support from his parents if needed. A few months later, his wife became pregnant and eventually delivered a healthy son. Because of her concern about the effects of medication during pregnancy, her medication was tapered and then stopped. The player's wife met with the psychiatrist twice monthly. She remained optimistic and confident during and after the pregnancy and became a happy and caring mother. She elected to start taking her medication again, and the psychiatrist followed her for another year, during which time she maintained a stable mood, low anxiety, good energy, and high functioning.

Tip 3: Trigger the Relaxation Reflex

Cardiovascular exercise is a reliable way to trigger the body's relaxation reflex through the reduction of accumulated muscle tension and the release of certain calming brain chemicals that are long acting. Brisk walking with a partner several times per week is a good place to start. Individuals should also become aware of their breathing. Stress breathing is shallow, rapid, and uneven, whereas relaxation breathing is deep, smooth, and slow. Various breathing techniques (e.g., patterned relaxation breathing, nasal hyperventilation, clearing breath) are described in Chapter 2, "Mental Preparation." Massage, music, movies, meditation, muscle stretching, napping, and meals are also reliable triggers of relaxation.

Case Study: Fitness Test Phobia

A first-year college soccer player was concerned about passing the team's fitness test at the end of the first week of preseason practice. Even though she had followed the fitness plan given to her by the team's strength coach all summer and had always done well in distance running and sprints, she was still concerned. She was apprehensive because she had heard that the head coach often made decisions about playing time based on fitness test performance. She was less concerned about the distance test, but she knew that she would get anxious and tight on the "beep test" (a 20-meter shuttle run).

Intervention: The sports psychiatrist developed a pretest routine for the player that included controlled prolonged expirations and dropping of her arms and shaking out of her tension. In addition, if the athlete's anxiety rose, she was to go immediately into a triple-clear breathing pattern of 4 counts in though the nose and then 6 out thorough the month, followed by 4 in and 8 out, then 4 in and 12 out. During the test, she would breathe with long, smooth, strong exhalations that were synchronized with arm movements and stride. The prolonged exhalations were followed by passive, easy inhalations without the use of her chest or neck muscles. This approach saved energy and did not allow the buildup of carbon dioxide as the shuttle run got faster. Instead, she stayed ahead of the rising demand for oxygen and clearing of carbon dioxide by maintaining the long expiration cycles. She practiced these breathing techniques daily for a week, and at night visualized light and easy running on the test. In addition, she practiced the test a few times with these routines and a partner. She did well and gradually built her confidence. She passed the test, finishing in the top 25% of the team.

Tip 4: Think Positively and Look Calm and in Control

A person's mind and body have repetitive patterns of thinking, emotion, facial expression, posture, and movement that are associated with good stress control and life balance. Also, actions follow thoughts, and certain facial expressions, such as a light smile, are associated with better emotional control. Maintaining a calm and confident outward appearance can help in creating a faster pathway out of a stress cycle.

Case Study: Choking in Tryouts

A freshman high school student decided to try out for a premier club lacrosse team but was worried that she might choke in tryouts as she did the year before. She noted her tendency to get anxious and tight in high-pressure situations and then make mistakes. Once she made a mistake or two, she would get down on herself and quickly lose confidence.

Intervention: The sports psychiatrist asked the athlete to identify her main strengths as a lacrosse player. She said she was a midfielder with good stick and passing skills, excellent field awareness, and above average speed and athleticism. When asked to identify a word phrase that would describe her play when relaxed and confident, she said that it would look "easy and rhythmic," that she would "just flow." Next, she was asked to put an anxious look on her face and then shift to a confident one. She was able to produce the anxious look quite easily but had trouble creating a confident expression. To get a better sense of a confident expression, the athlete and psychiatrist did an image search on the computer for "confident lacrosse player." Of the many images that surfaced, she eventually selected one that connected strongly with her and printed it out. She practiced the expression daily, starting first with a loose lower face and then progressing to a light smile of confidence. In addition, she visualized completing all drills and scrimmages with calm and confidence for 3–5 minutes nightly during the week before the tryouts. She attended the first two tryouts and felt that she had stayed relaxed and made few mistakes. A few days later, she accepted the offer of a roster spot on the team.

Tip 5: Develop a Support Network

Most individuals need a support network comprising several people who can be trusted and who are readily available to provide sound advice. One main purpose of a circle of support is to have people to talk with about stressors and to help put those stressors into perspective. A support network might include a combination of family, friends, and colleagues. An individual can learn from the example of and seek advice from people in his or her network, particularly those who seem to manage stress well. If establishing a network is not possible or effective, an individual can seek assistance from a spiritual advisor, physician, or therapist.

Case Study: Caught in the Middle

A third-year high school lacrosse player sought assistance from a sports psychiatrist because he had not recovered completely from a fractured leg that he sustained in a game 1 year earlier. The player complained of persistent pain and tightness that inhibited his running and fitness. Because he was unable to get back to full speed, he had not played in any games. In a discussion with the player's mother on the phone before the initial appointment, the psychiatrist discovered three other major stressors: 1) a contentious divorce of the player's parents resulting from an extramarital affair, with continued fighting between his mom and dad; 2) an older brother with cerebral palsy who had many medical problems and recurrent surgeries; and 3) the athlete's difficulty with higher-level math and science courses. Discussion of these stress areas with the athlete produced anger, disappointment, and sadness, and a feeling of being trapped in the conflict between his parents. When asked whom he could rely on to help him with his situation, he said that there was no one.

Intervention: The player seemed open to the idea that he needed a support network because his situation was complicated. For his academics, he agreed to use a tutor and a neighbor who was good in science and math. For the conflict between his parents, he agreed that separate meetings with them might increase their awareness of how much pressure he felt to take sides. Regarding the time he was expected to spend with his older brother, the athlete openly talked about feeling guilty about wanting to be with his own friends, but not being comfortable doing that because his mother seemed so stressed. Once the mother was informed of his feelings, she agreed to seek assistance and better explore community resources for her older son. Finally, the coach of the athlete's club team was contacted and said he had suspected that family stress was negatively impacting the player's recovery. Because the coach had a good relationship with the player and had known him for 6 years, he agreed to drive him to some of the games so they could talk. After a few months, the player became much more engaged in his rehabilitation program. An enhanced stretching routine resulted in improved flexibility and diminished pain and tightness. As the months passed, he began to regain the speed and athleticism that had always been a strong part of his game.

Tip 6: Take Regular Breaks From the Demands of Sports

The mind and the body operate in high-stress periods using energy that is stored in the chemical systems of the brain, muscles, liver, and certain glands. These chemical supplies can be depleted if recovery breaks are not strategically inserted into each day, month, and year. Short breaks (20–30 minutes) every 6–8 hours are often enough to allow for energy resupply. Longer breaks (days to weeks) with a complete work disconnect are often helpful after prolonged periods of exertion. Breaks should have different tasks and patterns than the demands of athletic training and competition and should trigger enjoyment, humor, laughter, and relaxation.

Case Study: Take a Nap

A fourth-year professional defensive lineman was seen by the sports psychiatrist in the training room while receiving treatment for a deep thigh bruise. When asked how things were going, he said he was always exhausted and had become more irritable toward his wife and 2-year-old daughter. After 9–10 hours of practice, meetings, and films, he said he was tired and needed a break. However, when he got home, he said his wife wanted him to play with his daughter, who had not seen him all day. He resented these requests and would often storm off mad to his basement retreat. The problems with that approach were that tension with his wife would last for hours and he tended to stay downstairs and skip dinner.

Intervention: The player was encouraged to have a discussion with his wife about the demands of his workdays and how energy draining and sometimes boring the activities were. He agreed to ask her for 30–45 minutes for a quick recovery nap as soon as he got home in exchange for joining the family upstairs afterward for play and dinner. She agreed to try this, and after a week, they were both surprised with how cheerful and energetic he was with his daughter and how much more they enjoyed family meals together.

Tip 7: Improve Time Management Skills

Time management skills can be improved by breaking down the day into smaller time blocks and accomplishing at least one task during each. Completing one small task (or a small part of a larger task) in each time block is preferable to failing to complete a larger task that day.

Case Study: Academic Procrastination

A third-year college soccer player was referred to a sports psychiatrist by his head coach because of academic stress and threatened loss of eligibility. The athlete described himself as an average student who was generally disinterested in most subjects and did not like sitting in class, reading textbooks, or taking notes. He especially did not like researching or writing papers, but three of his four current classes had paper writing requirements. In addition to disliking most subjects, he described a pattern since high school of waiting until the last minute to study for tests, complete projects, or write papers. He had not taken advantage of the free tutoring services offered by the athletic department's academic support center. In fact, he did little during his 10-hours-per-week required study time at the center. He had no history of specific learning or attention difficulties and no current substance misuse. He did tend to stay up quite late (2–3 A.M.), gaming, watching television, or surfing the Internet, and spent most of his time after practice hanging out with his teammates or members of the women's soccer team.

Intervention: Because most of his classes were in the morning (9 A.M. to noon) and practice did not start until 3:00 P.M., the athlete agreed to block out 2 hours of academic time after classes. He agreed to go directly to the academic support center and work twice a week with English and history tutors. In addition to this prepractice time, he identified 7:00–10:00 P.M. four times a week as additional time that he would use to work on his assignments. Finally, he agreed to shift his bedtime to midnight or earlier so that he could get a solid 7–8 hours of sleep. With this structured time and additional support, he began to catch up with his work and turned in some overdue papers. Going forward, he was able to stay ahead and his confidence soared. At the end of the semester, he expressed surprise at how much he had learned and how much he had enjoyed the one-on-one time with his tutors. In addition, he felt that this new disciplined approach had carried over to soccer. He noted improved skills in several areas because of extra work he had done with an assistant coach.

Tip 8: Stay Informed, Get the Facts, and Ignore Rumors

Incorrect information can lead to false perceptions or opinions, unnecessary thinking, and heightened emotions that drain energy. Individuals can benefit from seeking out the source of rumors and regularly getting updates on a situation even if little change has occurred. Small bits of information can lead to new solutions.

Case Study: The Coach's Opinion Matters

A first-year college softball player sought assistance from a sports psychiatrist after the winter break because of concern that the new coach had developed a negative opinion of her. She felt that during the fall, the coach had been disinterested in her because she was not athletic and lacked speed; however, she felt that this assessment did not make sense because she knew that the old coach had recruited her for her defensive skills and her power. She had become disappointed and resentful, could feel herself giving up, and was recently thinking of transferring to another school. She had not discussed her views or feelings with any members of the coaching staff or team members.

Intervention: The player was advised to identify an assistant coach who was approachable and had been on the staff of the prior coach. She arranged to meet with this coach and ask for some feedback on areas in which she was doing well and areas in which she could improve. The assistant coach was very supportive and encouraging and said that the entire staff was very positive about her potential to contribute to the team's success in the upcoming season and thought that she had a good chance of starting if she continued to work on her defensive skills and base running. She left the meeting with a completely different view of her situation and wished she had connected with the coach sooner.

Tip 9: Consider a Spiritual or Religious Solution

Spiritual views may help individuals to see problems in different ways and may enhance natural creativity. Solutions to stress are often just around the corner if a person stays positive and allows enough time to pass.

Case Study: A Bible Study Group

While receiving treatment for an ankle sprain during the first week of the season, an undrafted first-year free-agent professional football player was visited by a sports psychiatrist in the training room. To the athlete's surprise, he had made the practice squad, but he did not feel accepted or respected by his teammates. He described himself as a quiet type with a strong spiritual base but was wondering if he would fit in with this particular team.

Intervention: The player was not aware that the team had a chaplain-led Bible study group that met each week at a veteran player's home. Later that day, he sought out the chaplain and agreed to attend the next meeting. In addition, he had a nice conversation with the chaplain about the spiritual commitment of many of the team's players and coaches. After attending several Bible study groups, he felt more connected with the team and more comfortable with his role on the practice squad.

Tip 10: Avoid Excessive Sedatives and Stimulants

The use of alcohol, marijuana, nicotine, and caffeine often increases during periods of high stress. Sedatives and stimulants are often used together and can lead to risky dose escalations in short periods of time. These agents may bring temporary relief but can often lead to insomnia and rebound anxiety. During times of stress, individuals should limit alcohol to three drinks per day and monitor their stimulant intake. As little as 500 mg of caffeine (4–6 cups of coffee) or 10–15 mg of nicotine (10 cigarettes, one-half can of snuff) per day can interfere with sleep duration and quality and raise stress.

Case Study: Stimulant Drinks, Excessive Alcohol, and Postgame Insomnia

A third-year defensive professional football player was referred by the team athletic trainer to a sports psychiatrist for evaluation of insomnia after he had asked for sleep medication for use after a midseason game. He described a long-standing pattern of difficulty with unwinding after a game and of having trouble falling asleep before 2–3 A.M. This pattern dated back to his second year of college and seemed to be getting worse, because lately he could not fall asleep until daybreak. He often watched movies in the middle of the night. When asked about the use of stimulants and alcohol, he acknowledged using two liquid stimulant drinks pregame to raise his intensity level and then drinking four or more mixed drinks at clubs with his teammates after the game to help him unwind. Because he had just become a starter after adding a second energy drink, he was reluctant to cut back. He had received one 10-mg zolpidem tablet to help him sleep after the last game and felt that it had helped.

Intervention: The psychiatrist explained how high-dose stimulants and heavy drinking interfere with sleep and energy. The player and psychiatrist concluded that the player's intensity level was naturally on the high end and that he was sensitive to the arousal effects of caffeine and the sleep-blocking potential of alcohol as it was wearing off. He agreed to stop using one of the stimulant drinks and to reduce his alcohol use for a few weeks. He understood that taking a sleeping pill was risky and did not make sense if he was aggravating a sleep problem with excessive stimulants and alcohol. After a few weeks, he noted improvement because he was able to fall asleep earlier. Also, because he did not need to be at the team's facility until noon postgame, he could sleep in. Other unwinding strategies were suggested, and he substituted light music for movies after returning home at night.

Tip 11: Have Fun at School, Practice, and Competitions, and Develop an Enjoyable Hobby

Individuals need to have fun in work and play. They benefit from experiencing laughter and humor throughout the day. If academics and athletics are not fun, then a person should change the mix of people in his or her social network (e.g., by adding someone who is calm and can lighten the mood). After practice or during time off, athletes can benefit from involvement in a hobby that uses different skills and that is not as high pressure or results oriented. Activities can be more enjoyable if shared with others.

Case Study: Not Fun Anymore

A high school senior tennis player who had already accepted a college scholarship sought assistance from a sports psychiatrist because he was not enjoying practices anymore and dreaded going to out-of-town tournaments. Over the 2 years he took to find a college, he noted increased performance pressure, reduced enjoyment during extra practices, and building resentment that tennis had taken time away from his friends and his other love, writing.

Intervention: When asked the last time he had enjoyed practice and competition, he at first said a few years ago, but then commented that it might have been even longer due to the constant struggle to maintain his junior tennis ranking and the need to play in so many high-profile tournaments with so much travel and missed time from home, school, and his social network. The psychiatrist asked if the player had any videotapes of his playing, and he said that his parents had always videotaped his matches but that he had never looked at any of them. He agreed to look back though some of the videos to see if he could determine when he had lost his joy of playing. To his surprise, he had to go all the way back to age 10 to see himself enjoying tennis on the court. He was so impressed with his natural exuberance that he decided to try to imitate his younger self in the next few practices. At the following session, his demeanor had completely changed and he seemed more at ease and cheerful. When asked about the change, he cited the video and a change in perspective and approach that had occurred after watching it. He had decided that college was not going to be all about tennis and that he was going there to become a better person and a writer as well. He had already canceled participation in an upcoming tournament and was going to hang out with an old friend whom he had not seen in some months. Finally, he committed to resume his writing, something else at which he excelled but without the same pressure levels.

Tip 12: Develop Positive Routines, Record Positive Moments, and Visualize Success

Individuals can benefit from starting and ending each day with patterned but flexible routines that last 15–30 minutes. An awakening routine that raises energy and prepares the person for the activities of the day might include exercising, stretching, reading, going outside, listening to invigorating music, watching the news, or eating a nutritious meal. A midday routine, such as a meal, social conversation, or walk, can be used to recover lost energy and maintain focus and concentration. An end-of-day routine is needed to shift from action to calm and to prepare for sleep. This routine might include listening to soft music, reading, calling a support network member, or meditation. At the end of the day, it is often useful to formally register the positive moments. Reviewing them in detail helps the sights, sounds, and positive emotions to be fully imprinted. Another useful tactic is to spend some time visualizing success for the next day or for a longer period for an important project or life event. The individual should allow the images to be strong and clear.

Case Study: Awakening Routine

A top-prospect professional baseball middle infielder in his third year on a minor league team began asking the sports psychiatrist questions after a spring training clubhouse presentation on energy production and maintenance. He described early morning sluggishness that did not wear off until 1–2 hours after practice had started. He expressed concern about the mistakes that he was making and worried that he might lose his spot on the 40-man roster if this pattern did not change. He reported always having been a night owl, staying up until 2 or 3 A.M. most nights, watching television or communicating with his friends. Even though he fell asleep easily and was getting 5–6 hours of sleep, he did not awaken easily. He described his morning routine as hitting the snooze button on his alarm three times before rushing out the door for morning practice. He always felt rushed and poorly prepared for the day. He was tired of waking up on the practice field. He did not use tobacco or other stimulants and was not a heavy drinker.

Intervention: The player agreed that he needed 8 or more hours of sleep and was therefore open to shifting his bedtime back to 11:00 P.M.

He also agreed that he needed to do something to wake himself up at his hotel room before driving to the facility. Because he was not a breakfast eater, he decided he would keep a supply of energy bars and cold bottled water and consume one each as soon as he woke up. Then he would do three 60-second heart rate–raising exercises in succession (push-ups, jumping jacks, low weight repetitions), with only 1-minute recovery time. Finally, he would take a cool shower before leaving the hotel. Once he got to the facility, he would eat some cereal and yogurt with fruit and ride an upright exercise bike for 5–7 minutes before getting fully dressed and going outside 10–15 minutes before practice. After trying this routine for a week, he noted a significant rise in his overall energy level, and he was gradually able to move his bedtime to his goal of 11 P.M. He felt more prepared for practice, and his early morning mistakes diminished.

Conclusion

Every athlete has a characteristic stress response that develops during high-demand periods. This response usually consists of anxiety, depression, anger, physical pain or somatic dysfunction, or some combination. The specific pattern can be easily identified by showing Figure 3–1 to the athlete and asking him or her to determine which pattern better fits his or her experience and rating his or her reactions on a scale of 0–10. Stress drains energy and changes sleep and, if unchecked, can result in burnout or illness. Fortunately, stress recovery breaks and the body's relaxation system can effectively counterbalance the disruptive effects of stress. Consultation with a sports psychiatrist or other mental health clinician skilled in alternative medicine or performance enhancement training techniques can usually help to identify the unique features of each individual's stress and relaxation responses. An individualized, empowerment-based stress control plan that improves functioning and performance can be easily developed and implemented. Because relationship stress is a common problem for athletes and coaches, focusing on improving communication and trust and creating shared time is important.

Key Clinical Points

- The common stressors of sports participation (daily practice, injury, travel, repetition, performance expectations, lack of privacy, media attention, family separation) can lead to temporary stress reactions that interfere with athletic performance and quality of life.

- The four common stress reaction patterns are anxiety, depression, anger, and somatic response. Each of these is typically accompanied by changes in sleep, energy, eating, and substance use. Some athletes have one dominant pattern, whereas other athletes have mixed symptoms.

- A natural (hard-wired) relaxation system exists in the body as a natural counterbalance to the stress system. Breathing, breaks, meditation, prayer, music, reading, massage, power naps, exercise, and stretching are good ways to activate relaxation and reduce stress. These activities should be done every morning and evening.

- Effective stress control includes three basic strategies: 1) identifying, organizing, prioritizing, and addressing existing stressors and demands; 2) reducing the current stress response through social support, counseling, short-term medications, and increasing positive moments and successes; and 3) identifying and working through background factors, such as trauma, loss, personality style, and mental disorder, that make stress more likely, intense, and frequent.

- The athlete's long-term happiness, satisfaction, and contentment come from activating positive emotions, getting lost in the love of the game, establishing supportive relationships, finding something meaningful in what he or she does, and working hard for each accomplishment.

References

Asmundson GJG, Taylor S: It's Not All in Your Head: How Worrying About Your Health Could Be Making You Sick and What You Can Do About It. New York, Guilford, 2005

Childre D: Freeze Frame: One Minute Stress Management: A Scientifically Proven Technique for Clear Decision Making and Improved Health. Boulder Creek, CA, Planetary Publications, 1998

Hackett TP, Cassem NH (eds): Massachusetts General Hospital Handbook of General Hospital Psychiatry, 2nd Edition. Littleton, MA, PSG Publishing, 1987

Loehr J, Schwartz T: The Power of Full Engagement. New York, Free Press, 2003

Rollnick S, Mason P, Butler C: Health Behavior Change: A Guide for Practitioners. London, UK, Harcourt, 2000

Strain JJ: Psychological Interventions in Medical Practice. New York, Appleton-Century-Crofts, 1978

Weil A: Breathing: The Master Key to Self Healing (Audio Disc). Boulder, CO, Sounds True, 1999

Chapter 4

Energy Regulation

Athletes at all competitive levels need energy, wakefulness, motivation, and psychomotor vigilance (focus) to perform optimally. Energy needs to be readily available in the muscles for rapid or sustained movement and in the brain for focus and sustained attention.

The body has three main energy systems that operate with one another in integrated ways, depending on the available levels of oxygen, food, and stored nutrition. The first is the phosphate system, which does not require oxygen or food and which supplies energy immediately to muscles for short activity bursts of 10–15 seconds (e.g., a sprint in track, a long pass in football, or stealing a base in baseball). The energy in this system is stored in muscle cells in adenosine triphosphate (ATP) and replenished rapidly for short periods by linkages to creatine phosphate.

The second energy system is the anaerobic glycolysis system, which is activated once the energy in the phosphate system is exhausted. At this point, the muscles and brain rely on the breakdown of glucose without adequate oxygen. When glucose is broken down in the absence of oxygen, the ATP is restored, but lactic acid builds up and the muscles eventually burn and fatigue. This system is good for 1–2 minutes of high-intensity activity (e.g., an 800-meter run in track, sustained movement up and down the court in basketball, a 200-meter freestyle swim).

The third system is the aerobic metabolic system, which involves the breakdown of simple sugars, fats, or proteins in the presence of oxygen. This system restores the supply of ATP without lactic acid production and prefers circulating simple sugars first and fats second over proteins. Simple sugars, such as glucose, fructose, or galactose, come from recently ingested food or from stored glycogen in the muscles or liver. Fats, which come from either recently ingested fatty acids or stored fat molecules in the subcutaneous tissues or visceral organs, are broken down by β-oxidation to restore ATP. The aerobic metabolic system can supply energy for several hours of sustained medium- to high-intensity activity without resupply and thereby enables an athlete to run a half marathon or play an entire soccer match.

Athletes learn, depending on the variable requirements of their specific sport, how to produce and maintain adequate energy supplies for practice, for competition, or over a long preseason and season. They accomplish this primarily through regulation of 1) nutrition and hydration; 2) energy, alertness, fatigue, and sleep; 3) chronic fatigue and burnout prevention; and 4) stimulants and stimulating activities. In this chapter, I discuss the significance of each of these areas to energy management in sports, emphasizing the different requirements of endurance sports, such as distance running, cycling, triathlons, and cross-country skiing; burst sports, such as track sprints, field events, and weight lifting; and mixed endurance and burst sports, such as soccer, lacrosse, and football. Additionally, I discuss the body's natural circadian system; the timing of breaks, rest, and sleep; and the prevention of chronic fatigue and burnout.

Nutrition and Hydration

The foundation of energy supply and release in the body comes from food, fluid, and electrolyte balance. Different sports tax the body's energy systems in different ways. Endurance sports require moderate amounts of energy over long time periods and therefore use a combination of circulating and stored carbohydrates and fat. Because carbohydrate stores can be depleted in only a few hours, carbohydrate resupply is necessary to prevent fat energy system activation. A typical marathon or ultramarathon runner will load on complex carbohydrates, such as breads, cereal, pasta, or whole grains, and hydrate before long training runs or races, then resupply with carbohydrates and fluids throughout the run. Different runners have different requirements; some need more fuel than others. Even before the aerobic carbohydrate system is exhausted, the fat system is activated and can supply energy for up to 24 hours of continuous exercise. In contrast, sprint sports rely on the phosphate and anaerobic glycolysis systems for energy. Precompetition carbohydrate loading is not as important unless athletes are competing in multiple events on the same day, as is common in track and field, diving, and swimming. Mixed endurance and sprint sports require an energy base for continuous movement, as well as carbohydrate, fluid, and electrolyte balance for the sprint component. For example, in a typical soccer game, an outside midfielder over 90 minutes may run 5–7 miles and, on top of that endurance base, may make 20–30 sprint runs forward in the attack or backward to defend. Therefore, conserving energy through mini-breaks (slowing down) on the field and resupplying with an energy or electrolyte drink during injury stoppage or at half-time are critical.

For athletes in any sport, carbohydrate and electrolyte resupply are important and should be done promptly before the next training session. Immediate resupply with a 4:1 ratio of carbohydrate to protein grams within 2 hours after exertion increases insulin release and therefore carbohydrate storage. Waiting longer than 2 hours can result in reductions of storage of up to 50%. For hydration after exercise, especially on hot days when significant fluid loss occurs, 20–24 oz of a sports drink per pound lost is necessary and should occur within 30 minutes. Therefore, weighing before and after practice is a critical routine in fluid management. Protein resupply is not as necessary for energy maintenance, but it is important to build new muscle and repair damaged tissue from high-intensity or sustained movement. Although solid foods can be used for nutritional resupply, many athletes tolerate and more quickly absorb liquids and can follow them later with solid food and an activity break or rest.

Case Study: I Just Ran Out of Energy

A recent high school graduate and highly ranked junior tennis player attended an elite tennis academy to train for a year in hopes of getting a scholarship to college or perhaps turning professional. At her home high school, she had practice and matches after school and usually ate a midday lunch that she brought from home. She had never been a breakfast eater. When she arrived at the tennis academy, she was surprised at how much time was spent with fitness, practice, and matches, with both early and late sessions as the norm. The morning session was the most intense, lasting 2 hours. Almost immediately, she noted that after the first hour her energy level dropped significantly. She became frustrated that she couldn't keep up and that she made more mistakes than typical. Even though she was encouraged to wake up early and eat a light breakfast before practice, she preferred to sleep in. After the coaches noticed her energy drop, she was sent to a sports nutritionist, who suggested a simple breakfast of fruit, yogurt, and an energy bar. She was referred to a sports psychiatrist for evaluation after she had struggled unsuccessfully for a week to introduce this early morning nutrition.

Intervention: Although she slept well and awoke well rested, the player did not feel that she fully awakened until she got moving on the court. The psychiatrist discussed with the athlete the importance of resupplying her depleted fluids and carbohydrate stores after a long night's sleep. She agreed to set her alarm for an hour before practice and to immediately drink a half bottle of cold water and eat a piece of fruit and a small yogurt. To accelerate her awakening, she also introduced some simple cardiovascular activation by doing jumping jacks for 60 seconds, resting for 5 minutes, and repeating. After the first week, she noted that she was more awake at practice and felt better through most of the morning, but she still experienced a fade in her energy in the last 30 minutes of the morning session. She addressed this by eating a small energy bar as she was leaving for morning practice. This mixture of whole grains, seeds, fiber, nuts, and dried fruits supplied her with sufficient energy without gastrointestinal upset. Over time, she became a regular breakfast eater and introduced more varied foods.

Case Study: I Was Drained at Mile 30

Having successfully completed several marathons, a graduate student distance runner decided to further test his endurance by running a 50-mile race. He trained over a 6-month period and even vacationed in the area of the ultramarathon to acclimatize to the higher altitude. He learned with the longer distances to resupply his fluids and food to sustain his energy. Unfortunately, the race took place on an unusually hot day, and around mile 30, he became nauseated and listless. He stopped for a scheduled break to consume a 16-ounce energy drink and a small snack, but he felt only a little better. A more experienced runner saw him and told him he needed salt and recommended eating some saltine crackers. After eating a dozen crackers and walking around, he began to feel better. After 5 minutes, he resumed his run and finished the race.

Intervention: A review several weeks later of the runner's excess sweating and fluid replacement revealed that he had replaced his fluids adequately but not his salt. Over the first 30 miles, he mainly drank water and ate small carbohydrate snacks. Even though more balanced electrolyte solutions were available, he found from past experience that they were too heavy and sat in his stomach, making him uncomfortable when running. The following year, he ran the same race, but this time he alternated drinking water with diluted electrolyte solutions. In addition, at several of his scheduled refueling breaks, he made sure to resupply his carbohydrates and salt.

Case Study: It's Too Hot to Have Two Practices a Day

A drafted rookie professional football lineman was seen by a sports psychiatrist in the training room at the end of the first week of training camp. The psychiatrist asked how the player felt about his performance. The athlete replied that he was doing well in the morning practices but felt that his energy level was far too low in the afternoon practices. A review of his postpractice routine showed that he replaced his fluids with an electrolyte drink based on his lost weight. In addition, he went to the cafeteria and got a lunch to go but waited to eat until he had taken a 45-minute nap.

Intervention: The player's concerns were discussed with the head athletic trainer, who felt that the athlete was waiting too long to resupply his carbohydrates and that this delay, along with a reduced ability to rehydrate adequately, was limiting his energy. After the next morning practice, the player was instructed to immediately consume a nutritional drink that contained carbohydrates and protein for resupply. Additionally, he was to consume sufficient water or electrolytes to replace his lost weight. Almost immediately, he felt better after practice and instead of going to his room first to take a nap, he went to the cafeteria and ate his meal there before napping in his room. This revised resupply routine completely corrected his lower energy in the second practice.

Energy, Alertness, Acute Fatigue, and Sleep

Ideal levels of energy, alertness, and focus for athletic practice and competition are derived from two complex brain systems that work in tandem. The first system, for wakefulness and alertness, comprises a series of circuits in the brain stem that rise through the midbrain to the cortex. The second system, for sleepiness and sleep, comprises circuits that arise from the forward part of the midbrain and connect with other circuits in the cortex and the lower brain (Hans et al. 2005; Postolache and Oren 2005; Stiller and Postolache 2005). The sleep system is linked to changes in light patterns through the visual system in a reoccurring circadian rhythm. Under ideal circumstances, these two systems operate in opposition to each other: the wakefulness system activates to full capacity from the morning into the evening and night while the sleepiness/sleep system is suppressed; just as the wakefulness system begins to deactivate from a full day's activity pattern, the sleep system activates with darkness and rising melatonin levels to promote adequate continuous sleep that restores energy, refreshes psychomotor vigilance, and consolidates learning in preparation to meet the next day's demands.

Unfortunately, these systems do not consistently work in tandem and do not always individually activate effectively or efficiently. When this lack of synchrony occurs and energy and alertness levels fall, then mental and physical fatigue develop. Fatigue is best described as a low-energy state that is accompanied by reduction or impairment of 1) alertness, 2) sustained attention, 3) logical reasoning, 4) mental quickness, 5) motor coordination, and 6) reaction time. Acute fatigue in athletes has many causes, including a series of physically and mentally demanding tasks, boring or monotonous routines, irregular or long work hours, disrupted or inadequate sleep, travel and jet lag, competitive or life stress, injury and pain, poor performance and losing, and accumulating sleep debt. Fortunately, fatigue can be prevented through daily awakening, recovery, unwinding, and sleep-enhancing routines that maintain wakefulness and combat daytime sleepiness. Some of these strategies have already been described in the preceding chapters, but the essential ones for long-term success are sleep maintenance, morning activation, daytime refueling, brief recovery breaks, avoidance of high-dose stimulants and alcohol, monitoring and elimination of sleep debt, and ongoing stress control (Table 4–1).

Some sports interfere with the synchronized balance of the wakefulness and sleep systems because of the time and frequency of competition, the amount of travel, the length of a typical day, and the frequency and severity of injuries. For example, baseball games usually run near or through the natural end of the wakefulness cycle and are scheduled nearly every day, with travel in between. In addition, during baseball season, days are long, often exceeding 14 hours and ending after midnight. When the day is long and begins with low activity levels, producing and maintaining energy for that day can be difficult. Athletes in sports with these patterns sometimes resort to the use of stimulants to raise energy and to the use of sedatives, such as alcohol and sleep or pain medications, to ensure adequate wakefulness-sleep balance. When travel occurs across three times zones, performance on the next day is diminished. Studies in several sports, including baseball, football, and basketball, show that the traveling team incurs this jet lag disadvantage (Reilly et al. 2005).

The circadian rhythm of sleep is more strongly biological and therefore more difficult to disrupt. Many aspects of sports training and competition, however, can block sleep cycling and continuity. Some examples are late-night travel, awakenings from injury and pain, overstimulation from game preparation and intensity, emotional activation from winning or losing, watching TV in bed to unwind, stimulant use, and high-dose alcohol or nicotine use. Sleep is structured into repeating 90-minute cycles of non–rapid eye movement (NREM) and rapid eye movement (REM) (Stiller and Postolache 2005). When compared to a wakeful state, NREM sleep is characterized by reduced muscle tone, slow infrequent eye movements, and slow-frequency, high-voltage activity on electroencephalogram (EEG). In normal adults, 75%–80% of total sleep time is spent in NREM sleep. REM sleep is characterized by absent muscle tone; increases and decreases in respiration, blood pressure, and heart rate; rapid eye movements; dreaming; and rapid, low-voltage waves on EEG. At the beginning of sleep, most (90% or more) of a 90-minute sleep cycle is spent in NREM sleep. As sleep continues, REM sleep becomes longer. If an athlete sleeps a normal amount (i.e., 8–9 hours), he or she will typically awaken from REM sleep. If an athlete can sleep continuously through three or four 90-minute sleep cycles, he or she will achieve about 80%–85% restoration. Less than the ideal amount of sleep results in a sleep debt that can accumulate over days to weeks and result in difficulty awaking (sleep inertia) or temporary or prolonged fatigue. Fortunately, a sleep debt can be erased by one or two nights of longer sleep (i.e., 10–12 hours).

TABLE 4–1. Acute fatigue: causes, characteristics, and solutions

Causes	Characteristics	Solutions
Physically demanding tasks	Reduced alertness	Awakening routines
Boring or monotonous routines	Diminished sustained attention	Unwinding routines
Irregular or long work hours	Impaired logical reasoning	Sleep enhancement routines
Disrupted or inadequate sleep	Reduced mental quickness	Wakefulness maintenance
Travel and jet lag	Decreased motor coordination	Daytime refueling
Competitive or life stress	Slowed reaction time	Brief recovery breaks
Injury and pain		Avoidance of high-dose stimulants and alcohol
Poor performance and losing		Elimination of sleep debt
Accumulating sleep debt		Ongoing stress control

Sports and sports-related behaviors routinely interfere with sleep. The most common sleep interferences for football players are injury and pain, postgame activation or heavy alcohol use, and overactive thinking or worrying before bedtime. Surprisingly, obstructive sleep apnea is no more common in oversized professional football players than in the general population (Rice et al. 2010). In fact, the amount of body fat is not well correlated with sleep-disordered breathing. For baseball players, the reasons for insomnia are different. The most common interferences are postgame activation (e.g., game intensity, eating, exercise, watching TV or videos), fatigue with a circadian phase shift, worrying, jet lag, and stimulant use. In both these sports and others, insomnia is also common in individuals with anxiety, mood, and attention-deficit disorders.

Solutions to insomnia in athletes involve good sleep hygiene, stress control, and medications that work but do not affect next-day alertness, mental quickness, or motor coordination (Loehr and Schwartz 2003). Basic sleep hygiene strategies involve environmental control (i.e., room temperature, noise control, mattress size and comfort), avoidance of activating behaviors in the 2 hours before bedtime (eating, drinking, exercising, bright light exposure), and the introduction of relaxation routines (reading, books on tape, dim lighting, music, warm shower/bath, relaxation breathing) and white noise (e.g., fan, music, white noise recordings or machine). Medications are used to reset the sleep pattern and then are either discontinued or used as needed. The most common resetting medication is zolpidem 5 or 10 mg just before bedtime daily for 5–7 days. Zolpidem can then be used two or three times a week thereafter. Some individuals have chronic insomnia that results from the high demand of their sport or a psychiatric disorder. If these individuals are not regular consumers of alcohol, they can take zolpidem daily with few side effects. Other options for acute and chronic insomnia are trazodone alone (25–100 mg) 90 minutes before bedtime or trazodone and ramelteon 8 mg combined. The main caution with trazodone is that an individual must allow sufficient time (9 or more hours) for the medication to wear off, because its main side effect is morning sleepiness. Fortunately, trazodone usually wears off within an hour if the athlete has a strong awakening routine. Although trazodone is often the best choice for active thinkers or worriers, sometimes a short-acting benzodiazepine such as alprazolam 0.25 mg or lorazepam 0.50 mg in the late evening a few days a week can be helpful. For those individuals who do not respond to any of these medication strategies, a trial of quetiapine (25–75 mg) at bedtime can be initiated; this medication can be used to reset sleep and then can be taken as needed, which can be nightly for severe cases.

Case Study: Can I Have Some Sleeping Pills to Help Me Fall Asleep?

A late-career professional baseball pitcher (late-innings reliever) mentioned to the team physician during his preseason physical that he wanted a prescription for zolpidem to help him fall asleep at night. He had occasionally taken zolpidem in the past two seasons, if he thought he might pitch in a day game or if the team arrived late at a city and had to play the next day. He had no obvious high-stress state, did not report past insomnia, and denied tobacco, alcohol, or substance misuse. He was referred to a sports psychiatrist for an evaluation of his sleep.

Intervention: The player had been a major league pitcher for 13 years and was married, with twin girls who were in middle school. The family lived with his wife's parents in his hometown. During the off-season, he tended to fish and hunt, waking up late and going to his new lakeside cabin late in the afternoon. He would stay there until an hour after sunset, when he would go home to connect with his family. After his wife and kids went to bed, he would stay up until 2:00–3:00 A.M., watching television or movies. He did not mention any prominent stressors, except some concern about his daughters being in middle school and their being a little more oppositional and showing an interest in boys. He recognized that he had been going to bed too late and felt that he could use zolpidem to make sure he got enough sleep to be refreshed and ready to compete. He understood that he had shifted his sleep-wake cycle 3–4 hours forward and that it might take 5–7 days to comfortably get into a more normal rhythm. He agreed to try ramelteon, a melatonin agonist, for a week; to stop watching television 2 hours before bedtime; and to unwind with some light reading of sports magazines and the local newspaper. After a week, his sleep improved and he did not feel that he needed zolpidem. He continued taking ramelteon for most of spring training and then bought some melatonin to use if he had trouble falling asleep. During the season, he again requested zolpidem occasionally for use when traveling and before day games. He pitched well in relief and had no major problems with sleep. At the end of the season, he agreed to keep his sleep-wake schedule more like it was during the season.

Chronic Fatigue and Burnout Prevention

The demands of practice and competition—especially if continuous with few breaks, repetitious with little variability, and filled with travel and jet lag—can produce chronic fatigue or burnout (Loehr and Schwartz 2003). Elite athletes at increasingly younger ages are seeking better training and competition by moving to training academies or by training and competing year round. In addition, early specialization in one sport can cause daily high pressure and can sometimes take the joy out of all activities. College and professional athletes seek additional training during breaks to increase their chances of being on the starting lineup or moving to the next level. This level of commitment leaves little time for low-key socialization or the development of other interests or skills. Relentless patterned demand over time can drain vital energy and lead to a chronic low-energy state that is not improved by creativity, exploration, laughter, and easy fun. When individuals do not have adequate energy, they do not pursue exciting and novel experiences, and their positive emotional responses diminish.

A difficult task is to design a training program with enough intensity that athletes improve but with enough breaks and variability to keep training fresh and enthusiasm high. Experienced coaches seek input from their athletes and often vary the length of practice, give unexpected days off, and intersperse fun activities with practice sessions. Many coaches of field sports divide their teams into small groups and have them compete against one another in simple games that emphasize some of the skills of the sport. For example, soccer teams might play soccer volleyball, in which players on opposing teams try to head the ball back and forth over the net, moving their other team back if the ball falls to the ground. In baseball, a fun activity is a short round of pepper, in which a batter hits balls to a circle of players 20 feet away; players rotate in and out of play as they miss hits or make fielding errors. If inserted strategically, brief, easy, fun games such as these can energize a practice session and keep athletes alert and fresh.

Chronic fatigue can develop from yearlong training and competition, training boredom, inadequate sleep with a sleep debt, and lack of success. Most athletes come to realize the threat of chronic fatigue and make adjustments to prevent it. At the end of the sports season, most athletes take a 30- to 45-day recovery break. Although they often maintain some fitness work, they usually seek out other hobbies or interests. As their energy returns, they move back to sports-specific training. To combat training boredom, athletes like to vary their routines, doing different things on different days and even working with teammates, competitors, or athletes from other sports in the off-season in small groups to introduce both support and socialization. To ensure adequate sleep, many athletes discover routines that aid sleep and avoid activities that block sleep. They occasionally use medications, if available, to prevent poor sleeping patterns from becoming entrenched. In addition, they benefit from setting aside at least 1 day a week to catch up on lost sleep. Finally, lack of individual or team success can compound a low energy state and must be addressed. Individual athletes can set and pursue goals with determination and support. A team can seek outside consultation from other coaches or mental skills trainers, who take a fresh look at the team's performance and make sure it is optimized given the current talent levels. Good organizations conduct thorough improvement reviews of all aspects of leadership, coaching, player mix and commitment, and team culture at least once a year.

Case Study: After 5 Minutes, I Get So Fatigued I Can't Keep Up

A rising second-year college basketball player referred himself to a sports psychiatrist over the summer because of chronic stress and anxiety following a 3-year struggle to keep up with the running and fitness requirements of his sport. Beginning in eleventh grade, after he reached his adult height (6'8") and weight (210 lb), he began to have increasing difficulty keeping up with the running in practice and games without becoming very short of breath and fatigued. Because he was a dominant player, his high school coach gave him frequent breaks, which worked to help him through his last two seasons and to get him on the roster of a small Division I school. As he began the more rigorous workouts for college in the summer before his first year, he struggled even more with becoming quickly tired and feeling heavy in his legs. Because his college coaching staff was not as tolerant of permitting different fitness standards for him, they added on extra fitness sessions. These did not go well, and the player complained of general tiredness and shortness of breath when running sprints or on the court. One day at practice, he ran so much that he became dizzy and short of breath and complained of chest tightness. At this point, he was pulled from all training and sent for medical evaluation. After an extensive workup by a cardiologist and a pulmonary specialist, the athlete was diagnosed with mild exercise-induced asthma, but it was not severe enough to explain his extreme symptoms. He missed the entire season because the workup was quite detailed and involved several specialized cardiac and pulmonary function tests, including exercise treadmill testing. The player began using a preventive inhaler and worked individually with an athletic trainer, but he could not improve his fitness over his second semester. He consulted a sports psychiatrist for evaluation to see if stress was playing a role in his fitness limitations.

Intervention: At the first session, the player's resting and standing heart rates were determined using a wristwatch and heart monitor. Interestingly, he had a rise of 40 beats per minute from sitting to standing (70 to 110). After his heart rate returned to normal, he was asked to hyperventilate strongly for 45 seconds through his mouth. His heart rate again increased sharply from 70 to 105 beats per minute. After he recovered, he was taken out for a half-mile run that included flat, downhill, and then uphill sections. He did fine on the first quarter mile, but as he started up the hill, his breathing became labored and he complained of fatigue in his legs and stopped. At this point, his heart rate had risen to 185 beats per minute. His recovery was slow, taking almost 5 minutes for his heart rate to fall below 100.

The athlete's history was interesting in that he had been a chronic mouth breather since childhood due to allergic rhinitis, and he was unable to move much air through his nostrils. He was referred to an allergist, who prescribed nasal steroids and recommended using saline nasal spray when the player worked out indoors if he felt that the air quality was poor. While running, he would hyperventilate as soon as the metabolic demand increased; he partially corrected this by learning to shift his attention to expiration and pushing air out rather than inspiration and getting air in. As he made this change, he greatly reduced the inspiratory friction and noisiness of his breathing. The player worked on this different breathing approach with his athletic trainer and was gradually able to increase the intensity of his workouts to match those he would have if he returned to basketball. As his confidence increased, so did his workouts. He liked the idea of keeping his airways clear with the nasal sprays and of reducing the energy he used by pushing the air out to power his running and letting it more passively flow back in during inspiration. He also made sure to stay well hydrated and replace his lost salt, because he was a very heavy sweater. He decided to transfer to another school at a lower competitive level and try out for the team. A repeat of the hyperventilation and running tests with the altered breathing schemes produced quite different results, with increases in his heart rate that were far less than those at his first visit.

Case Study: All I Do Is Tennis—I Think I Need a Break

A highly ranked junior tennis player decided to move to a tennis academy in another state at the beginning of ninth grade to increase his chances of getting a tennis scholarship to a top Division I program. He separated from his family and moved into the academy's dorm and began training much more rigorously than ever before. In addition, he began taking online high school classes in the evenings after a full day of tennis and fitness. After 2 years of continuous tennis training and competition, he had become a much better player and was attracting attention from many top schools. While home on winter break, he mentioned to his parents that he thought he might be depressed because he didn't enjoy anything and had no energy. In fact, for the month before coming home, he had been shorting his studies and going to bed early, sleeping 10 or more hours.

Intervention: During his initial evaluation by a sports psychiatrist, the player said he was tired of the constant pressure, travel, and long days. At this point, he wasn't even sure he wanted to play tennis in college. He had some friends at the academy but felt so competitive with them that he couldn't get close. At times, he felt that the coaches played favorites and head games as a way to motivate the athletes to play better. When asked what he did for fun and to relax, he was unable to come up with much other than listen to music or go for a walk. In fact, on reflecting on the questions, he said he might not have laughed all year. After a second meeting with the psychiatrist, also attended by his parents, the athlete decided to move back home and train locally. In addition, the psychiatrist discussed the importance of taking formal breaks from tennis to allow him to recover mentally and physically. He decided to take a full day off from fitness and tennis each week and started guitar lessons. In addition, he committed to 30–60 minutes of guitar practice four nights a week. He reconnected with old friends from his neighborhood and school and started the process of getting his driver's license. After a few months, his energy and motivation rose and his outlook changed. He felt recharged and began looking forward to visiting colleges in the fall.

Stimulants and Stimulating Activities

Some athletes use stimulants as shortcuts to build energy. Unfortunately, this strategy is shortsighted, because energy systems can be decremented and stores depleted without proper attention to longer-term production and maintenance approaches. Energy levels often correlate with body temperature (Krauchi et al. 2005); as the body temperature drops, so do levels of alertness and motivation. Drops in body temperature occur naturally during sleep but also during inactive periods, such as while sitting on a couch watching television, at a desk roaming the Internet, or in bed reading. These low temperature–low energy periods can easily be reversed with bursts of cardiovascular activity, such as jumping rope or sets of pushups, or by consuming a hot or cold drink. Surprisingly, as little as 5 minutes on an exercise bike or treadmill can boost alertness and energy for hours because energy systems are activated and energy production soars (Youngstedt 2005). In contrast, although a temporary boost in alertness or energy does occur with nicotine use from oral tobacco or smoking, the burst is often very short lived and necessitates additional use. Without activities that turn on energy production, levels will drop as time passes. Other stimulating activities include getting outside into the light and fresh air. The temperature change quickly alters core temperature if full rapid breathing is used, and the light signal serves to activate energy systems. If getting outside is not possible, as is common in winter months, then the use of a light box can help; 20–30 minutes of exposure to high-intensity light (10,000 lux) can increase energy system activation for the day. Finally, breaks are important to energy restoration and release. A nap of 15–30 minutes in a lounge chair or on a couch is often sufficient to recharge energy systems (Monk 2005).

Despite the simplicity and short duration of stimulating activities, stimulants are nevertheless used to excess by athletes. The most common are nicotine, caffeine, and over-the-counter and prescribed stimulants. They are often used together in a stimulant stack to achieve a stronger and faster effect. The problem with stimulants is that they generate their effect by the release of circulating adrenaline (epinephrine) and by stimulating neural networks that use dopamine and norepinephrine. Repeated use of stimulants over days can deplete stores of these compounds, creating a ceiling effect, or can produce side effects in sensitive individuals. The most common side effects are increased muscle tension, gastroesophageal burning, jitteriness, impaired heat regulation, and insomnia. Each of these side effects uses energy, ensuring that depletion develops earlier. Stronger stimulants such as ephedrine, atomoxetine, methylphenidate, modafinil, or amphetamines can generate a consistent alerting or energizing effect if fatigue is present, but performance does not usually improve unless confidence is raised. If the stronger stimulants are used in combination with nicotine and caffeine, then side effects at some level are common. In summary, using stimulants in low dosages and in concert with stimulating activities is the best approach, because activities stimulate production of neurotransmitters and stimulants activate their release. In contrast, without a routine of activities that keep energy levels raised, stacking stimulants eventually leads to depleted energy supplies or side effects or both.

Case Study: It Takes Me 15 Minutes to Wake Up on the Field, and by Then I've Made Too Many Mistakes

A third-year professional football player who was competing for a backup offensive position, was seen by a sports psychiatrist in the training room before a morning practice. When asked how his camp was going, he said he was making too many mistakes at the beginning of practice and that he felt that the coaches were becoming frustrated with him. A quick review of his prepractice routine revealed that he skipped breakfast and came straight to the field for dress and taping. He typically got onto the field just as practice was starting. He acknowledged that he had always taken 30–45 minutes to awaken in the mornings, especially if rising before 7:00 A.M.

Intervention: The player agreed to leave his room 15 minutes earlier to create an awakening routine to ensure that he was ready to play when practice started. He began by going straight to the cafeteria and eating a breakfast of simple and complex carbohydrates. After getting to the training room, he dressed and then went to the upright bike for 5–7 minutes to raise his heart rate from 100 to 110. After he got taped, he went onto the field and did some simple sprints and stretches. By the time practice started, he felt completely awake. With these changes, the player's confidence improved.

Case Study: Can I Get Amphetamines to Help Me With My Alertness and Concentration?

A midcareer professional baseball player was referred to a sports psychiatrist by the athletic trainer for the evaluation of complaints of poor concentration and focus in the outfield and at the plate in the second half of the season. The athlete had talked to other players who had suggested that he try some strong coffee, but he had never drunk coffee because he did not like its taste and said it made him jittery. He had heard of players who had therapeutic use exemptions to take amphetamines, and he remembered from college that these had helped him stay awake and focus for hard tests. He had started noticing more difficulty focusing this season after shifting from an everyday outfielder to a backup or a late-innings replacement. He felt sure that a low dose of short-acting amphetamine would help with his energy and attention.

Intervention: The player's history did not reveal any pattern consistent with an attention deficit, mood, anxiety, or sleep disorder. He was healthy and injury free, did not take any medications, and was not a tobacco or alcohol user. He described low energy on the days he did not play and difficulty raising his energy on days that he did play. He had been unable to remain focused when fielding or hitting. The psychiatrist asked the athlete to review his pregame routine. Because he was single, he tended to awaken late, around 11:00 A.M., and then stay in his apartment watching movies or television or playing video games until he left for the clubhouse. He tended to get to the clubhouse later than in prior years, arriving about 1 hour before batting practice. After batting practice, he typically played cards with some of his teammates. His hitting routine during games consisted of timing the pitcher's pitches in the dugout when he was third up to hit and swinging a weighted bat when in the on-deck circle. To combat boredom when he did not play, he tended to chew gum or spit sunflower seeds. He still did his in-season weight lifting after the games.

The sports psychiatrist helped the athlete realize that his overall energy level was too low and that his entire pregame routine needed a makeover. The player agreed to get up earlier and go out for breakfast no later than 9:00 A.M. After breakfast, he would go for a walk or ride his bike around the harbor. He also decided to get to the ballpark no later than 2:30 P.M. and start his game preparation, whether playing or not, by spending 30 minutes using the exercise bike or treadmill. After that, he would go outside for a 10- to 20-minute run, alternating sprints one day with distance the next. Before the organized team stretch that preceded batting practice, he would go outside early and do some short sprints to get his heart rate up. After batting practice, he stopped playing cards and went to the whirlpool instead. If he was not playing, he would go into the clubhouse late in the game and ride the exercise bike for 5 minutes to prepare himself for being a defensive replacement. On days he was in the lineup, he decided to regularly go into the clubhouse and ride the exercise bike to raise his energy. Over the next few weeks, the player reported a steady rise in his energy and confidence. He understood that a therapeutic use exemption was not indicated in his situation.

Conclusion

Sports psychiatrists and other providers (e.g., team physicians, athletic trainers, strength and conditioning staff) can assist athletes in building and maintaining energy levels to help them perform at their peak. The athletes may benefit from learning skills that improve nutrition, hydration, alertness, energy, and sleep; stimulating behavioral routines; and burnout prevention techniques. Perhaps the most important of these is healthy sleep hygiene, which requires the development of strong awakening, refreshing, and unwinding routines. Far too many athletes skip breakfast and between-meal snacks, fail to achieve adequate rehydration and carbohydrate resupply, develop sleep debt, and use stimulants as shortcuts. Most, however, are very open to revising their daily patterns, which can be accomplished using motivational enhancement techniques in the training area or the office.

Key Clinical Points

- Three main energy systems—the phosphate, anaerobic glycolysis, and aerobic metabolic systems—operate to support burst activity, endurance, alertness, and mental quickness. These need to be supported through sound nutritional strategies and recovery breaks.

- Food, fluid, and electrolyte resupply must be individualized to the sport and athlete for optimal performance. Immediate resupply is critical following energy expenditure and the loss of fluids and electrolytes.

- The body's wakefulness and sleep systems work in tandem to maintain alertness and restore energy systems. Continuous sleep of at least 6 hours and sound awakening and unwinding routines are critical.

- Sleep debt and chronic fatigue are common in sports that require long days, daily practice and/or play, travel, and nighttime play, but can be corrected with a day off and catch-up sleep.

- Stimulants in combination (caffeine, nicotine, ginseng, prescription stimulants) are often used in sports as shortcuts for energy production when sleep has been interrupted or chronic fatigue has set in. Some stimulant use is helpful to energy production and maintenance, but stimulants work best when combined with behavioral routines such as awakening exercises, energy meals, breaks, and naps.

- Sleep or antianxiety medications are sometimes needed on a daily basis to reset a sleep-wake pattern that has become unbalanced. Common problems are jet lag, late-night play, poor sleep hygiene (eating, channel flipping, Internet surfing), and staying up too late. After an earlier sleep time is established, medication frequency can be reduced.

References

Hans PA, Dongen, V, Dinges DF: Sleep, circadian rhythms, and psychomotor vigilance. Clin Sports Med 24:237–249, 2005

Krauchi K, Cajochen C, Wirz-Justice A: Thermophysiologic aspects of the three-process model of sleepiness regulation. Clin Sports Med 24:287–300, 2005

Loehr J, Schwartz T: The Power of Full Engagement. New York, Free Press, 2003

Monk TH: The post-lunch dip in performance. Clin Sports Med 24:237–249, 2005

Postolache TT, Oren DA: Circadian phase shifting, alerting, and antidepressant effects of bright light treatment. Clin Sports Med 24:381–413, 2005

Reilly T, Waterhouse J, Edwards B: Jet lag and air travel: implications for performance. Clin Sports Med 24:367–380, 2005

Rice TB, Dunn RE, Lincoln AE, et al: Sleep-disordered breathing in the National Football League. Sleep 33:819–824, 2010

Stiller JW, Postolache T: Sleep-wake and other biological rhythms: functional neuroanatomy. Clin Sports Med 24:205–235, 2005

Youngstedt SD: Effects of exercise on sleep. Clin Sports Med 24:355–365, 2005

Chapter 5

Substance Use and Abuse

The patterns of use and misuse of and dependence on alcohol, illicit drugs, and prescription medications are different among athletes than among people in the community. Athletes more commonly use and misuse performance enhancers, such as stimulants, anabolic-androgenic steroids (AASs), peptide hormones, releasing factors, and antiestrogenic agents, than serious street drugs of abuse, such as heroin, cocaine, hallucinogens, and phencyclidine (PCP) (McDuff and Baron 2005). The substances most commonly used in the community—alcohol, caffeine, nicotine, and marijuana—are also the most commonly used in sports. In addition, for athletes, these substances are usually the ones that account for most positive urine tests; adverse substance-related events; and impairments with health, general functioning, and athletic performance. Interestingly, serious alcohol, illicit drug, and performance enhancement substance abuse or dependence is uncommon in active players. The exceptions are binge alcohol and smokeless tobacco dependence in male college athletes, and alcohol, smokeless tobacco, and narcotic pain medication dependence in male late-career or retired professional athletes.

There are practical reasons for the different substance use patterns in athletes. First, compared to the general population, elite athletes are a young, healthy, and thoroughly screened subpopulation with frequent, intense training and very high performance standards. Second, they are monitored closely for early signs of substance misuse through daily observation by athletic trainers and coaches, regular visits to team physicians, and random urine testing. For these reasons, they have lower rates of serious substance problems (i.e., abuse or dependence). Their rate of other substance misuse, however, is higher because they have additional reasons for using than nonathletes. Whereas both athletes and nonathletes use substances to party or relax or if they develop a substance use disorder (abuse or addiction), athletes additionally may use or misuse for injury recovery and pain control and for performance enhancement (Table 5–1).

Injury and acute or chronic pain in active and retired athletes present a special risk for misuse, abuse, or dependence on opiates and sedatives. In the National Football League (NFL), for example, about 60% of players sustain an injury during a typical season, causing 37% of those to miss one or more games and 10% or more of all players to be put on injured reserve status, thus ending their season (National Football League Players Association 2011). In addition, in a recent joint study of 644 former NFL players (average age=48; average years played=7.8), the NFL and the National Institute on Drug Abuse found that 52% used pain medication while playing (Barr 2012). Of those players, 63% acknowledged getting the medications from a nonmedical source, 71% reported pain medication misuse while playing, and 15% endorsed misuse in the past 30 days. Misuse is defined as taking the medication in dosages higher than prescribed or obtaining the medication from a nonmedical source such as a friend, a teammate, or the Internet.

Performance enhancers have a long use history in professional and international sports, and even though regular, random urine testing is conducted at most levels, athletes are still willing to risk getting caught, fined, or suspended to compete better. Therefore, the misuse of stimulants and sometimes steroids is encountered regularly in a sports psychiatry practice. The most common presentation of stimulant misuse is an athlete taking methylphenidate or amphetamines without a prescription or a therapeutic use exemption. The risk of getting caught is low because of the short half-life of these medications and the routine absence of postgame testing in U.S. professional sports. Anabolic steroids were more common in the 1980s and 1990s in U.S. professional sports, but with current testing and sanctions, the most common presentation is a player testing positive for a steroid from a contaminated nutritional supplement. Most professional leagues have responded to this problem by providing players with a list of known safe supplements and/or manufacturers (McDuff and Baron 2005).

The use of performance-enhancing substances by athletes is a high-profile issue that has resulted in several governmental hearings and investigations. AAS scandals have occurred in the Olympics, Tour de France, and U.S. football and baseball, and some highly publicized suicides have occurred in steroid-using young athletes. Each of these incidents has received such intense media and governmental attention that elite athletes are viewed as influencing younger athletes and even non-

---

TABLE 5–1. Substances and sports: reasons for use and misuse

Injury recovery and pain control	**Partying and relaxation**
Promote faster healing	Produce pleasure and escape
Speed up rehabilitation program	Fit in and boost confidence
Reduce swelling and stiffness	Reduce stress and relax
Improve range of motion	Raise energy and alcohol tolerance
Improve sleep and restoration	Seek sexual encounters
Relieve aches and pains	Socialize and reduce boredom
Reduce frustration and irritability	Reduce negative emotions
Substance abuse or addiction	**Enhance performance**
Manage a hangover	Improve concentration and focus
Negate a toxic effect	Reduce exhaustion and fatigue
Alleviate cravings	Increase strength and muscle mass
Relieve withdrawal symptoms	Improve endurance and oxygenation
Respond to substance urges	Raise intensity and aggression
Cover up negative emotions	Increase wakefulness and attention
Avoid interpersonal conflicts	Reduce weight and body fat
Respond to peer pressure	

---

athletes to experiment with or use alcohol, performance enhancers, and drugs of abuse at higher rates. In response to this criticism, a number of sports have enacted clear countermeasures since early 2000.

All U.S. intercollegiate sports, most U.S. professional sports, and the Olympics have credible urine testing programs. Most of these strongly target performance-enhancing substances and have variable levels of emphasis on drugs of abuse and alcohol. (Table 5–2 lists banned substances and methods by sport.) For example, among the U.S. professional sports, the NFL has a very strong policy for dealing with performance enhancers, alcohol incidents, and problem drinking, whereas Major League Baseball (MLB) has a less stringent policy regarding alcohol and drugs of abuse for major league players (40-man roster) than for minor league players (non–40-man roster). Most of these drug testing programs and substance use policies fall under the collective bargaining agreements of each professional sport, although the World Anti-Doping Agency (WADA) oversees the policies for the Olympics and other international sporting events. Antidoping campaigns for youth have been developed using high-profile athletes as spokespersons in the community. In addition, the World Anti-Doping Agency (2009) has developed a Teacher's Tool Kit

TABLE 5–2. Banned substances and methods, listed by sport

Substance or method	NCAA	WADA	NFL	MLB	NBA	NHL
β_2-Adrenergic agonists	Banned	Banned	Not specified	Not specified	Not specified	Numerous agents banned (WADA list)
Alcohol	Banned, rifle only	Banned, numerous sports	Treatment and sanctions for alcohol abuse or events	Treatment for alcohol abuse and dependence	Not specified	Not specified
Anabolic-androgenic steroids	Numerous agents banned	Numerous exogenous, endogenous, and isomers/metabolites banned	Numerous agents banned	Numerous agents banned	Numerous agents banned	Numerous agents banned (WADA list)
Antiestrogenic agents	Banned	Banned	Banned	Banned	Not specified	Numerous agents banned (WADA list)
β-Blockers	Banned, rifle only	Banned, numerous sports	Allowed	Allowed	Allowed	Allowed
Blood doping, oxygen transfer	Banned	Banned	Not specified	Banned	Not specified	Not specified

TABLE 5–2. Banned substances and methods, listed by sport (*continued*)

Substance or method	NCAA	WADA	NFL	MLB	NBA	NHL
Drugs of abuse	Heroin, marijuana	Narcotics and glucocorticosteroids during competition	Amphetamines and analogs, cocaine, MDMA, opiates, PCP, opioids (preseason only)	Cocaine, LSD, marijuana, opiates, PCP, MDMA (minor leagues only; with reasonable cause only for major leagues)	Amphetamine and analogs, cocaine, LSD, opiates, PCP, MDMA	Numerous agents banned
Gene doping	Not specified	Banned	Not specified	Banned	Not specified	Not specified
Hormones, growth factors, and the like	Banned	Numerous agents banned	Numerous agents banned	Numerous agents banned	Not specified	Numerous agents banned (WADA list)
Manipulation, adulteration	Banned	Banned	Banned	Banned	Banned	Banned
Masking agents	Banned	Banned	Banned	Banned	Numerous agents banned	Numerous agents banned (WADA list)
Nutritional supplement contamination	Banned	Banned	Banned	Banned	Not specified	Not specified

TABLE 5–2. Banned substances and methods, listed by sport (*continued*)

Substance or method	NCAA	WADA	NFL	MLB	NBA	NHL
Stimulants	Numerous agents banned, including caffeine	Numerous agents banned during competition	Numerous agents banned	Performance-enhancing	Numerous agents banned	Allowed
Therapeutic use exemptions	Allowed	Allowed	Allowed	Allowed	Allowed	Allowed

Note. LSD=lysergic acid diethylamide; MDMA=3,4-methylenedioxymethamphetamine, or Ecstasy; MLB=Major League Baseball; NBA=National Basketball Association; NCAA=National Collegiate Athletic Association; NFL=National Football League; NHL=National Hockey League; PCP=phencyclidine; WADA=World Anti-Doping Agency.

that targets all children, not only athletes. This broader preventive targeting is based on the following beliefs: 1) instilling antidoping and fair-play values will reduce experimentation; 2) understanding performance-enhancing substance use may reduce the likelihood of supplement or medication use to alter physical appearance or body image; and 3) anti-doping values such as honesty; health; excellence in performance; fun and joy; teamwork; respect for rules, self, and others; courage; community; and solidarity can be applied to all areas of life.

Substance use in sports can logically be divided into the following three categories: 1) *legal substances*—alcohol, tobacco, and prescription medications; 2) *illicit substances*—marijuana, opiates, cocaine, amphetamine analogs, lysergic acid diethylamide (LSD), and PCP; and 3) *performance enhancers*—stimulants, anabolic steroids, hormones, and releasing factors. Although substances can be separated in this way, ample clinical and survey evidence indicates that regular use of one substance makes use of another substance in the same or a different category more likely. For example, alcohol use, tobacco use, and marijuana use tend to cluster, whereas anabolic steroid use clusters with growth hormone and insulin-releasing factor, as well as with prescription medications, including sedatives, stimulants, and narcotic analgesics. One study of male college athletes showed that users of performance enhancers, including legal supplements, were more likely than nonusers to be problem alcohol and illicit drug users and to demonstrate higher sensation seeking (Buckman et al. 2009). In a study comparing male and female college athletes to nonathletes, male but not female student athletes were more likely than nonathletes to have engaged in past-year heavy (binge) drinking (39.5%) and to have used performance-enhancing drugs (55.8%), any banned drugs (9.7%), nutritional supplements (45.7%), and smokeless tobacco (32.2%) (Yusko et al. 2008). Interestingly, the past-year use of drugs of abuse by male and female athletes was significantly lower than that by male and female nonathletes. However, this finding should be considered with the fact that male athletes used drugs of abuse twice as often during the off-season (30.9%) as during the season (15.5%). In contrast to male athletes, female athletes were significantly less likely than non-athletes to be heavy drinkers and users of drugs of abuse and weight loss products. Like male athletes, however, female athletes used drugs of abuse at far higher rates during the off-season (21.5%) than during the season (5.1%).

In this chapter, I review and present case studies on the use, misuse, and abuse of the most common substances—alcohol, cannabinoids, legal stimulants (caffeine, nicotine, over-the-counter [OTC] medications)—encountered in a sports psychiatric practice, as well as the less common but higher-profile group of performance enhancers (banned stimulants, steroids, hormones, and releasing factors). I discuss each substance category separately, emphasizing patterns of use, reason for use, risks of use, effect on performance, and reduction or cessation strategies.

Alcohol

Beverage alcohol is the most common substance used by athletes of all competitive levels who are seen in sports psychiatry (Martens et al. 2006). A sports clinician learns about athletes' alcohol use in multiple ways, including the following: 1) from a staff member or coach who smells alcohol on an athlete's breath at meetings or during treatments; 2) from a positive random test for urine alcohol when done as part of a broader panel for drugs of abuse; 3) following an alcohol-related event, such as a fight, citation for underage drinking, or an arrest; 4) via a call from a family member or a mention of concern during a family or couple's session; 5) by observing or hearing a mention of a hangover; 6) by overhearing conversations about severe intoxication (passing out, blacking out, arguments, inappropriate behaviors) by players in team meetings, at practices, or on road trips; and 7) through discovery during an evaluation for poor performance, interpersonal conflict, insomnia, anxiety, or stress.

Because alcohol use in general and binge use in particular are common among high school, college, and professional athletes and coaches, constant monitoring for risky or heavy use is essential. An important goal is to detect risky patterns of use early, so preventive interventions can be made. A sports clinician needs to gain the trust of athletic trainers and coaches so they will feel comfortable mentioning their concerns and sharing their observations. In addition, the clinician should spend time with athletes in the early morning, especially after certain nights when heavy drinking is more likely (e.g., after a game).

Although serious cases of alcohol dependence are seen in athletes, this problem is uncommon in active players. Reasons include the relative young age of the population, the high performance demands, and the lack of free time to engage in regular drinking. More severe drinking problems can surface in the off-season, when the days and nights are less structured, but these are uncommon as well. Instead, alcohol tends to negatively impact functioning and performance in sports because of binge drinking episodes with or without severe intoxication.

When a sports clinician first learns of a pattern of episodic heavy drinking through a mention by a team staff member or direct observation, the clinician should make informal contact with the athlete. This best occurs in the training room, on the practice field, or in an office at the end of the day. After a general discussion of the athlete's current self-confidence, injuries, or stress levels, the clinician can shift the discussion to areas known to be affected by binge drinking, such as sleep, energy, or concentration. If the athlete mentions a concern in any of these areas, then more direct questions about drinking patterns can follow. At this point, the clinician should attempt to keep the athlete's defensiveness low by using motivational interviewing strategies (open-ended questions, affirmations, reflective listening, summary statements). Once an athlete's trust has been gained, he or she is generally open to feedback about anything that might improve his or her performance.

More formal alcohol use evaluations are warranted when serious alcohol-related events occur. Such an evaluation is best done in an office near the training room for college and professional athletes or in a private off-campus office for high school athletes. The athlete is asked to provide a detailed history of the event, such as an arrest for driving while intoxicated, and this information is compared with media and police reports. The clinician gathers the specifics of the day or evening—including when drinking started, where it took place, who was present, what beverage was consumed, what the alcohol content was, and how much was consumed—to try to estimate the blood alcohol level at the time of the event (Table 5–3). Most athletes are surprised to learn that the body can get rid of only one drink per hour and that the blood alcohol level is higher in people with an absence of food in the stomach, of lower weight, with a higher percentage of body fat, of female gender, and after drinking distilled spirits (Appendix 5–1, Fact Sheets 1 and 2).

The clinician then takes a detailed history of the athlete's current and past substance use, starting with alcohol. The best way to begin is by asking about the athlete's general pattern of use in a typical week, with the goal of first uncovering how many drinking days as opposed to how much on a drinking day. For athletes in different sports, heavy drinking days commonly occur around their playing schedule; for example, most college teams have a 48- to 72-hour pregame no-drinking policy, which affects drinking patterns. Other important facts that should be obtained in a player's history include the family's history of problem drinking; the likelihood of hangovers, fights, and unprotected sex; and the athlete's natural sensitivity to alcohol's intoxicating effects. Low sensitivity to alcohol's intoxicating effects means that the body's recognition systems for intoxication are not as active, allowing these athletes to rapidly drink four to six standard drinks before they note any impairment. By that point, the brain's subcortical excitement centers have activated and cortical judgment centers have turned off so that heavier and riskier drinking is more likely. On the other hand, high sensitivity to alcohol and

TABLE 5–3. Blood alcohol content[a] by number of drinks[b], gender, and weight

		Body weight (lb)								
Drinks	Gender	90	100	120	140	160	180	200	220	240
1	M	–	.04	.03	.03	.02	.02	.02	.02	.02
	F	.05	.05	.04	.03	.03	.03	.02	.02	.02
2	M	–	.08	.06	.05	.05	.04	.04	.03	.03
	F	.10	.09	.08	.07	.06	.05	.05	.04	.04
3	M	–	.11	.09	.08	.07	.06	.06	.05	.05
	F	.15	.14	.11	.10	.09	.08	.07	.06	.06
4	M	–	.15	.12	.11	.09	.08	.08	.07	.06
	F	.20	.18	.15	.13	.11	.10	.09	.08	.08
5	M	–	.19	.16	.13	.12	.11	.09	.09	.08
	F	.25	.23	.19	.16	.14	.13	.11	.10	.09
6	M	–	.23	.19	.16	.14	.13	.11	.10	.09
	F	.30	.27	.23	.19	.17	.15	.14	.12	.11
7	M	–	.26	.22	.19	.16	.15	.13	.12	.11
	F	.35	.32	.27	.23	.20	.18	.16	.14	.13
8	M	–	.30	.25	.21	.19	.17	.15	.14	.13
	F	.40	.36	.30	.26	.23	.20	.18	.17	.15

Note.   F=female; M=male.
[a]Subtract .015 every hour after drinking.
[b]One standard drink=12 ounces beer; 5 ounces wine; 1.5 ounces hard liquor.
Source.   Modified from National Highway Traffic Safety Administration 2000.

serious hangovers often serve as protective factors against recurrent binge drinking.

Heavy alcohol use on just one occasion (defined as five or more standard drinks for a larger man or four or more drinks for a larger woman) can interfere with athletic performance in multiple ways in the short term. First, for some individuals, alcohol is a strong diuretic and therefore can lead to dehydration that may take 24 or more hours to correct. Second, alcohol is known to temporarily interfere with carbohydrate and energy metabolism and may adversely affect aerobic performance by as much as 10%. Third, alcohol in excess causes hangovers and if severe can lead to reduced prepractice or pregame hydration and nutrition, slowed reaction time, inattention, and impaired learning. Fourth, alcohol intoxication impairs judgment, which can lead to falls, fights, or arrests. It is common enough to see an athlete injured in a fight or a fall; sustain a severe bruise; or break a finger, hand, wrist, or tooth. An arrest may result in detention, missed practices to attend administrative or legal hearings, or suspension from practice or games if team or league rules are violated. Fifth, heavy drinking is a common cause of poor sleep quality or overt insomnia. Athletes, like other people, need at least 6 but usually 8 or 9 hours of *continuous* sleep to wake up refreshed with restored energy. As alcohol is metabolized after a night of heavy drinking, it tends to awaken the brain and interfere with normal sleep cycling, often leading to early awakening. This reduces the next day's energy and can reduce attention, reaction time, and motor coordination.

Alcohol's long-term negative effects on performance result from excessive weight gain and from health consequences. Importantly, alcohol has no nutritional value but contains 7 calories per gram, just behind fat for the most calories per gram of any food group. In addition, mixers or fortified alcoholic beverages can result in even greater caloric intake, which causes athletes to add unwanted fat and leads to impaired performance. Also, the increased likelihood of unprotected sex can result in sexually transmitted diseases or an unwanted pregnancy, which can in turn produce unneeded stress or require treatment with antibiotics that can have side effects such as loss of appetite or nausea. Because most athletes are young, more serious negative health effects, such as liver injury or gastric bleeding, are not common.

Case Study: Limiting Partying

A 19-year-old single professional baseball player, who was drafted out of high school, was seen by a sports psychiatrist in the third week of spring training after testing positive for alcohol on a routine team urine drug test. He readily admitted that he had stayed out late the night before the test, drinking with a few of his teammates. He estimated that he drank about 12–14 standard drinks over a 6-hour period, but said he did not drive. He experienced restless sleep, had a mild hangover, and felt slow the next day. He also recalled that several of his fellow players and one of his coaches commented on how bad he looked. He described a developing pattern since leaving home of twice-weekly trips to the bars with late nights and drinking to intoxication. He did not see this lifestyle as a problem and in fact thought he was doing well and was hoping to be assigned to the higher-level rookie team as a starting catcher. The psychiatrist elicited information about the athlete's drinking pattern that night and estimated that at the player's weight (200 lb), his peak blood alcohol level was around .15–.17.

Intervention: The psychiatrist and player discussed the pros and cons of heavy drinking and the potential impact it could have on athletic performance. The player knew little of alcohol's negatives and had not even considered that the coaches could easily identify him as one of the "party boys" and might hold the behavior against him. He agreed to limit his drinking to four drinks on 1 night a week. He also agreed to regular monitoring of his performance progress as a player and his intended changed drinking pattern. The psychiatrist saw the player once more during spring training and informally four more times during the season. The athlete reported light social drinking and steady improvement in his defense, handling of the pitching staff, and hitting.

Case Study: Multiple Alcohol-Related Events

The assistant athletic trainer, after regularly smelling alcohol in the training room during the first month of the season, asked the team psychiatrist to have an informal conversation with a midcareer relief pitcher. The clinician located the player in the clubhouse and engaged him in casual conversation. Because the player's arrest during the off-season for drinking and driving had been publicized in the media, the psychiatrist brought up this topic, asking about the circumstances of the athlete's arrest, the status of his driver's license, and his upcoming court date. The player acknowledged bad judgment in not calling a cab and stated that he had considered not drinking at all for a while, noting that he often got into confrontations with others when intoxicated. He added that his attorney's preference was for him to stop drinking, at least until his court date. The psychiatrist briefly discussed with the player the risks to his career of not bringing his best to the ballpark, and the player agreed to talk further in the days ahead.

On the next road trip, the athlete had another alcohol-related incident. He got into a verbal altercation with a security guard after returning to the hotel late from a bar and not being able to find his room key. He was so obnoxious and loud that the athletic trainer was called. A few days after returning from the road trip, the player had another incident at a restaurant near his apartment. While waiting to get another drink, a guy at the bar who recognized the athlete asked him what he was looking at. The player responded in a provocative manner, and the guy walked over and got into his face, which aggravated the player into hitting the stranger. The next day, the psychiatrist saw the athlete in the training room while he was receiving treatment on his bruised and swollen pitching hand. The player immediately said that he had consumed only a few beers but that the other guy was drunk. He recognized in retrospect that he should have walked away.

Because of this series of three alcohol-related incidents in 3 months, the athlete was open to the idea that he had a problem controlling his drinking and that his behavior could threaten his career. He agreed to an evaluation with the team assistance program counselor, who specialized in problem drinking.

Intervention: The counselor thought the player had a serious problem and recommended intensive outpatient treatment three times a week while in town and twice-weekly phone sessions while on road trips. Surprisingly, the athlete engaged quickly and fully in his outpatient group and began attending Alcoholics Anonymous meetings at the treatment program and then in the community. He committed to complete abstinence for the remainder of the season and was able to succeed. After a month, he reported feeling more rested, energetic, and confident and noted that his pitching coach demonstrated more interest and support.

Marijuana and Other Cannabinoid Mixtures

Marijuana is the most commonly used illicit substance among adolescents and young adults in the United States. In one study, about 35% of high school seniors and about 50% of college students endorsed past-year use (Saugy et al. 2006). The active compound in marijuana is delta-9-tetrahydrocannabinol (THC), although the flowers, leaves, and stems of a mature hemp plant contain more than 60 additional cannabinoids, which may explain the variable effects of different plants. THC generates its effects by attaching to cannabinoid receptors located on the surface of neural networks that influence pleasure, concentration, thinking, planning, movement, coordination, sensory patterns, and time perception (Campos et al. 2003).

As mentioned at the beginning of this chapter, college and professional athletes have lower marijuana use and abuse rates than nonathletes, especially during the season, when drug testing is active. Because use rates in male and female college athletes increase substantially during the off-season (doubling in males and quadrupling in females), clinicians can presume that similar increases occur in professional athletes when no testing is done. The fact that THC has a half-life of 1 week or more makes detection of its use far easier than other substances such as cocaine, opiates, or amphetamines. Therefore, in recent years, some athletes who are drug tested have begun to use herbal alternatives to marijuana. K2 and Spice are commonly used brands of synthetic cannabis that are sold in head shops and gas stations or over the Internet. These products are a potpourri of dried shredded plant materials, packaged as mild, moderate, and strong options. Presumably, synthetic cannabinoids are added to the plant mixtures to produce a high similar to that of marijuana. However, different products sold as spice products may contain other active compounds that produce different effects and side effects. These substances were banned in March 2011 by the U.S. Food and Drug Administration (FDA) for 1 year to allow further study of their negative effects and health risks (U.S. Drug Enforcement Administration 2011).

The most common reasons stated by athletes for using marijuana are relaxation, sleep, anger control, and pain relief (Appendix 5–1, Fact Sheet 3). Most athletes do not describe many negative effects, but these effects typically develop over long periods of time. Clinically, the most common negatives are declining motivation and interest; irritability, especially if anger or depression is already a problem; altered motor coordination; slowed reaction time; and impaired complex learning (Crean et al. 2011). As the THC content increases in marijuana, serious effects, such as panic, paranoia, or hallucinosis, increase in likelihood. Serious side effects during intoxication include vomiting, dizziness, headaches, visual disturbance, agitation, impaired thinking, and hallucinations. In states where medical marijuana laws have been passed, there has been an influx of very high-potency cannabis that may produce different effects than the variety with lower THC content. An herbal alternative, such as K2 or Spice, is even riskier because of the variability of the products (U.S. Drug Enforcement Administration 2011).

Case Study: Life-Threatening Reaction to Synthetic Cannabis

An early career professional baseball player was taken to the emergency room in an ambulance after a few of his teammates called 911. The group was playing cards in a hotel room after dinner when this player left to get some food. About an hour after he returned, he started to behave strangely, becoming more agitated, paranoid, and incoherent in his speech and saying something about bright lights. He also was sweating profusely, breathing rapidly, vomiting, and complaining of chest pain. When he arrived at the emergency room, he could not give a coherent history and appeared to be hallucinating. His pulse and blood pressure were elevated, but his temperature was normal. A serum toxicology screen was negative. His other lab tests, including a comprehensive metabolic panel, complete blood count, and urinalysis, were normal. An intravenous tube was inserted, and the patient was given diazepam to help him relax and stay in bed. After 4 hours of observation, he began to think more clearly but he had no memory of the night's events. He was eventually released back to his hotel room to be observed by his roommate for the rest of the evening.

Intervention: The following day, the athlete was seen by the team psychiatrist. The clinician could tell that the player was afraid he would get in trouble if he talked, so the clinician reassured him that his cooperation would be viewed positively. He admitted smoking a marijuana substitute with another player, who told him that he would not test positive on the team's urine drug screen. The athlete appreciated receiving a fact sheet on synthetic cannabis from the physician and vowed never to smoke anything like that again. He was followed through the remainder of the season and had no reoccurrences of his symptoms or other indications of a substance use or mental disorder.

Case Study: Persisting Psychosis From Marijuana

A veteran professional basketball player from another city was taken by his parents and girlfriend for an evaluation with a sports psychiatrist during the off-season because of his agitation, irritability, thought disorganization, hyperreligiosity, paranoid delusions, inability to sleep, and disinterest in eating or taking fluids. These behaviors had started the day after his return from a 1-week trip to Jamaica with his girlfriend and several other couples from his team. According to the girlfriend's report, he did fine until the last few nights when he became unable to sleep and instead kept saying that he needed to go buy a Bible. When asked why, he said that he had done some bad things in his life and he needed to read and pray. On the flight home, he was constantly mumbling and quoting biblical passages. After he got to his parents' house, he worsened and began wandering about the yard. He was driven from his home 2 hours away for a psychiatric evaluation. He had never before experienced any period like this and did not drink, smoke, or use drugs. In addition, he had not been under high stress, was healthy, and did not take any prescribed or OTC medications. He had no personal or family history of mood, anxiety, sleep, or psychotic disorders.

Intervention: The athlete was not able to give an organized history, but he listened as his family and girlfriend described what they had observed. Because he had not slept in 3 nights, his sleep problem became a priority. He reluctantly agreed to an office urine screen, which was positive for marijuana and negative for all other drugs of abuse. When asked if he had smoked while on vacation, he glanced away. His girlfriend felt that marijuana was a possibility because several of the other couples were known marijuana users. The parents agreed to get hotel rooms nearby, and the player was given quetiapine 25 mg for sleep and agitation. The clinician instructed him to take one tablet as soon as he got to the hotel and one or two more at bedtime and then to return in the morning.

Although the athlete looked better the next morning, he was still preoccupied with his shortcomings and was convinced that something bad might happen to him. The player seemed apprehensive to be in the psychiatrist's office alone, so his family was asked to sit in. The athlete's father, who stayed with him the first night, said that his son slept 6 continuous hours before tossing and turning until sunrise. The player was instructed to get some exercise (walk around a track at a local high school), eat regular meals, and stay well hydrated. He seemed surprised to learn that his fear and insomnia might have been triggered by marijuana. On the second day, he was told to take quetiapine 25 mg twice daily and 50 mg at bedtime and return again.

At the third meeting, the athlete looked less fearful and said he felt less guilty and ashamed about his past. He said he had slept even better the second night. Alone, he acknowledged smoking a small amount of marijuana on two occasions while on vacation but said the drug was very strong and made him immediately anxious and self-conscious. Over the next 2 days, he improved enough to go home. The clinician instructed the athlete to continue his daily exercise and to socialize only with his family and girlfriend over the next few days. He and his parents checked in by phone each morning. It took 2 full weeks for him to slowly return to his normal self. He tolerated quetiapine three times a day without difficulty and eventually tapered off his daytime doses. He continued taking 50 mg at bedtime for another week and then took them as needed. His symptoms completely resolved by the fourth week after his initial symptoms. He has had no similar symptoms over the past 6 years since the incident and has vowed never to try marijuana again.

Case Study: Marijuana, Motivation, and Irritability

A rising third-year high school varsity standout running back and linebacker was brought by his mother to a sports psychiatrist for an evaluation just before the beginning of the fall semester. She and the coach noted that the player had shown declining motivation for football and school that dated back to the previous spring. In addition, they described increasing irritability at home and at summer practice. The evaluation was triggered by an incident at practice in which the player got into a fight with two other players and then got in the face of his position coach who tried to break up the fight. The athlete described a declining interest in football and frustration with being one of the few black players on the team. He felt that the coaches and captains were always riding him, even though he had played offense and defense in every varsity game his first 2 years. He was strongly considering quitting. He stated that he did not drink but had become a regular user of marijuana in the middle of the previous semester. He felt that marijuana was the only thing that kept him calm and that helped him deal with his mother's drinking and his responsibility of caring for his two younger brothers who were always getting picked on by older white guys at the park next to his house. He was convinced that he would have hurt someone badly if not for smoking. A urine drug screen was positive for marijuana and negative for other drugs.

Intervention: The athlete agreed to weekly visits to work on stress and anger control and also committed to try to stop smoking marijuana. He expressed an interest in having his mother come to a joint session to discuss her drinking and irresponsibility, but he didn't think she would agree. After 3 weeks his urine test was negative, but the following week it was positive again. He stated that he got angry at practice, quit the team, and went back to smoking. Over the next 3 weeks, he struggled to stay clean; was becoming angrier at his mother and teachers; and could not sleep, being awakened by vivid dreams with violent content. He agreed to try risperidone 0.5 mg at bedtime, and a meeting with his mother was scheduled. During the family session, his mother started by saying that she had a drinking problem and she needed help to quit. She was referred to another therapist and quickly became abstinent. This change, along with the risperidone treatment, seemed to tip her son back in the direction of abstinence. Although he did not rejoin the football team, he decided to run outdoor track in the spring. He remained in treatment for the following year and is doing well in school and sports.

Legal and Banned Stimulants

Stimulants alone or in combination are commonly used by athletes to increase alertness, boost energy, raise intensity or aggression, improve concentration, lose weight, and treat attention-deficit disorder or excessive daytime drowsiness (Avois et al. 2006; Docherty 2008). The most common stimulants encountered in clinical sports practice are caffeine, nicotine, ginseng, and OTC amphetamine analogs (ephedrine, synephrine, phenylpropanolamine). Prescription medications (methylphenidate, amphetamine, modafinil, atomoxetine) and illicit drugs (cocaine, methamphetamine) are less commonly used but are more likely to produce adverse effects or lead to sanctions or suspensions. Stimulant use is most commonly identified during an evaluation of insomnia, anxiety, fatigue, poor concentration, or overheating, or because of requests for medications (nicotine replacement or varenicline to stop using smokeless tobacco, or stimulants for poor focus and concentration). Athletes at the collegiate or professional level frequently use two or more stimulants, and often in high dosages, but are unaware of these agents' synergistic effects (Appendix 5–1, Fact Sheets 4 and 5). Clinicians need to realize that athletes' levels and patterns of use during the season are typically much higher than during the off-season or preseason (e.g., spring training camp).

Caffeine

Caffeine, a naturally occurring plant alkaloid, is a central nervous system stimulant that was first isolated from coffee in 1820. It is legal and used by nearly 90% of the U.S. adult population, usually in coffee, tea, sodas, energy drinks, supplements, OTC pills, and prescription medications. It is, therefore, the most common stimulant seen in sports psychiatry practices. Although the vast majority of athletes use low doses without any negative effects, some take 500–750 mg/day or more and do have adverse effects, especially if the individuals are stimulant sensitive (Reissig et al. 2009). When evaluating caffeine intake, the clinician needs to ask about all possible sources and to quickly compute the daily amount and record the time of the last dose because dependence can develop and withdrawal can occur.

Case Study: Coffee, Heartburn, and Sleep Problems

A veteran baseball player asked to meet with a sports psychiatrist after a spring training clubhouse talk on stimulant use. The athlete said he had been a regular coffee drinker since college and noted that in recent years he had become increasingly reliant on it to raise his energy level on road trips. He typically drank 2 strongly brewed cups of coffee before breakfast and then several more after getting to the ballpark around 2 P.M. If he felt his energy dip, he would usually have another cup before batting practice, and in the last two seasons he had also added an energy drink an hour before the game. He was consuming about 800–1,000 mg of caffeine each day. He did not use other stimulants but described feeling wired after a game and would often have one or two mixed drinks with vodka to unwind after he got home. Over the last year, he noted restless sleep and more heartburn upon awakening; his primary care physician had started him on an antacid.

Intervention: The athlete expressed an interest in giving up coffee completely but wanted to keep a reduced amount of caffeine in his daily routine. He decided to purchase some 100-mg caffeine tablets for use in the morning. He had never been a breakfast eater, so he decided to eat some fruit and a breakfast bar before starting a combined 15-minute period of treadmill work and light stretching. After doing this routine for several weeks, he noticed that he was hungry after his morning workout, so he added a bowl of whole grain cereal or oatmeal to his breakfast. To boost his energy after arriving at the ballpark, he started consuming some fruit juice and yogurt before going outside for a fast walk or a light jog. Before batting practice, he would pedal the upright exercise bike for 10 minutes and then go outside for a good stretch. If still fatigued before a game, he would drink a cup of ginseng tea, as a teammate had recommended. He was able to completely stop drinking coffee and had greatly reduced his caffeine intake. His heartburn diminished, he was able to unwind more easily after games without alcohol, and his sleep and energy improved.

Nicotine

Nicotine is a naturally occurring plant alkaloid that is found in the leaves of the tobacco plant. Although cigarette smoking is not common among athletes in any sport, smokeless tobacco use is quite common in rodeo, baseball, and power sports such as football, wrestling, lacrosse, and hockey, with up to 30%–40% of male athletes using it during the season (Eaves et al. 2009; Severson et al. 2005). An easy way of identifying nicotine-dependent users is to find out if the first dip is within 30 minutes after awakening or if a last dip is just before lights out. Two especially good ways of generating interest in quitting smokeless tobacco are to give a team presentation discussing the pros and cons of use and introducing cessation medications or to have the team dentist give regular oral examinations looking for gum disease or precancerous lesions (leukoplakia). Although nicotine replacement is useful for reducing cravings and withdrawal symptoms, behavioral change is necessary for success in quitting. Two effective strategies are to pair an athlete who wants to quit with another who has already quit and to identify what substitute behaviors will replace dipping. Another helpful technique is to use oral substitutes, such as toothpicks, sugarless gum, seeds, candy, or a mouth guard. Although varenicline was originally approved for use with cigarette smokers, it can also be helpful for smokeless tobacco users. Sometimes the higher dosage of 1 mg twice daily is not needed, and dosages as low as 0.5 mg twice daily may be sufficient. The best time to quit for baseball players is during the off-season; however, football players seem more open to quitting at any time. Additionally, older athletes with children seem to be most ready to quit.

Case Study: Using Medication to Help Stop Long-Term Snuff Use

A married veteran professional baseball player with two school-age children approached the team's psychiatrist in the last month of the season because of an interest in stopping a long-standing pattern of moist snuff use. During the season, he would start dipping soon after awakening and typically take his last dip just before bedtime. He used a brand with high nicotine content (more alkaline) and used nearly one can of dip a day, a very high dosage. Although he enjoyed the energy boost and relaxation, he had noticed over the past few years much less relaxation, more gum irritation, and general annoyance with the nastiness of the habit. He had tried nicotine replacement without success and wanted to try varenicline after seeing a commercial for it on television.

Intervention: The player was given a prescription for varenicline to start at home after the season ended. He was instructed to begin taking 0.5 mg in the morning for 7–10 days and then add a second dose in the late afternoon. He was also given a second prescription for 1 mg twice daily in case he wanted to raise the dosage. He stayed in touch by phone and gradually cut down over the first 2 weeks and quit dipping during the third week. At the fourth week, he raised his dosage to 1 mg in the morning and kept 0.5 mg in the afternoon. He did not dip during the entire off-season, even during his hunting and fishing trips and before and after workouts, when he used to dip. He stopped the medication after 2 months and remained abstinent through the very end of spring training the following year, when he slipped, but not to prior levels. Instead, he usually used other oral substitutes, such as gum and seeds, but he especially liked the oversized, flavored Australian tea tree toothpicks. As the next season ended, the player asked for another varenicline prescription, expressing confidence that he could stop this time for good.

Case Study: Quitting Snuff Use With Behavioral Strategies

A veteran football player asked to meet the team's psychiatrist during training camp for assistance with quitting moist snuff, stating "I'm sick of it, and so is my wife." He had tried unsuccessfully to quit on his own during the off-season but could only go for a week or two before restarting. He was pleased, however, that a can now lasted him 4 days rather than 2. He had never tried nicotine replacement or varenicline but was not interested in either.

Intervention: He was given a fact sheet with common behavioral strategies for quitting. He told his wife, a few of his teammates, and the head team physician and athletic trainer of his goal to quit and asked for their support. He was taught some simple relaxation and activating breathing patterns to deal with cravings and was seen twice weekly throughout camp and the beginning of the season for support and as an additional strategy. He did decide to use an occasional oral substitute of a tart gum that was available in the training room. He managed to quit snuff use that season and never went back to dipping.

Over-the-Counter Amphetamine Analogs

OTC amphetamine analogs are typically purchased by athletes from health foods stores or over the Internet to lose weight, intensify workouts, combat fatigue, and increase game intensity. The most common analogs are ephedrine, synephrine, phenylpropanolamine, and pseudoephedrine. They are typically combined with caffeine (40–300 mg), ginseng, or excitatory amino acids. Before the FDA's ban on the sale of ephedrine and ephedra-containing supplements in the United States in April 2005, many of the products contained a stimulant stack of high daily doses of ephedrine (10–80 mg) and caffeine (100–800 mg) and low to moderate doses of synephrine. In addition, many athletes using these products were also smokeless tobacco users and coffee drinkers. Since the FDA ephedrine ban, the analog supplements now typically contain lower doses of ephedrine (≤10 mg/day) and caffeine but higher doses of synephrine and ginseng. Regardless, these supplements carry the same risk as any potent stimulant, especially if stacked. Common side effects are palpitations, jitteriness, insomnia, heat injury, cardiac arrhythmias, chest pain, and stroke. During regular rounds in the locker room, sports clinicians can learn which supplements are most used, as well as provide players with up-to-date information on the supplements. Players should be cautioned repeatedly, especially during hot weather, about the potential for stimulants to additively trigger serious heat or cardiovascular side effects.

Case Study: Stimulant Stacking

An overweight college football lineman was pulled off the practice field on a hot day early in the season because he was complaining of dizziness and chest discomfort. He was noted to be flushed and hot to the touch, and his heart rate was 130. He was not sweating. He was immediately taken to the training room. His oral temperature was 103.5 degrees, and his blood pressure was 150/94. He was placed into an ice bath, and intravenous fluids were started. After a few hours, he began to feel better, and the team's psychiatrist visited him later in the day to explore his use of stimulants. The player acknowledged using an OTC supplement for weight loss and exercise intensification, but he did not know what was in it. He had been taking two tablets three times a day throughout the summer.

Intervention: The supplement was taken from the player's locker and the label inspected. As the clinician suspected, the supplement contained high-dose ephedrine (10 mg/capsule, for a total of 60 mg/day) and high-dose caffeine (100 mg/capsule, for a total of 600 mg/day). In addition to taking the supplement, the player was a moderate coffee drinker (200–300 mg/day of caffeine) and had been exercising with a long-sleeve shirt to induce sweating. The clinician educated the athlete about the risk of this approach to weight loss and the toxic effects of high-dose stimulants. The player agreed to stop using the supplement and made an appointment to see the team's nutritionist.

Prescription Stimulants

In recent years, increasing numbers of athletes have come to college or professional sports teams already having a diagnosis of adult attention-deficit disorder or, less commonly, excessive daytime sleepiness due to narcolepsy or central or obstructive sleep apnea. They typically have been prescribed short-acting methylphenidate, amphetamine salts, modafinil, or armodafinil by a family physician or primary care sports medicine physician of their prior team. These athletes tend to take higher doses of their medications just before practice or a game but surprisingly not as much before class, studying, meetings, or key social events.

In addition, more athletes are asking to be assessed for problems with focus, sustained attention, attention shifting, distractibility, and poor daily organization and planning. Many professional leagues have instituted standards for these evaluations, addressing the credentials of the evaluator and the content of the evaluation. For an athlete to continue or begin taking a prescribed stimulant that is on the banned list of performance enhancers, he or she must submit an application for a therapeutic use exemption to a league authority, and a review structure must occur. The application typically consists of a copy of the evaluation for a new request, or a summary of the treatment and response from the previous year for a renewal. Sometimes, copies of the treatment notes and prescriptions are also requested for renewals, and a minimum number of face-to-face meetings in a year are required (usually two to four). When a therapeutic use exemption is granted, it is usually good for a full year or the remainder of that year's playing season if granted late.

The most common clinical issue seen in athletes taking prescription stimulants is a tendency to use short-acting formulations in higher than needed doses to boost practice and game intensity. The clinician's best approach for this situation is to change the prescription to a long-acting formulation, taken in the morning upon awakening after a light or full breakfast, and then to raise the dosage slowly over 4–8 weeks while watching for improvement in the athlete's impulsivity, motor restlessness, forgetfulness, focus, and sustained attention during practice, play, meetings, film watching, studying, and social interactions with teammates, family, and friends. If the athlete's medication wears off before the end of the workday, the clinician can prescribe a second but perhaps lower dose of a long-acting agent, to be taken between 12:00 P.M. and 2:00 P.M. Athletes should be advised to eat both breakfast and lunch before taking the medication, because its appetite suppression can cause some players to lose weight over the course of the season. Less common side effects include headache, motor tics, insomnia, and anxiety. A day off from these medications is not necessary in adults, but athletes typically reduce their dosage in the off-season, when their days are not as filled.

Case Study: Overstimulation From Short-Acting Amphetamine Salts

A midcareer minor league baseball player who transferred from another organization had a 3-year history of treatment for adult attention-deficit disorder, inattentive type. He had been taking amphetamine salts 30 mg at 3:00 P.M. and an additional 30 mg at 6:00 P.M. for night games. He was pleased with the improvement in his sustained attention during workouts, batting practice, and fielding, but noted that he had more difficulty falling asleep after games and often watched television or played video games until 2:00 or 3:00 A.M. He was reluctant at first to change his medication because he was pleased with his performance, but he agreed to try 20 mg of long-acting amphetamine salts around noon, followed by a single 30-mg dose of short-acting amphetamine salts at 6 P.M. After a week, he noted that he had an easier time unwinding after games and was typically asleep by 1:00 A.M., only 10–20 minutes after lying down. In addition, his wife, without prompting, noted that he had become a better listener and was more patient with their infant son and dog. At the end of the season, the player agreed to try the long-acting amphetamine salts 20 mg twice daily if needed for full days, and then to switch at the beginning of spring training to long-acting amphetamine salts 20 mg upon awakening and 10 mg at 2:00–4:00 P.M.

Anabolic-Androgenic Steroids and Other Muscle Mass Builders

A diverse group of substances, most notably the AASs and their precursors, are taken by some athletes at all competitive levels in many sports to boost performance by increasing muscle growth and sometimes decreasing body fat to raise lean body mass (Catlin et al. 2008; Horn et al. 2009; Parkinson and Evans 2006). These substances have been banned for athletes, as have peptide hormones and analogs, β_2-adrenergic agonists, and antiestrogenic agents. Antidoping policies also address additional groups of substances, such as diuretics, other masking agents, and local anesthetics, as well as specific methods, such as enhancement of oxygen transfer, chemical and physical manipulation, and gene doping. Detection of each of these substances and methods requires extremely sophisticated scientific techniques and irrefutable chains of custody for specimen collection, labeling, transport, storage, testing, and retesting. Because most of the substances are synthetically made and have many chemical analogs, testing technology and methods are challenged to keep up with the increasing numbers of novel compounds. Many other substances are present in such small quantities or have so many active or inactive metabolites that developing a scientifically sound methodology that can withstand legal challenge is both difficult and expensive.

The largest and most well-known group of mass-building substances includes the AASs and their precursors (prohormones), chemical analogs, or related compounds that produce the same effect in the body as the natural major male hormones, testosterone and dihydrotestosterone (Appendix 5–1, Fact Sheet 6). The performance-enhancing effects from AASs result from enhanced protein synthesis in muscle cells, which builds mass, and the masculinizing properties commonly associated with the development and maintenance of male secondary sexual characteristics. This group of substances primarily comprises synthetic analogs of testosterone. Most sports ban 40–50 of these compounds plus any unknown but related analogs for which detection is not yet possible. When one AAS is taken in extremely high doses in repetitive cycles or when several are taken together in high doses (stacking), then muscle mass and strength increase far beyond that possible through natural means.

Although most people associate AAS use with elite athletes, the typical users are noncompetitive body builders or even nonathletes who want to be more muscular or look better. Because of intense media attention regarding multiple high-profile cases of AAS use in professional and international sports, including baseball, football, body building, wrestling, track and field, and cycling, stronger antidoping programs have been developed at elite and lower competitive levels. Due to the rising rates of previous-year AAS use in youth from the mid-1990s (1%) to the mid-2000s (2.5%) and the high lifetime use rates in 2009 for high school–age boys (4.3%) and girls (2.2%), serious concern has developed about side effects and dependence. Estimates suggest that up to 30% of AAS users will develop a dependence disorder, and AAS use appears to be strongly associated with abuse of and dependence on other substances, especially alcohol, opiates, and sedatives (Kanayama et al. 2009).

Because many athletes and nonathletes have used AASs in cycles over many years or even decades, small studies and case reports of persistent medical and psychiatric side effects in some long-term users are increasing. Although most current or past AAS users are healthy because they are still young, the concern about future health is justified and supported by both experimental and naturalistic studies. Presently, the most commonly described lasting medical effects involve 1) the cardiovascular system (hypertension, cardiomegaly, myocardial ischemia, dyslipidemia, clotting abnormalities, and cerebrovascular accidents); 2) the neuroendocrinological system (hypogonadism, prostate hypertrophy but not cancer); 3) the hepatic system (cholestasis, tumors, rupture); and 4) premature death (Horn et al. 2009). The most common long-term neuropsychiatric effects are 1) mood disturbances (hypomania or mania), 2) impulse control difficulties (aggression and violence), 3) primary addiction, and 4) multiple-substance addiction. All of the long-term effects may not be known until the current heavy lifetime users move into the fifth or sixth decades of life and more observations can be made (Kanayama et al. 2008, 2009).

Although not as well known, available, or frequently used as the AASs, other substances can enhance athletic performance through similar or different mechanisms. Peptide hormones and related substances, such as human growth hormone, human chorionic gonadotropin, and insulin-like growth factor, increase muscle size and strength, improve muscle definition, reduce fat, aid in tissue repair, increase protein synthesis, and stimulate general growth. Erythropoietin, on the other hand, stimulates red blood cell production, thereby improving endurance and aiding muscle recovery. Hormone antagonists and modulators, such as the aromatase inhibitors, selective estrogen receptor modulators, other estrogenic substances, and myostatin modifying agents, are chemically and physiologically different from AASs but also have in common with AASs the enhancement of performance by building muscle size and strength. They also are used because they reduce some of the side effects of AASs, including breast enlargement. β_2-Adrenergic agonists act as bronchodilators at lower dosages, enhancing performance by increasing airflow and oxygenation, but are directly anabolic at higher dosages, promoting muscle growth and reducing body fat. Some inhaled medications are permitted during competition if they are used to treat exercise-induced asthma or bronchospasm. As detection methods for AASs have improved, shifts to these less common substances appear to be increasing because no practical or validated urine or blood tests exist for these agents.

Case Study: Stopping AAS Use

A 30-year-old married financial advisor and amateur body builder was referred by his attorney to a psychiatrist for an evaluation after being arrested at a local post office while attempting to pick up a shipment of anabolic steroids and benzodiazepines. He had a 10-year history of annual cycling on and off anabolic steroids in preparation for summer body building competitions. At the time of his evaluation, he was in the build-up phase, adding mass and weight by working out twice daily, consuming extra calories, and stacking several different anabolic agents. He had come to dislike this stage because he felt so large and bloated. He much preferred the cutting stage that followed, when he completely changed his nutritional plan to drop his body fat and shape his physique. After a decade of doing this annually, he felt that he was addicted to the roller-coaster process of getting bigger and then cutting. He marveled at how good he felt about himself when he competed or went to the beach. He had already weighted the positives of use against the negatives, including his current legal trouble, the strain in his marriage, and some changes in his health, such as testicular shrinkage, gynecomastia, and polycythemia (his hematocrit was 58%).

Intervention: He wanted to stop using AASs but thought that doing so would be very difficult. A 4-week plan for tapering off steroids and using diazepam was implemented. He was seen weekly in the psychiatrist's office, and his wife came to several early sessions to express her concerns and offer support. He assembled a support network consisting of two co-workers who were in substance recovery and a long-time friend. These three men also attended a meeting at the psychiatrist's office to discuss their roles in the process. As a result of that meeting, the body builder decided to start going to Narcotics Anonymous (NA) with his coworkers. No urine testing was done, because it would have been sent to a reference lab and was too expensive. Instead, serial hematocrits were obtained to ensure a gradual decline. The tapering plan went fine, and the patient's mood, which had been apprehensive and irritable, improved greatly. He was able to institute a balanced plan of cardiovascular workouts and strength work at a new gym that did not trigger urges to shift back to his old workout pattern. After 6 months, he felt comfortable that he had changed, and he shifted to once-monthly meetings with the psychiatrist along with twice-weekly NA meetings. At his legal hearing, he was given probation before judgment, with required abstinence and 50 hours of community service. A year after his arrest, he was abstinent for steroids and sedatives and was doing well at work and at home.

Case Study: Steroids and Unusual Injuries

A veteran professional tennis player who was engaged to be married asked to meet with a sports psychiatrist in the middle of the season because of insomnia and irritability. He described difficulty falling asleep and staying asleep for the previous several months and tied these problems to several injuries that kept him from playing and the recent hospitalization of his sister for pelvic surgery. His irritability began in the off-season, and he connected this to the stress of making plans for a fall wedding. He strained his quadriceps early in the season while running and was plagued by the injury for months. In addition, he had been bothered by nagging wrist pain over the past 2 weeks, and this injury was just recently diagnosed as an avulsion fracture of one of his wrist bones. While discussing his injuries and his off-season workouts, the topic of his added weight and muscularity surfaced. He did feel that the extra mass from his new workout routine increased his power but may have contributed to his "season of injury," and he also felt that he had lost some speed and flexibility.

Intervention: Although the athlete never acknowledged using anabolic steroids in the off-season, the clinician strongly suspected use of these drugs. The player was seen regularly through the end of the season for stress control and was given as-needed zolpidem for sleep. The athlete discussed with the psychiatrist his frustration with his injuries, concern about his sister, and relationship with his fiancée. They talked through his past workout routines and how the last year had deviated from his usual. He agreed that his frame could not carry the greater mass, and he knew from talking with the athletic trainers that his injuries were very uncommon. Without openly discussing steroids, it was clear that he had decided against any further use. The following season, he struggled to regain his old form but he persisted and is now performing well.

Conclusion

Sports psychiatrists must be skilled at evaluating and treating the common substances of abuse, such as alcohol, marijuana, caffeine, and nicotine, and the less common group of performance enhancers, such as stimulants, steroids, and other body mass builders. In addition, clinicians need to know the pattern and prevalence of each category for high school, college, and professional levels of competition, as well as typical changes in these patterns from in-season to off-season. The group of performance enhancers requires additional technical knowledge of urine drug testing, policy and sanctions, and short- and long-term health risks. Because athletes may be reluctant to open up to sports providers who work for the team or the league, clinicians also need skills at developing rapport and trust, enhancing readiness to change, improving performance, and finding substitute behaviors. Most of the time, substance interventions in sports require a team approach, which involves coordination with team physicians and athletic trainers, family members, coaches, agents, league officials, and general managers or athletic administrators (McDuff et al. 2005). Typically, leverage to change can be acquired from the legal or administrative problems associated with substance misuse.

Key Clinical Points

- Athletes use or misuse substances for four main reasons: 1) partying and relaxation, 2) performance enhancement, 3) injury recovery and pain control, and 4) abuse or addiction.

- Substances used in sports can logically be divided into three categories: 1) legal (alcohol, tobacco, and prescription medications); 2) illicit (marijuana, opiates, cocaine, amphetamine analogs, LSD, and PCP); and 3) performance enhancers (stimulants, anabolic steroids, hormones, and releasing factors).

- Alcohol misuse is easy to detect if athletic trainers, physicians, coaches, family members, and sports psychiatrists communicate regularly about the odor of alcohol, hangovers, alcohol incidents, interpersonal conflict, poor sleep, and declining performance.

- Alcohol interferes with athletic performance in the following ways: 1) dehydration, 2) altered energy production, 3) hangovers, 4) insomnia, 5) weight gain, 6) injury from fights and falls, and 7) stress.

- The use of marijuana substitutes (synthetic cannabinoids) such as Spice and K2 is increasing because they are not detected in routine urine testing. They are quite toxic, however, with risks of severe anxiety, paranoia, perceptual distortions, and brief psychotic episodes.

- The combined use of legal and banned stimulants (stimulant stacking) is common in sports and results in a higher risk of stimulant side effects, such as heat injury, anxiety, insomnia, weight loss, and heart palpitations.

- Oral tobacco use is much higher among athletes than in the general population, but quitting is possible through behavioral change and medications (nicotine replacement and varenicline).

- The authorized use of prescribed stimulants for attention-deficit disorder, narcolepsy, sleep apnea, and excessive daytime sleepiness is increasing. The short-acting formulations are more likely to be misused and cause stimulant side effects.

- Anabolic-androgenic steroid use in U.S. professional and international sports is decreasing because of more aggressive and sophisticated urine testing. However, use of alternative compounds, such as human growth hormone, androgen receptor modulators, peptide hormones, insulins, and hormone antagonists, is increasing because they are harder or impossible to detect.

- The long-term general and psychiatric health of chronic AAS users is becoming clearer as they get older. AAS addiction occurs in 30% of regular users.

References

Avois L, Robinson N, Saudan C, et al: Central nervous system stimulants and sport practice. Br J Sports Med 40:16–20, 2006

Barr J: Painkiller misuse numbs NFL pain. Available at: http://sports.espn. go.com/espn/eticket/story?page=110128/PainkillersNews. Accessed January 12, 2012.

Buckman JF, Yusko DA, White HR, et al: Risk profile of male college athletes who use performance-enhancing substances. J Stud Alcohol Drugs 70:919–923, 2009

Campos DR, Yonamine M, de Moraes Moreau RL: Marijuana as doping in sports. Sports Med 33:395–399, 2003

Catlin DH, Fitch KD, Ljungqvist A: Medicine and science in the fight against doping in sport. J Intern Med 264:99–114, 2008

Crean RD, Crane NA, Mason BL: An evidence-based review of acute and long-term effects of cannabis use on executive cognitive functions. J Addict Med 5:1–8, 2011

Docherty JR: Pharmacology of stimulants prohibited by the World Anti-Doping Agency (WADA). Br J Pharm 154:606–622, 2008

Eaves T, Schmitz R, Siebel EJ: Prevalence of spit tobacco use and health effects awareness in baseball coaches. J Calif Dent Assoc 37:403–410, 2009

Horn S, Gregory P, Guskiewicz KM: Self-reported anabolic-androgenic steroid use and musculoskeletal injuries: findings from the Center for the Study of Retired Athletes health survey of retired NFL players. Am J Phys Med Rehabil 88:192–200, 2009

Kanayama G, Hudson JI, Pope HG: Long-term psychiatric and medical consequences of anabolic-androgenic steroid abuse. Drug Alcohol Depend 98:1–12, 2008

Kanayama G, Brower KJ, Wood RJ, et al: Anabolic-androgenic steroid dependence: an emerging disorder. Addiction 104:1966–1978, 2009

Martens MP, Dams-O'Connor K, Beck NC: A systematic review of college-student athlete drinking: prevalence rates, sports-related factors, and interventions. J Subst Abuse Treat 31:305–316, 2006

McDuff DR, Baron D: Substance use in athletics: a sports psychiatry perspective. Clin Sports Med 4:885–897, 2005

McDuff DR, Morse E, White R: Professional and collegiate team assistance programs: services and utilization patterns. Clin Sports Med 4:943–958, 2005

National Collegiate Athletic Association: NCAA Study of Substance Use Habits of College Student-Athletes. Indianapolis, IN, National Collegiate Athletic Association, January 2006

National Football League Players Association: NFLPA injury report finds increases during 2010 season. Posted January 28, 2011. Available at: https://www.nflplayers.com/Articles/player-news/nflpa-injury-report-finds-increases-during-2010-season. Accessed February 5, 2012.

National Highway Traffic Safety Administration: Addressing Alcohol-Impaired Driving: Training Physicians to Detect and Counsel Their Patients Who Drink Heavily (Report No. DOT HS 809 076). Washington, DC, National Highway Traffic Safety Administration, July 2000. Available at: http://stnw.nhtsa.gov/people/injury/alcohol/impaired_driving. Accessed February 5, 2012.

Parkinson AB, Evans NA: Anabolic androgenic steroids: a survey of 500 users. Med Sci Sports Exerc 38:644–651, 2006

Reissig CJ, Strain E, Griffiths RR: Caffeinated energy drinks: a growing problem. Drug Alcohol Depend 99:1–10, 2009

Saugy M, Avois L, Saudan C, et al: Cannabis and sport. Br J Sports Med 40:13–15, 2006

Severson HH, Klein K, Lichtensein E, et al: Smokeless tobacco use among professional baseball players: survey results, 1998 to 2003. Tobacco Control 14:31–36, 2005

U.S. Drug Enforcement Administration, Office of Diversion Control:National Forensic Laboratory Information System Special Report: Synthetic Cannabinoids and Synthetic Cathinones Reported in NFLIS, 2009-2010. Springfield, VA, U.S. Drug Enforcement Administration,September 2011, p. 1. Available at: http://www.deadiversion.usdoj.gov/nflis/2010rx_synth.pdf. Accessed February 5, 2012.

World Anti-Doping Agency: Teacher's Tool Kit, Version 2.0, Teen Unit 2. April 2009. Available at: http://www.wada-ama.org/Documents/Education_Awareness/Toolkits/WADA_TTK_Teen_2009_EN.pdf. Accessed October 12, 2011.

Yusko DA, Buckman JF, White HR, et al: Alcohol, tobacco, illicit drugs, and performance enhancers: a comparison of use by college athletes and nonathletes. J Am Coll Health 57:281–290, 2008

Fact Sheets on
Substance Use and Sports

Fact Sheet 1—Alcohol Use and Sports

Fact Sheet 2—Alcohol Use and Athletic Performance

Fact Sheet 3—Marijuana Use and Athletic Performance

Fact Sheet 4—Stimulant Use and Athletic Performance

Fact Sheet 5—Stimulant Use in Sports

Fact Sheet 6—Major Categories of Mass-, Strength-, and
Endurance-Building Substances

Fact Sheet 1: Alcohol Use and Sports

Extent of use (males ages 21–29)	Social use past month (70%) Binge use past month (45%)[a] Heavy use past month (15%)[a]
Reasons for use (% citing reason)	Socialization (75%) Feel good/relax/escape (15%) Deal with stress (3%) Improve performance (0%) Other (unwind, fall asleep, reduce anger)
Reasons for cutting down or quitting (% citing reason)	Health concerns (25%) Against beliefs (15%) Hurt my performance (10%) Don't like it (10%) No desire for effect (7.5%) Prior bad experience (5%)
Factors affecting blood alcohol level	Body weight (lower levels for heavier persons) Body fat (higher levels in persons with more body fat) Time (higher levels the shorter the period; body only clears one drink an hour) Food (higher levels with an empty stomach) Type of drink (lower levels for beer than for wine than for distilled spirits, even with the same alcohol content per drink)
Short-term effects (within hours to next day)	Impairs coordination and judgment Reduces social and sexual inhibitions Slows reaction time May increase sadness, guilt, frustration, or aggression Impairs sleep quality Results in passing out or blacking out
Negatives for performance	Injury (fights, accidents) Empty calories (weight gain with poor nutrition) Dehydration (diuretic effect—not easily corrected) Hangover (slowed reactions, reduced energy, headaches, vomiting) Insomnia (poor concentration, low energy and motivation) Other drug use (more likely when drinking)

[a]Binge use=five or more drinks on the same occasion at least once in past month; heavy use=five or more drinks on the same occasion for 5 or more days in past month.
Source.   National Collegiate Athletic Association 2006.

Fact Sheet 2: Alcohol Use and Athletic Performance

Effect			Drinking timetable	
	0–12 hours	12–24 hours	24–48 hours	Regular heavy drinking
Positive alcohol effects (≤4 drinks per occasion)	Relaxation Unwinding Pleasure Destressing Socialization Break from routine	Stress control	Stress control	Few after 30+ days
Negative alcohol intoxication effects (≥5 drinks per occasion)	Disinhibition Dehydration Aggression Raised emotional intensity Slowed reactions Incoordination Change in sleep Impaired judgment Thrill seeking Passing out Blacking out	Hangover Dehydration Reduced reaction time Injury Altered carbohydrate metabolism Poor sleep Reduced learning	Hangover Reduced reaction time Injury Irritability Poor sleep Reduced learning	Same as for 24–48 hours, plus family, team, relationship, legal, and financial stress

Fact Sheet 2: Alcohol Use and Athletic Performance (continued)

Effect	Drinking timetable			
	0–12 hours	**12–24 hours**	**24–48 hours**	**Regular heavy drinking**
Negative effects on performance	Fights and injury Driving under the influence Drunk driving offenses Partner aggression Moodiness Insomnia	Lateness Inattention Low energy Slower reaction time Moodiness Injury risk Insomnia	Lateness Inattention Low energy Slower reaction time Injury risk Insomnia	Same as for 24–48 hours, plus poor nutrition
Negative effects on health	Injury Stress	Injury Stress	Injury Stress Sexually transmitted diseases	Hypertension Chronic insomnia Liver injury Weight gain Sexually transmitted diseases Mood changes Stress and anxiety Anger and conflicts

Source. McDuff and Baron 2005.

Fact Sheet 3: Marijuana Use and Athletic Performance

Background	Studies have found that cognitive impairments resulting from smoking marijuana can last up to at least 28 days after an individual last smoked the drug. The more a person had smoked before abstinence, the more profound this impairment, with marijuana smokers with lower IQs faring worse than their higher IQ peers, even if the latter had routinely smoked more of the drug.
Extent of use (males ages 18–25)	Social use last year (20%) Any use past month (15%) Daily use (5%)
Reasons for use (% citing reason)	Socialization (60%) Feel good/relax/escape (30%) Deal with stress (5%) Improve performance (1%) Others (improve sleep, reduce anger, reduce pain)
Reasons for quitting or avoiding	Health concerns (35%) No desire for effects (15%) Against beliefs (10%) Don't like it (10%) Illegal (7.5%) Afraid of getting caught (5%)
Short-term effects	Impaired coordination Difficulty with problem solving Difficulty with thinking Distorted perceptions Problems with learning and memory Increased appetite/overeating
Long-term effects (emotional and behavioral)	Anxiety Irritability Anger Insomnia Reduced appetite Lower motivation and achievement Moodiness Poor coping Slowed reaction time Addiction
Long-term effects (health)	Increased heart rate Irregular heart rhythm Increased heart attack risk Increased upper airway, lung, and upper digestive tract cancer risks

Fact Sheet 3: Marijuana Use and Athletic Performance *(continued)*

Recognizing use	Smell in clothing
	Absences
	Lateness
	Tiredness
	Low energy
	Poor effort or motivation
	Suboptimal memory and learning
	Easily frustrated/angered
	Partner conflict

Source.   Crean et al. 2011; National Collegiate Athletic Association 2006; Saugy et al. 2006.

Fact Sheet 4: Stimulant Use and Athletic Performance

Commonly used stimulants

Caffeine

Where found and how much	Average American adult consumption: 200 mg/day Coffee (50–100 mg/cup) Tea (30–80 mg/cup) Caffeinated soda (40–60 mg/can) OTC caffeine (100–200 mg/tablet) Pain killers (32–100 mg/tablet)
Positive effects	Alertness in fatigued state, increased muscle contractions, increased endurance
Negative effects	Headaches, anxiety, tremors, insomnia, poor appetite, dependency, arrhythmias
Recommendation	Limit use to <200 mg per day Avoid use with other stimulants

Nicotine

Where found and how much	Cigarettes (.5–2 mg/cigarette) Chewing tobacco (.5–5 mg/chew) Snuff (40–60 mg/can) Pipe (.5–3 mg/bowl) Cigar (10–40 mg/cigar)
Positive effects	None demonstrated, but subjective increased energy and relaxation reported
Negative effects	Lung/oral cancer, dependence, anxiety, tremors, insomnia, nausea
Recommendation	Don't start Limit use to <10–20 mg/day—then quit

OTC stimulants (ephedrine, synephrine, phenylpropanolamine)

Where found	Cold preparations Dietary supplements Internet
Positive effects	Increased alertness in fatigued state
Negative effects	Anxiety, tremors, insomnia, nausea, vomiting, loss of appetite, dependency
Recommendation	Avoid completely, especially if using caffeine and/or nicotine

Fact Sheet 4: Stimulant Use and Athletic Performance *(continued)*

Prescription stimulants **(methylphenidate, amphetamines, modafinil, asthma medications)**	
Medical uses	Attention-deficit disorder, narcolepsy, depression, asthma
Positive effects	Treatment of the above problems Increased performance if fatigued
Negative effects	Anxiety, tremors, insomnia, irritability, loss of appetite, dependence
Recommendation	Take only if prescribed by a physician Inform team athletic trainer/physician
Illicit drugs **(cocaine, crack, methamphetamine, prescription stimulants)**	
Routes of administration	Ingestion, smoking, intranasal, injection, chewing
Positive effects	Self-perception of enhanced ability, sense of pleasure and well-being
Negative effects	Anxiety, tremors, insomnia, weight loss, paranoia, sudden death, dependency, aggression, infection, depression, psychosis, hypomania, sexual dysfunction
Recommendation	Do not use these drugs, which are illegal and violate drug policy Seek help from team psychiatrist

Source. Avois et al. 2006; McDuff and Baron 2005; Reissig et al. 2009.

Fact Sheet 5: Stimulant Use in Sports

Stimulant	Common sources (amounts)	Reasons for use	Negative effects
Nicotine	Tobacco: cigarettes (0.5–2 mg/cigarette), snuff (40–60 mg/can), chew (.5–5 mg/chew), cigars (10–40 mg/cigar) Nicotine medications: gum (2–4 mg/piece), lozenges (2 mg/lozenge), patch (7, 14, or 21 mg/patch), nasal spray (10 mg/mL), inhaler (4 mg/cartridge)	Relaxation Alertness Arousal Calmness Stimulation Concentration Pain relief	Gum disease Oral sores/cancer Insomnia Heartburn Irritability Shakiness Loss of appetite Vivid dreams Addiction Anxiety
Caffeine	Coffee (50–100 mg/cup), tea (30–80 mg/cup), soft drinks (40–60 mg/can), energy drinks (80–500 mg/can), alcohol energy drinks (100–200 mg/can), pain medications (32–100 mg/tablet; e.g., Excedrin: 65 mg/tablet), caffeine pills (100–200 mg/tablet), chocolate	Energy boost Relaxation Loss of appetite	Stomach pain Insomnia Anxiety Headaches Withdrawal and dependence
Ginseng	Teas, tinctures, extracts, tablets	Energy Increase sexual functioning Concentration	Nausea, diarrhea Headaches Insomnia Irritability Restlessness Hypertension

Fact Sheet 5: Stimulant Use in Sports (*continued*)

Stimulant	Common sources (amounts)	Reasons for use	Negative effects
Amphetamine and analogs (methamphetamine, ephedrine, synephrine)	Amphetamines—prescription medicine for attention-deficit disorder, narcolepsy, weight loss Ephedrine—natural plant chemical banned in United States for strokes and heart problems but available online and in other countries Synephrine—substitute for ephedrine; often combined with caffeine and aspirin Methamphetamine—illegal drug of abuse that can cause severe addiction	Weight loss Energy lift Concentration Decongestant Euphoria Aphrodisiac Wakefulness	Rapid heart rate Hypertension Arrhythmias Weight loss Anxiety Insomnia Agitation Dizziness Stomach upset Headaches Overheating Paranoia
Cocaine	Illegal drug of abuse that can cause severe addiction	Euphoria Energy Sexual arousal	Anxiety Depression Exhaustion Addiction Stroke Heart attack

Fact Sheet 5: Stimulant Use in Sports *(continued)*

Stimulant	Common sources (amounts)	Reasons for use	Negative effects
Methylphenidate	Prescription medication for the treatment of attention-deficit disorder	Concentration Impulsiveness and hyperactivity Decreased distractibility Studying	Weight loss Motor tics Insomnia Headaches Mood changes Arrhythmias
Modafinil	Prescription medication for excessive daytime sleepiness from narcolepsy, nighttime shift work, or obstructive sleep apnea	Wakefulness Energy boost Studying	Insomnia Heartburn Dry mouth, thirst Flushing Sweating

Source.   Avois et al. 2006; Docherty 2008; McDuff and Baron 2005; Reissig et al. 2009.

Fact Sheet 6: Major Categories of Mass-, Strength-, and Endurance-Building Substances

Substance category	Performance effects	Negative health effects
Anabolic-androgenic steroids (AAS)		
Exogenous[a]	Increases endurance	Acne
1-Androstenedione		Aggressiveness
Boldenone	Promotes fat loss	Baldness
Danazol	Increases muscle recovery	Breast enlargement (males)
Gestrinone		
Methandrostenolone	Increases muscle size and strength with exercise	Clitoral enlargement (females)
Nandrolone		
Stanozolol		Hair growth (face and body—females)
Tetrahydrogestrinone		Hypertension
And many others		Impotence (males)
Endogenous[b]		Liver dysfunction
Androstenediol		Mania
Androstenedione		Muscle strains/ruptures
Dihydrotestosterone		Prostate enlargement
Dehydroepiandrosterone		Stunted growth (adolescents)
Testosterone		
Metabolites and isomers		Tendon tearing
4-Androstenediol		Testicular atrophy
5-Androstenedione		
Epi-dihydrotestosterone		
Epitestosterone		
19-Norandrosterone		
And others		
Other anabolic agents		
Clenbuterol		
Selective androgen receptor modulators		
Tibolone, zeranol, and zilpaterol		

Fact Sheet 6: Major Categories of Mass-, Strength-, and Endurance-
Building Substances *(continued)*

Substance category	Performance effects	Negative health effects
Peptide hormones, growth factors, and related substances		
Erythropoiesis-stimulating agents (e.g., EPO)	Increases endurance capacity with exercise (EPO)	Acromegaly and arthritis
Chorionic gonadotropin		Cardiomyopathy and heat failure
Luteinizing hormone (males)	Increases muscle recovery (EPO)	Deep vein thrombosis (EPO)
Insulins and corticotropins	Stimulates growth	Diabetes and hypercholesterolemia
Growth hormone	Enhances muscle definition	Facial nerve paralysis
Insulin-like growth factor	Increases muscle size and strength	Heart attack and stroke (EPO)
	Reduces body fat percentage	Myopathies and osteoporosis
	Aids muscle tissue repair	Pulmonary embolism (EPO)
	Increases protein synthesis	Softening of connective tissue
	Reduces protein breakdown	Stomach irritation and ulcers
	Masks AASs and reduces effects	Weakening of injured muscles and bones
β_2-Adrenergic agonists		
All banned except salbutamol (below 1,600 µg/24 hours) and salmeterol	Improves aerobic exercise	Anxiety, dizziness, and headaches
	Reduces fat	Arrhythmias and muscle cramps
	Enhances muscle growth	Insomnia and mood instability
Hormone antagonists and modulators		
Aromatase inhibitors	Causes anabolic effects	Abdominal discomfort
Selective estrogen receptor modulators	Increases strength	Flushing
Myostatin function modifiers	Reduces AAS side effects	Reduced libido
		Verbal slurring

Fact Sheet 6: Major Categories of Mass-, Strength-, and Endurance-
Building Substances *(continued)*

Substance category	Performance effects	Negative health effects
Diuretics and other masking agents		
Furosemide and spironolactone	Prevents detection of banned substances	Cramps and headaches
Thiazides and triamterene		Electrolyte imbalances
Probenecid, epitestosterone, and others	Causes weight loss	Heart and kidney failure
		Hypotension and dizziness

Note. EPO=erythropoietin.
[a]Not naturally produced.
[b]Produced in the body.
Source. Catlin et al. 2008; Kanayama et al. 2008, 2009; McDuff and Baron 2005.

Chapter 6

Injury Recovery and Pain Control

Injuries are routinely encountered in collision, contact, and noncontact sports, although they vary considerably in type, location, frequency, mechanism, and severity by sport, gender, level of play, cycle of the season, and intensity of practice and competition. Sports psychiatrists need to have broad knowledge of common and serious injuries to 1) assist with their management, 2) address emotional and motivational barriers to recovery and return to play, and 3) connect injured athletes with the proper practitioner or approach if the recovery is not going well. In general, injuries are three or more times higher in games than practices, two times higher in preseason practices than in-season practices, and more likely in games for men's sports than women's sports. Of reported injuries, 80% are new injuries rather than recurrent ones or complications of prior ones. Lower-extremity injuries account for about 50% of all injuries, whereas upper-extremity injuries account for about 20% and head/neck and trunk/back injuries account for about 10%–12% each. Ankle ligament sprains are the most common injury, accounting for about 15% of the total. Contact with another player is the most common injury mechanism, accounting for nearly 60% of game injuries and 40% of practice injuries. Of course, in some sports, including football, wrestling, ice hockey, and men's lacrosse, contact is an integral part of practice and play, and indeed these sports are the ones with the higher injury rates. The exceptions to this trend are women's soccer and women's gymnastics, which also have high overall injury rates for both practice and games or meets. Interestingly, injuries in noncontact sports are more common in practices than in games (Hootman et al. 2007; Huffman et al. 2008; Rechel et al. 2008).

129

Even though new or recurrent injuries are seen and treated daily, about 70% are mild to moderate in severity and do not result in much lost time. Others are more severe, resulting in significant missed time (21 days or more typically), requiring surgery and prolonged rehabilitation periods, ending a season, or raising the risk of recurrent injury or long-term complications. These more severe injuries, such as catastrophic brain or spinal cord damage, complete ligament tears, fractures, heatstroke, or concussion, are closely monitored by sport, gender, level of play, and recurrence rates. In high school, the most common severe injuries are fractures (36%), complete ligament tears (15%), and incomplete ligaments tears (14%); and the most common locations for injury are the knee (29%), ankle (12%), and shoulder (11%) (Darrow et al. 2009). Of these severe injuries, nearly 60% result in medical disqualification for the season. The most common sports with severe injuries are football, wrestling, girls' basketball, and girls' soccer. The severe overall injury rate for boys' sports is significantly higher than the overall rate for girls' sports, but when the same sports are compared (soccer, basketball, baseball/softball), girls' rates are higher (basketball) or the same (Table 6–1). Recurrent injuries account for only 10% of all injuries, but they are three times as likely to result in a decision to end athletic participation. Therefore, recurrent or first-time severe injuries make the rehabilitation process more variable and complex and highlight the importance of return-to-play decisions.

Through each of the four stages of injury and recovery, athletes experience negative emotions and fluctuating motivation and confidence (Table 6–2) (Galambos et al. 2005; Gordon 2010; Hamsom-Utley et al. 2008; Ivarsson 2011; Kvist et al. 2005; Webster et al. 2007). During the acute injury and stabilization stage, an athlete's pain, insomnia, apprehension, and uncertainty should be monitored. During the rehabilitation and recovery stage, an athlete needs to be observed for persistent pain, insomnia, stress, frustration, anger, motivation, social interactions, complications, and range of optimism or pessimism. In the return-to-play stage, important concerns include fear of reinjury or of injuring others, return of confidence, and injury prevention. Finally, if athletes are not able to return to play promptly or must leave the sport permanently, then they may experience depression, chronic pain, anger, and grief. In this chapter, I describe the role that sports psychiatrists can assume in injury management, return to play, and departure from sports. I emphasize important strategies for integrating treatment with the athletic trainers, physicians, and other medical staff; describe differences by type of injury, sport, and level of competition; and provide cases to highlight the most important clinical issues. A practical four-stage model will be used to

TABLE 6–1. Comparison of high school and college injury rates by gender

Sport	Boys/men		Girls/women	
	Practice	Games	Practice	Games
College baseball/softball	1.9	5.8	2.7	4.3
High school baseball/softball	.9	1.8	.8	1.8
College basketball	4.3	9.9	4.0	7.7
High school basketball	.9	1.8	1.4	3.6
College soccer	4.3	18.8	5.2	16.4
High school soccer	1.6	4.2	1.1	5.2
College football	9.5	35.9		
High school football	2.5	12.1		
College wrestling	5.7	26.4		
High school wrestling	2.0	3.9		
College volleyball			4.1	4.6
High school volleyball			1.5	1.9

Note. Injury rates are reported as injuries per 1,000 athletic exposures (i.e., a single practice or game).
Source. Darrow et al. 2009; Hootman et al. 2007.

identify high-risk athletes, facilitate recovery and return to play, prevent reinjury, and manage prolonged competitive absences or retirement.

Common and Less Severe Injuries

Participation and injury rates are rising in youth, high school, college, and professional sports. Possible explanations for the rise in injury rates, despite improvements in equipment, changes in rules, increases in injury prevention training, and expanded availability of athletic trainers and sports medicine physicians at practices and games, include the increased size of athletes and increases in the speed and intensity of play. In the National Football League (NFL), for example, offensive linemen, who are the largest players, have increased 40 lb over the past two decades from an average of 280 lb to nearly 320 lb. In professional hockey, one longitudinal study showed that compared with players in the 1920s and 1930s, current players were, on average, 17 kg heavier and 10 cm taller, with in-

TABLE 6–2. Stages of injury recovery: athlete emotions and critical issues

Areas of focus	Stages of injury recovery			
	Acute injury	Rehabilitation and recovery	Return to play	Departure from the sport
Reactive emotions	Hurt Anxiety Fear Disappointment Sadness Doubt Annoyance	Frustration Anger Stress Doubt Quitting Tension	Anxiety Fear Guardedness Intensity Doubt	Depression Uncertainty Resentment Loss/grief Loss of function Career change Self-doubt
Contemplative emotions	Apprehension Uncertainty Embarrassment Shame Pressure Confusion Concern	Optimism Pessimism Hopelessness Certainty Distrust Distraction Guilt Apathy	Fear (reinjury) Fear (injuring others) Tentativeness Intensity Confidence	Resentment Remorse Regret Jealousy Contempt
Critical issues	Pain control Sleep Energy Information Support	Persistent pain Boredom Social isolation Complications Motivation Substance use	Range of motion Speed/quickness Endurance Confidence and focus Soreness	Chronic pain Loss of function Financial strain Lifestyle change Career and identity Substance use

creased body mass index ($+2.3$ kg/m^2) and upper-body strength, and a suggestion of increased aerobic capacity (maximal oxygen consumption) (Montgomery 2006). Similar increases have occurred in other men's sports at high school, college, and professional levels, especially football, basketball, and lacrosse. Fortunately, most injuries are mild or moderate, resulting in no missed time or only a few missed days of practice. In this section, I describe some of the most common injuries for men's and women's sports across competitive levels (Table 6–3) and provide case examples that illustrate sports psychiatry's and psychology's supportive and facilitative role.

Ankle Sprains

Ankle ligament sprains are the most common sports-related injury (Nelson et al. 2007). They occur in sports that require quick turning and jumping in tight spaces around other athletes. Ankle sprains account for 20% of injuries in high school sports and 15% of injuries in college sports. Most (90%) result from ankle inversion or rolling onto the outer foot, straining the lateral (outside) ligaments. The highest rates of ankle injuries for males occur in basketball and football and for females in basketball and volleyball. In similar sports for males and females, males had higher injury rates in practice, whereas females had higher rates in competition.

Treatment of minor ankle sprains is conservative, consisting of rest, ice, compression, and elevation (RICE). Once the swelling and pain have diminished, athletes can begin regular range-of-motion and strengthening exercises. In addition, some athletes feel more confident walking in a compression sleeve or a brace, especially when they have recurrent injuries. Low doses of anti-inflammatory medications are sometimes used for pain control. Ankle sprains are annoying and frustrating, especially if boots or crutches are required and practice is missed. A sports psychiatrist can support recovery by inquiring about the injury and encouraging adherence to immobilization, elevation, and icing at home. If no ligaments are torn, then a rapid return to play can be projected. Reinjury in the first few workouts or practices can be diminished by the temporary use of a compression sleeve or by taping.

Case Study: It Hurts So Bad, Something Must Be Torn

A freshman varsity soccer player rolled her dominant ankle while dribbling on goal in practice on an uneven field. She fell to the ground, started crying, and could not continue. She was taken off the field by two teammates. She had never been injured before, and because she had been practicing well, she was hoping to get some playing time in the next

---

TABLE 6–3.   Common, less severe injuries

Ankle sprains

Shin splints

Hamstring strains

Knee strains and patellar tendinitis/tracking problems

Shoulder and elbow strains and tendinitis

---

game at the end of the week. When examined by the athletic trainer at the end of practice, there was minimal swelling, no point tenderness, full range of motion, and no laxity. The athlete, however, reported severe pain throughout the exam and did not feel that she could walk to the bus to go home. She was given a pair of crutches and told to ice several times before bed and elevate while sitting and sleeping. She was driven home by an upperclassman. The next day, she returned to the training room before practice but said she doubted she could go full speed.

Intervention: While standing with the head coach, the sports psychiatrist, who was working with the team to improve cohesion and communication, asked the player about her injury based on what the athletic trainer had said. The athlete understood that no ligaments were torn but said it was still painful to run and turn. She seemed upset that she might not be ready for the next game. She did not participate in practice, but rather was encouraged to sit and engage in range-of-motion work, alternating with some light running. She was complimented by the coach and team captain on her recent hard work and creative play and reassured that she would recover quickly. After practice, she met with the athletic trainer, who recommended a compression sleeve along with continued rest and ice. The next day, she seemed much more confident and was able to participate in most drills at a reduced speed. She made a quick recovery and was brought in at the end of the next game when the team had a comfortable lead.

Shin Splints

Medial tibial stress syndrome (MTSS), commonly called shin splits, is a common repetitive-use injury seen in sports that involve significant running and pounding, as in cross-country running or soccer; jumping or pounding on hard surfaces, as in gymnastics, volleyball, and basketball; or repetitive muscular contractions of the lower leg, as in swimming or cycling (Galbraith and Lavalee 2009). MTSS typically manifests as exertional lower-leg pain (middle distal tibia) that is thought to result from tendinitis, periostitis, muscular strain or dysfunction, or tibial stress reaction. This injury is usually diagnosed from history and examination, which requires looking above or below the source of the pain for flat feet; abnormal gait; weakness, imbalance, or reduced flexibility of muscles; skeletal (i.e., knee, pelvis, and lower spine) abnormalities; or inadequate footwear. X-rays or imaging studies may be necessary to distinguish MTSS from a more serious diagnosis of stress fracture.

Acute treatment of MTSS usually consists of complete rest, ice, anti-inflammatory medications for pain, and local treatments such as ultrasound, electrical stimulation, phonophoresis, or whirlpool baths. Sub-acute treatment involves an alteration of the training regimen, such as substituting biking or swimming for running; the introduction of stretching and strengthening exercises; manual therapy to correct imbalances or inadequate range of motion in the kinetic chain; and new footwear and/or orthotics. Sports psychiatrists need to be familiar with the common signs and symptoms of MTSS, as well as the usual treatments. This is especially necessary when working with athletes in youth or high school sports, where access to a certified athletic trainer or a sport-trained or experienced physician may not be common. In addition, assisting coaches with examining training regimens for excessive intensity and inadequate rest or variability is a critical skill. Finally, familiarity with more serious diagnoses, such as stress fractures and exertional compartment syndrome, is important.

Case Study: It Could Be a Stress Fracture

A tall high school senior cross-country runner began complaining of increased middle and lower left tibial pain the week following a highly competitive invitational cross-country race on a very difficult and hard-packed dirt course. Although he had struggled with some tibial discomfort since the early part of the season, his pain had become much more severe since the race. His coach suggested that he take a break from running and substitute swimming, but the athlete wanted to train for the upcoming county championships because he was in his senior year and his team had a chance to win or place. He had not seen an athletic trainer because his school did not have one available to his sport. Also, because his parents worked late, he had not been able to see his primary care provider.

Intervention: The coach asked the sports psychiatrist who had been working to improve the team's mental preparation and strategy to speak to the athlete. The youth had run hard over the summer, running more than ever before (35–50 miles a week), and had trained especially hard in the 2 weeks before the invitational, with much more interval work, hoping to run his best time ever. He had pushed himself on the course during the recent race, noting that the ground was especially hard due to the recent lack of rain. When examined, he had tenderness and a raised area over his midtibia, and his pain increased with standing and with dorsi and/or plantar flexion. He was strongly encouraged to stop all training and to see a sports medicine physician, to which the athlete agreed. The coach called the psychiatrist later that night to say that the athlete's parents did not know of a sports physician in their network, and a referral to one was facilitated. Unfortunately, he was diagnosed with a stress fracture and was unable to run for the rest of the year. He was, however, quite proud of the fact that he had bested his old time by more than 2 minutes, even though the course was one of the toughest in the state.

Hamstring Strains

The sudden onset of posterior thigh pain, often with an audible pop, that occurs during high-speed running is common in the history of athletes who sustain hamstring strains (Heiderschreit et al. 2010). The pain typically results from a sudden stretching or tearing of some muscle fibers, intramuscular tendons, or the aponeurosis of the long head of the biceps femoris. This muscle originates from the ischial tuberosity and inserts onto the lateral condyle of the tibia and the head of the fibula and is involved in knee flexion and hip extension. Hamstring strains of the biceps femoris are very common at all competitive levels in sports that involve rapid acceleration, including track, football, baseball, softball, basketball, and soccer. As an example, a 10-year study of professional football players in the NFL showed hamstring strains of the biceps femoris were the second most common injury in training camp, after knee strains (Heiderschreit et al. 2010). Strains involving the other two hamstring muscles (semimembranosus and semitendinosus) are usually more severe, and are most common in sports involving kicking, such as dancing or martial arts.

After a running hamstring strain occurs, athletes usually experience pain with jogging, walking, standing, or sitting; reduced strength and range of motion; swelling or bruising; and point pain with examination (palpation or resistance testing). Most strains result in missed time from practice and/or competition, ranging from a few days for mild injuries to 3 or more weeks for moderate injuries. The reinjury rate is high, with more than 30% of athletes sustaining another strain within a year (Heiderschreit et al. 2010). The most common risk factors are hamstring weakness, fatigue, and tightness; imbalances in strength between hamstring and quadriceps; and pelvic and core strength and coordination difficulties. Acute management involves rest, ice, compression, elevation, pain control, and local treatments. For more severe injuries, muscle relaxants and sleep medications may also be used.

Sports psychiatrists may assist athletic trainers and team physicians by ensuring that an athlete's pain is controlled and that the athlete has adequate sleep in the first few nights after injury. Because most athletes who sustain a running-related hamstring strain have had a prior injury, they tend to have a good sense of what regimens work best for them. Even so, they are often reluctant to ask for short-term medications for pain and sleep. Once the athlete's pain resolves and strength and range of motion improve, attention shifts to preventing reinjury and monitoring disappointment and frustration levels. Unfortunately, because many recurrent injuries are seen in the 2-week period following the initial injury, disappointment and frustration are common. Additionally, a rehabilitation program that addresses the modifiable risk factors must be established and followed for the long term. Psychiatrists can support and encourage athletes to put in the extra time and energy required for a well-rounded injury prevention program.

Case Study: If This Keeps Happening, Then My Career Is Over

A second-year professional football wide receiver kept missing substantial practice and game time due to recurrent right hamstring strains. He missed four games during his first year, and six during his second year. He was extremely frustrated and discouraged, feeling that he was jinxed. When the sports psychiatrist asked about his prevention program, the player said he was just trying to avoid those activities that would likely trigger reinjury until he got to the end of the season.

Intervention: The psychiatrist was familiar with two veteran players, one a receiver and the other a defensive back, who had early career histories similar to this younger player's. After every practice, the two veterans engaged in a 30- to 45-minute organized routine of core and pelvic strengthening, as well as extensive stretching. In conversations over several seasons with the team psychiatrist, both players said they had picked up various aspects of their prevention program from athletic trainers, chiropractors, strength and conditioning staff, and physical therapists, and they would be willing to speak to the injured player. Over the next week, the younger player had lengthy discussions and demonstrations with both veterans. He began to put together the framework of his program and committed to develop it and work hard in the off-season. By the time he returned to training camp, he seemed cheerful and confident. He had worked out harder than ever before and felt like his prevention work had paid off. Over the next two seasons, he had no recurrent injuries and felt that he had reestablished his career.

Knee Sprains and Patellar Tendinitis/Tracking Problems

Knee ligament sprains and patellar tendinitis and tracking problems are common in both contact and noncontact sports. Ligament sprains occur from contact, turning, pivoting, twisting, landing, or repetitive use, and are commonly seen in football, soccer, basketball, lacrosse, field hockey, volleyball, cheerleading, and gymnastics. Less serious (grade 1) sprains of the medial collateral or lateral collateral ligaments usually occur in competition with contact and result in pain and swelling directly over the stretched or partially torn ligament but may also include some general joint swelling and restricted range of motion. These sprains can occur as isolated injuries or as part of more complex injuries that also involve the anterior and posterior cruciate ligaments. Medial collateral ligament (MCL) sprains may also be accompanied by meniscal tears because the MCL is attached to the medial meniscus. Sprains or partial tears of anterior and posterior cruciate ligaments usually occur from pivoting or landing from a jump. Less serious (grade 1) sprains produce knee pain, swelling, reduced range of motion, and a sense of knee instability. Most minor knee ligament sprains are treated with ice, ultrasound, reduced activity, compression, knee bracing, anti-inflammatory medications, and range-of-motion exercises, and usually result in 1–2 weeks of missed time.

Patellar tendinitis and patellofemoral syndrome are repetitive-use injuries that most often occur in sports involving running, such as soccer, lacrosse, cross-country, basketball, and field hockey. These injuries are also seen in collision or contact sports, such as football or rugby, that require significant lower-body lifting or strain from repetitive contact during drills with other players or equipment. Patellar tendinitis is most common in jumping sports, such as volleyball, basketball, and soccer, and results in pain with activity and pain directly over the tendon. Patellofemoral syndrome is more common in young athletes, women, or those with valgus deformities of the knees (knock-knees) or weak medial thigh or hip muscles, and in athletes who overtrain (e.g., runners who run excessive miles). Treatment involves a reduction in the intensity of training, ice, nonsteroidal anti-inflammatory medications, and stretching and strengthening of the hip and thigh muscles.

Case Study: I Don't Think Any of the Coaches Like Me

A second-year college basketball player was seen midseason by a sports psychiatrist in the training room while receiving treatment for patellar tendinitis and a sprained MCL. These conditions had gradually worsened since the beginning of the fall semester and were now limiting her ability to participate fully in practice. She started the season as a forward and had been playing 20 or more minutes a game, but now she was playing only late in games when the team was ahead. When asked about her confidence, she said it was the lowest it had ever been.

Intervention: Brief conversations with the head coach, athletic trainer, and team physician revealed that they felt that her injuries were not so severe that she could not practice. The coach had written her off and had begun to focus on the development of two freshmen. The discussion with the team physician led to the addition of a lidocaine patch to her regimen of anti-inflammatory medication and a compression sleeve. This did ease her pain and allowed more intensity in practice. Weekly meetings with the psychiatrist helped her work through her disappointment, and her confidence, as well as the quality of her play, gradually increased. Her minutes of play time increased but not back to the level at the beginning of the season. Over the spring term, she thought carefully about her role on the team and decided to transfer to another conference. She completed 2 more years at the new school as a starter and a solid contributor to the team.

Case Study: I Can't Even Run, So How Can I Play Soccer?

A rising junior college soccer player visited a sports psychiatrist for an evaluation of pain with running and frustration with chronic injuries. She had been diagnosed with patellofemoral syndrome but had been unable to find a solution. About 5 minutes after beginning a fitness run, she would develop sharp pain on the lateral aspect of her right knee and be unable to continue. This problem had developed late in the spring season, but she was able to play through it. She knew that if she didn't arrive at fall practice in fit condition, she would not be able to keep her starting position as an outside midfielder. She had gone to a sports orthopedist, who made the diagnosis and sent her to a physical therapist. She was given some stretching and strengthening exercises but had not developed a consistent routine.

Intervention: After the athlete discussed the history of the injury and the frustration with its limitations on her summer training, the psychiatrist performed a simple assessment of the athlete's lower-leg flexibility. Notably, her calf, hamstring, and hip extensors were extremely muscular and tight on both sides but more so on the right. In addition, her quadriceps was much more dominant laterally on the right (her kicking) leg. She was sent to a certified athletic trainer who showed her a simple routine for stretching her lower-leg and hip muscles and strengthening her medial quadriceps. She went to see him three times a week for 2 weeks and then continued the routine on her own. After 4 weeks, she resumed running without pain and adopted an extensive postrunning stretching routine. As her mileage and intensity increased without return of pain, her confidence soared, and she started her fall season well.

Shoulder and Elbow Strains and Tendinitis

Minor shoulder and elbow strains and tendinitis are common in sports involving throwing, passing, serving, rotation, punching, and spiking, as in javelin throw, baseball, softball, volleyball, water polo, swimming, boxing, badminton, tennis, cricket, and football (Bonza et al. 2009; Chumbley et al. 2000). The most common shoulder strains are from overuse or sudden action stress of the rotator cuff muscles (i.e., supraspinatus, infraspinatus, subscapularis, and teres minor), producing muscle stretching or tearing and tendon stretching or inflammation. Symptoms include a chronic dull ache, sudden pain, muscle spasm, tenderness over the spot of the strain, difficulty with overhead movements, and trouble sleeping. Treatment is the same as for other strains and includes rest, ice, local liniments, ultrasound, and anti-inflammatory medications in the acute period, followed later by range-of-motion, stretching, and strengthening exercises. The most common elbow strains also result from overuse and occur in racket sports, such as tennis, racquetball, or squash; throwing sports, such as baseball, softball, and cricket; and other lower-arm rotational sports, such as bowling, rowing, skiing, boxing, and swimming. The most common overuse strain locations are either 1) lateral (tennis elbow), which results from acute forearm-wrist extensor muscle and tendon stretching or tearing; or 2) medial (golfer's elbow), which results from forearm-wrist flexor muscle stretching and tendon inflammation or chronic strain with secondary muscle weakness, fatigue, and imbalance and tendinopathy with degenerative tissue changes. Although acute overuse responds quickly (within days) to rest, ice, local treatments, and anti-inflammatory medications, chronic overuse may require longer-term (over months) muscle and tendon strengthening and rehabilitation.

Case Study: I'm Sick of Doing Cuff Exercises

A right-handed minor league starting pitcher in his third year finished the prior season on the disabled list because of a chronic rotator cuff strain. He had pitched more innings than ever before, but as he got into mid-August, he began to have posterior shoulder pain with throwing. Magnetic resonance imaging (MRI) did not reveal any tears, but he was shut down for the season and put on a shoulder rehabilitation and cuff strengthening program. When he left for the off-season, he was to continue his cuff program, but he did not. When he returned to spring training, he felt confident and prepared, but his shoulder began hurting again after the first week. His frustration caught the attention of the athletic trainers, and he was referred for sports psychiatric evaluation.

Intervention: He immediately acknowledged his mounting frustration and said that he had never been injured before the previous year. He had dominated hitters in college and as a professional and had just assumed that off-season rest would solve his rotator cuff strain. The psychiatrist reviewed the importance of the four rotator cuff muscles to throwing and discussed how naturally weak they are compared with the other shoulder muscles. The athlete understood the importance of cuff strengthening but had not developed a good routine. He agreed to talk to one of the other pitchers who had struggled with the same issues. Following this discussion and an additional interaction with the athletic trainers, he began a regular cuff strengthening and shoulder stretching program. After 2 weeks, he had significantly improved and began a graduated throwing program. He seemed much more committed to maintaining his shoulder strength and flexibility.

More Serious, Rare, and Catastrophic Injuries

The most serious, rare, or catastrophic injuries are most likely to occur in males competing in collision sports (Huffman et al. 2008). However, not all serious injuries result from player-to-player contact and can occur as a result of a sport's movement demands, such as turning or jumping, which can produce ligament tears in the ankle and knee, or throwing, which can result in ligament tears in the shoulder and elbow. Although catastrophic injuries are rare, they must be reviewed carefully to ensure that rule and equipment changes are made as quickly as possible to protect player safety. Beginning in 1977, the National Collegiate Athletic Association (NCAA) initiated a tracking system for catastrophic football injuries that now monitors recreational, high school, college, and professional levels of competition. Catastrophic injuries are defined as brain or spinal cord injury or skull or spine fractures that involve some disability at the time of the injury. This surveillance and research system is now conducted as part of the National Center for Catastrophic Sports Injury Research at the University of North Carolina, Chapel Hill. In 2009, nine athletes had cervical cord injuries with incomplete neurological recovery (Mueller and Cantu 2010). Seven of the nine occurred at the high school level, and most involved defensive players in games. Also in 2009, nine athletes had sports-related brain injuries with incomplete recovery, and 24 had head or neck injuries with complete recovery. All nine of the brain injuries with incomplete recovery occurred in high school sports, whereas the 24 with complete recovery were mainly in high school and college. Although the catastrophic injury rate is low (0.46 per 100,000 high school players and 1.33 per 100,000 college players), the rates for 2007, 2008, and 2009 were the highest of the past decade. In this section, I discuss some of the most common serious injuries (Table 6–4) and provide management tips and case studies to highlight integrated psychiatric and medical treatment.

Brain Injury, Paralysis, and Concussion

Whereas skull, brain, cervical spine, and spinal cord injuries with complete or incomplete neurological recovery, such as paralysis, are rare, less severe brain injuries, such as concussion, are much more common and their rates seem to be rising. In college athletes, for example, concussion rates rose 7% per year over a 16-year period from 1988 to 2004. The highest rates occur in certain high school sports, such as boys' and girls' soccer and girls' basketball, and specific college sports, such as men's football, ice hockey, wrestling, and lacrosse and women's ice hockey, soccer, and lacrosse. Although some of the increase in rates is definitely due to better reporting, some of the increase is due to a rise in game intensity (e.g., concussion most often occurs in sports with player-to-player contact) (Hootman et al. 2007; Huffman et al. 2008).

TABLE 6–4.   More serious, rare, and catastrophic injuries

Brain injury, paralysis, and concussion

Eye and dental injuries

Dehydration and heat illnesses

Fractures

Muscle, tendon, and ligament tears (ankle, knee, elbow)

Back pain

Knee disruptions

Shoulder separations and dislocations

Concussion in sports has received increased attention over the past decade. A concussion is a temporary loss of brain function that usually results from a blow to the head and consequent oscillating movement of the brain inside the skull, causing tissue bruising, blood vessel rupture, and/or nerve injury. Concussions occur with or without a loss of consciousness and are sometimes categorized as *simple* if they resolve in 7–10 days or *complex* if longer. Nearly all sports at all levels of competition now require that a player who shows any symptoms, signs, or behaviors associated with concussion (Table 6–5) must be removed from play for that game and not return to practice or play until cleared by a medical provider. The NFL, for example, has instituted a regimented protocol for return to play after concussion (National Football League 2011, 2012). First, the player must be symptom free at rest and during an exercise challenge. Second, the player must repeat the computerized Immediate Post-Concussion Assessment and Cognitive Testing (ImPACT) and have the results compared to baseline. Finally, the player must be cleared by a neurologist experienced in head injury and not directly affiliated with the team. This protocol was instituted in part because of the concern about the development of chronic traumatic encephalopathy (CTE), a progressive neurodegenerative brain disease that leads to dementia and is seen in persons with repetitive brain trauma. Alarmingly, a half dozen or more former NFL players with histories of recurrent concussion and premature death have had postmortem findings of CTE (Boston University Center for the Study of Traumatic Encephalopathy 2012).

Strategies to reduce the likelihood of catastrophic brain and spine injuries and concussion have centered on changing rules (i.e., tackling technique in football), improved coaching techniques, increasing certified athletic trainer and physician availability during games, improved screening of those with prior head injuries, enhanced conditioning, and innovations in equipment design. Specifically, coaches instruct in proper blocking and tackling fundamentals; athletes improve conditioning to increase neck

TABLE 6–5. Common acute concussive and postconcussive symptoms

General	Head/neck	Emotional/cognitive	Neurological
Nausea/vomiting[a]	Ringing in ears[a]	Poor concentration	Confusion[a]
Feeling "foggy"[a]	Blurry vision[a]	Decision problems	Amnesia[a]
Sleepiness/insomnia	Headache	Sadness/depression	Slurred speech[a]
Fatigue	Light/noise sensitivity	Anxiety	Poor balance[a]
Memory difficulty	Neck stiffness	Irritability	Dizziness
Loss of appetite	Unequal pupils		Numbness/tingling

[a]Acute concussive symptom.

strength and make sure that equipment fits; officials aggressively enforce rules that ban the use of the head as a battering ram; and players who have signs and symptoms of concussion do not return to play that day and until they are back to normal and have been medically cleared.

Case Study: A Severe Concussion in High School Kept Me From Playing for Months

A third-year college soccer player was referred toward the end of the season for evaluation because of her reluctance to return to play following a mild concussion a few weeks earlier. During a game, the player was struck in the side of the head with a kicked ball. She came out of the game complaining of disorientation, nausea, dizziness, and headache. She did not return to play. Over the next week, she reported persistent headaches, dizziness with movement, poor concentration, light and noise sensitivity, and poor sleep. She went to practice but did not participate. She had previously sustained a severe concussion in her third year of high school while going up to head a ball, then had fallen hard to the ground and struck the back of her head. She had moderately severe postconcussive symptoms over the next 4 months and also developed moderate depression that was treated with an antidepressant and psychotherapy. This prior injury occurred during a high-stress time of family conflict.

Intervention: During the evaluation, the player expressed concern about returning to play, making reference to her high school concussion and depression. She felt that she was on the edge of depression all year because her playing time had been minimal compared to her second year, when she started every game. She had become convinced that her head coach no longer valued her as a player, and she felt powerless to change that view. She reported daily headaches, poor concentration in class and while studying, and light sensitivity. She felt that the athletic trainer and the coach were pushing her to come back to practice and that they did not believe her symptoms were as severe as she was reporting. Because the athlete had not seen a physician, the psychiatrist referred her to a sports medicine specialist experienced in concussion. In light of the seriousness of her concussion in high school and the fact that there were only two games left in the season, he recommended that she end her season. She was so relieved by his recommendation that her affect brightened considerably. Three weeks later, she had an end-of-season meeting with the head coach, who was more supportive than expected. She then developed her goals for the spring and sent them for review and input. She identified three areas to improve her play as a central defender and seemed upbeat about making them happen.

Rare Injuries (Neck and Spine Injuries, Eye and Dental Injuries, Dehydration, and Heat Illnesses)

In addition to neck and cervical injuries, certain injuries, such as eye and dental injuries, dehydration, and heat illnesses, are rare or unusual but have the potential for serious consequences (Huffman et al. 2008). Although most rare injuries allow return to play within a week, some result in surgery, significant missed time, chronic pain or disability, or even death. In high school sports, rare injuries are most common in boys, with the highest rates occurring in football, wrestling, and baseball (Huffman et al. 2008). The most common of these rare injuries were neck and spine (62%), followed by dehydration and heat illness (19%), eye injuries (12%), and dental injuries (7%). Neck and cervical injuries and dental injuries had the highest proportions of significant missed time (greater than 21 days) or a season-ending effect. Although dehydration and heat illnesses are not often considered injuries, they are common in sports played outdoors in the summer (e.g., football) or intense indoor sports (e.g., wrestling). Because of some high-profile heat injury deaths of professional football and baseball players, substantial attention is paid to the hydration status of all athletes, especially those who have had prior heat illnesses or are taking medications that increase metabolism and decrease sweating.

Case Study: It May Take a While to Get Over the Fear

A right-handed senior college softball pitcher was seen before the season in anticipation of returning to play for her final year. Her previous season ended when, after getting hit directly with a batted ball, she sustained a severe fracture to her left orbit and required extensive reconstructive surgery. In addition to the fracture of her orbital ridge, she also experienced bleeding into the anterior chamber of her eye, which caused permanent damage to her iris's ability to contract in response to bright light. This injury necessitated that she wear sunglasses and, for the first time ever, corrective lenses in that eye because of a mild reduction in her visual acuity. She sought assistance to overcome her fear of getting hit and of not being able to control her pitches, especially her rise ball, which she liked to throw inside to right-handed hitters.

Intervention: The psychiatrist obtained a detailed history of the circumstances of the injury, surgery, and residual deficits. Since the injury, the player's softball activity had been quite limited out of concern for the nonreactive pupil. After being cleared to play by a neuro-ophthalmologist a month before, the player began reconditioning herself physically and throwing off the mound without live hitters. She was concerned that she would be so afraid of getting hit that she would alter her mechanics or not be able to field her position.

In the initial meeting, the psychiatrist had her work on three basic mental skills: relaxation, attention narrowing, and visualization. For relaxation, the player mastered long, progressive, clearing breaths. She started by breathing in through her nose and then clearing out slowly and evenly through her mouth for at first 8, then 10, and finally 12 counts. She was naturally good at this because she had been a singer in high school. After 10 minutes of practice, she was able to do this breathing automatically. Next, she learned a visual narrowing skill using a single breath cycle. To start the cycle, she cleared all the air out through the mouth, then took a full nasal inhalation to a count of 4, allowing her gaze to shift out to the wall broadly. As she exhaled through her mouth to a count for 8, her gaze narrowed to a small 1-cm spot on the wall. As she got to 6 in her count, she broke her gaze from the spot and shifted her attention from sight to "feel" (to a small quarter-sized area just above her navel). She repeated this over and over, shifting to different small spots on the wall with each breath cycle. With each repetition, she noticed how much sharper her visual acuity became as she expired. The psychiatrist helped her to extrapolate this practice over to pitching by suggesting that she use one breath cycle to pick up the pitching signs and then, after going through her prepitch routine, use another breath cycle to pick out her target on the mitt. She was intrigued by this use of two breath cycles to complement what had always been a well-developed and confident pitching routine. Finally, she worked on developing a daily visualization routine. At night before bed, she relaxed by breathing, then closed her eyes and visualized a series of pitches using her narrowed-gaze facilitation of acuity. She agreed to practice each of these skills daily at home and return in 2 weeks. After 2 weeks of work and some successful pitching to live hitters, she began the season with confidence.

Fractures

Sports-related fractures are common in adolescents and adults (Court-Brown et al. 2008; Swenson et al. 2010; Wood et al. 2010). In both groups, fractures are usually low-energy events, and they involve the upper extremities about 80% of the time. Most occur in the finger phalanges, distal radius and ulna, and metacarpals in adolescents, and these plus the clavicle in adults. Not surprisingly, most sports-related fractures occur in males, with the most common sports being football, rugby, and skiing in adolescents in one British study. In U.S. high school sports, fractures required surgery only 16% of the time; nevertheless, 34% of the athletes with fractures lost greater than 21 days' time and 24% received medical disqualification for the season. Of all severe injuries in high school athletes (i.e., those resulting in at least 21 days of lost time), fractures were the most common diagnosis (36%), followed by complete ligament sprains (15%) and incomplete ligament sprains (14%) (Darrow et al. 2009; Swenson et al. 2010). Fortunately, high-energy fractures in collision and contact sports are infrequent, but when they do occur, they are more likely to involve the lower extremity. These fractures usually require surgery and can also end an athlete's season and sometimes career.

Case Study: I Can't Stand to Hit With This Forearm Protector

A right-handed college outfielder was hit by a pitch and sustained a simple midshaft fracture of his left ulna in the third game of the season. He was placed in a short arm cast for 4 weeks and could not play. The injury was especially frustrating because he was a senior and was expecting to be selected in the upcoming draft. When he returned to hitting off the tee, he noted consistent forearm pain, which was treated with anti-inflammatory medications. He progressed quickly to live hitting but could not get his old form back and did not feel as confident in the batter's box. He was seen by the psychiatrist 1 day after batting practice.

Intervention: Although he knew he needed and wanted to wear forearm protection, the player found it uncomfortable and distracting. He also noted a drop in his confidence on high and inside pitches and had been unable to pull the ball with power to left field as before. He described soreness but no pain. He was encouraged to speak to the athletic trainer and was given a less bulky protector that he liked much more. In addition, he reviewed his prepitch routine, making sure his attention shifted smoothly from visual to feel (i.e., out to the pitcher and in to his stance, hands, and core). With this emphasis and the new protection, he no longer focused as much on his forearm and slowly regained his form and power. Although he was drafted in a lower round than he might have been before his injury, he has progressed through the minor leagues and has seen some play at the major league level.

Muscle, Tendon, and Ligament Tears

Severe muscle and tendon tears are not common but occur in the calf, hamstrings, quadriceps, hip flexors, biceps, triceps, rotator cuff, and latissimus dorsi of the back. These tears may heal on their own, but if the tendon or muscle is torn completely or the muscle is pulled away from its origin or insertion, then surgery is usually required. Collision sports, such as football, rugby, and hockey, are most likely to produce severe tears requiring surgery and prolonged rehabilitation and restrengthening programs. Throwing or serving sports, such as baseball, softball, tennis, and volleyball, tend to produce shoulder or elbow tears.

Severe ligament tears are common in the ankle, knee, shoulder, and elbow. Ankle tears are the most common and are seen in most sports that involve running, jumping, pivoting, or quick changes of direction. Many of these tears will heal after a period of immobilization and strengthening, but surgery may be necessary if instability persists. One of the most difficult ankle injuries to overcome is a high ankle sprain in which the syndesmotic ligament between the tibia and the fibula is partially or completely torn. Initial treatment involves immobilization for 4–6 weeks in a boot or a cast if the ankle joint is stable or the insertion of a screw to join the tibia and fibula together with a longer period of immobilization.

Shoulder ligament tears are far less common than ankle tears. They can occur with contact, as in the case of an acromioclavicular separation, or from a throwing, grabbing, or reaching injury, as in rotator cuff tears. In more severe acromioclavicular separations of the shoulder, the joint capsule is disrupted and the ligaments that hold the clavicle to the acromion process of the scapula are torn. In these cases, surgical repair is necessary for long-term stability and return of function. In rotator cuff tears, pain or loss of velocity and control for throwers often tips the decision in the direction of a surgical repair.

Elbow ligament tears typically occur in the medial (ulnar) collateral ligament of overhead-throwing athletes, such as pitchers in baseball, quarterbacks in football, servers in tennis and volleyball, and throwers in water polo. This ligament is subjected to extreme force when the shoulder is externally rotated and the throwing motion accelerates forward. The original surgical procedure for this tear, developed by Frank Jobe, M.D., in 1974, has been termed the "Tommy John procedure" after the first pitcher to undergo the replacement of his ulnar collateral ligament with a tendon graft from elsewhere in the body. This surgery, although successful in returning elite athletes to prior competitive levels, often takes a full 12 months of rehabilitation. However, with subsequent modifications to the original procedure, including transposition of the ulnar nerve, few adverse consequences develop, especially if a graduated rehabilitation program is followed. Rehabilitation from this surgery, as for many other ligament repairs, requires patience and persistence, because minor setbacks are common. The main role of the sports psychiatrist in these cases is to follow the athlete through the entire injury and return-to-play process, offering at first pain control and sleep assistance, then motivational support, and finally assistance in overcoming fear of reinjury.

Case Study: Don't Rush Recovery

An early career professional tennis player was already being seen by a sports psychiatrist for mental skills training when he suffered a severely sprained ankle in competition. He was seen by a local sports orthopedist and noted to have substantial swelling and instability and was therefore put into a boot for 2 weeks. He was told that he had a partially torn ankle ligament that would require 4–6 weeks to fully recover. After 2 weeks, the swelling had resolved, the boot was removed, and the athlete started graduated, nontennis fitness and ankle range-of-motion and strengthening activities. As the player improved, he accelerated his activities faster than recommended, trying to get ready for an upcoming tournament. On his own, he added daily tennis drills, running, and plyometrics at the beginning of the third week. This resulted in a return of his pain and postworkout swelling. During one of the athlete's regular mental skills sessions, the psychiatrist recognized that the player had pushed his recovery much too fast and with too much intensity.

Intervention: The athlete was sent back to his orthopedist to be reexamined and for clarification of his injury and rehabilitation plan. He was instructed to make sure he understood which ligament was torn, what role it played in ankle stability in tennis, and what activities would raise the greatest risk of delayed injury. The orthopedist confirmed that although the player had improved, he had set back his recovery by pushing too hard and prematurely. The athlete learned that he had partially torn his anterior talofibular ligament (grade 2 sprain) on the lateral aspect of his ankle and that it should heal completely if he slowed down his rehabilitation and alternated activities. After this visit, the player followed the physician's instructions, and after 5 additional weeks had made a complete recovery and resumed competition.

Back Pain

Middle- and lower-back injuries are common in sports, especially those involving axial rotation (e.g., golf, tennis, diving, baseball, softball, discus, shot put, gymnastics), intense contact with twisting (e.g., football, rugby, basketball, wrestling), or weight loading (e.g., powerlifting) (Hoskins et al. 2009). Fortunately, most back injuries are not severe and involve temporary mechanical restrictions of the axial spine or muscular strain. These injuries usually resolve with rest, application of ice and/or heat, local treatments such as ultrasound, electrical stimulation, and massage; nonsteroidal anti-inflammatory drugs (NSAIDs) and muscle relaxants; and a modified strength and stretching routine.

Some back pain, however, is due to more serious causes, such as stress fractures, disk herniation, spinal stenosis, spondylolisthesis (slippage of one vertebral body over another), and foraminal narrowing with nerve root irritation. These conditions are more common in collision sports, and the rates and severity increase as the intensity of practice and competition increases. Retired professional athletes who played collision or contact sports also seem to struggle with the early onset of traumatic osteoarthritis and may develop chronic pain and functional disability as early as their third decade of life. These conditions require careful diagnostic assessment and specialized treatment, including local injections (epidural, facet, trigger point), spinal manipulation, aggressive active release therapy, and possibly surgery. Although surgery for more severe back pain, such as disk herniation, might constitute a threat to an athlete's career, case control studies of NFL and National Basketball Association players demonstrate that 75% return to competitive play rates (Hoskins et al. 2009).

Case Study: I'm Too Young to Have a Ruptured Disc

A midcareer professional golfer was referred by his primary care sports medicine physician to a sports psychiatrist for the evaluation of midback pain, frustration, irritability, insomnia, and marital strain. One month before, he had the sudden onset of severe midback pain radiating around his right flank while tossing a heavy medicine ball backward over his head during a preseason workout. This exercise, along with other new rotational strengthening activities, was part of a much more aggressive core and strength training program designed to increase his driving distance and club head speed. When the physician saw the golfer a few days after the injury, the athlete was unable to stand, bend, or turn without increased pain. He was sent for an MRI, and the results revealed a ruptured thoracic disc in the area of his pain. He was treated with a short course of prednisone, narcotic pain medications, muscle relaxants, physical therapy, and restriction from all sports-related activities. Over the next few weeks, he improved steadily and started some low-level cardiovascular training and light hitting at the driving range, trying to get ready for the first tournament of the season. As he increased his golf activities, however, his pain and muscle spasms returned and he could not get comfortable enough at night to sleep. At the time of his psychiatric evaluation, he complained of irritability, frustration, constant pain, restricted movement, and severe insomnia.

Intervention: His medication regimen was reviewed. He had been taking hydrocodone 7.5 mg as needed, diazepam 5 mg three times daily, and over-the-counter diphenhydramine 50 mg for insomnia. He did not feel that he was getting much pain relief or sleep and did not like the grogginess from diphenhydramine. He was very upset that he had worked so hard in the off-season and that now it looked like he could not compete. His constant pain and irritability had led to frequent arguments with his wife over petty issues. His pain medication was changed to hydrocodone 7.5 mg every 3–4 hours during the day and 15 mg at bedtime. In addition, an NSAID was added. His diazepam dosage was increased to 5 mg three times daily and 10 mg at bedtime. After a few days on this new regimen, he reported sleeping continuously for 6–8 hours, and his pain and back spasm were greatly reduced. With improvement in his sleep, he also noted that irritability diminished and he had improved interactions with his wife and physical therapist. At the same time these changes were made, he saw a spine surgeon who presented him the option of conservation treatment or surgery. He continued with conservation treatment even though it meant missing the first half of the season. During follow-up meetings, the topic of his marriage surfaced, and he noted that he had been having conflicts with his wife for several years about having children and the past actions of her parents and siblings. She subsequently attended several sessions, and each of these areas was explored and worked through. He eventually went back to a graduated fitness and golf regimen after tapering off his medications, but he ended up missing the entire season. He decided to go back to his old fitness regimen and is looking forward to a new year of competition.

Knee Disruptions

Complete or partial tears of one or more of the four supporting knee ligaments—the anterior cruciate ligament (ACL), the posterior cruciate ligament (PCL), the medial collateral ligament (MCL), and the lateral collateral ligament (LCL)—are common among severe injuries at all competitive levels and in both genders. By far the most common of these is a complete tear of the ACL. These tears require surgical repair and intense 6- to 9-month rehabilitation programs, but the injuries have good return-to-play rates, although not always a return to the same level. In college sports, ACL injuries are most common in women's gymnastics, soccer, and basketball and in men's football. When knee injury rates are compared by gender in the same sports, women consistently have rates three to four times higher than men in soccer, lacrosse, basketball, and baseball or softball. Several explanations have been offered for this, including 1) anatomical (the Q angle, from the top of the femur to the knee, is wider in women [17 degrees] than in men [14 degrees]), 2) hormonal (premenstrual effects caused by estrogen and progesterone), and 3) biomechanical (differences noted in women for jumping, landing, and pivoting). Although most ACL tears do not involve contact, those that result from player collision, especially in football, are more likely to be accompanied by torn PCLs and MCLs. These complex knee disruptions usually have longer rehabilitation periods, more complications, and lower return-to-play rates.

Case Study: I Was Stuck in the Hospital for 10 Days With Constant Pain

A rising fifth-year senior college offensive lineman was sent to another city to repair his torn ACL, PCL, and MCL 2 weeks after a contact disruption of his right knee during a spring football game. Also, because of chronic problems with his left knee (pain, swelling, and occasional locking), he was to have arthroscopic surgery for these problems at the same time. His surgeries, which went well technically, included patellar tendon repairs of his ACL and PCL, reconstruction of his right MCL, and trimming of a torn medial meniscus that had not shown up on the MRI. His left knee had small tears in lateral and medial menisci, some small interarticular bone fragments, and some cartilaginous defects on his medial and lateral femoral articulating surfaces. On the first postoperative day, he developed severe knee pain as well as unremitting, pounding right-sided headaches accompanied by nausea and light and noise sensitivity. He was given oxycodone 10 mg every 4–6 hours but reported little relief or sleep. He struggled through the knee pain and headaches for the entire week that he was at the hospital, calling the team athletic trainer several times each day. When he returned to the team, his knee pain was improved but his headaches and insomnia persisted. As a result, he was referred for psychiatric consultation and pain management.

    Intervention: This was the athlete's first surgery, and he was clearly very stressed by having it away from his team and family support systems. Although he had previously experienced some stress-linked migraine headaches during high school and college, they had never been as severe or lasted as long. His pain medication was changed to hydrocodone 7.5–

15 mg every 3–4 hours during the day and diazepam 10 mg at 6:00 P.M. and hydrocodone 15 mg at bedtime. On this regimen, his sleep improved and his headaches decreased in severity and were no longer continuous. Over the next 5 days, he slept well but experienced the variable onset of moderately severe, pounding, left- or right-sided headaches with nausea and light sensitivity that usually lasted 3–4 hours during the nighttime or daytime. In addition to experiencing headaches, he struggled with his early range-of-motion exercises, reporting intense pain. As a result, his pretreatment hydrocodone was increased to 15 mg and a neurological consultation was requested for the evaluation of persistent headaches. At the neurologist's suggestion, topiramate 25 mg/day was added and tapered up to 75 mg/day over the next 7 days. After these adjustments and some increased ambulation, the player's headaches finally diminished and his rehabilitation began to progress more smoothly. In retrospect, it became clear that the absence of support postsurgically played a major role in raising the player's stress level and that he improved as he regained his independence.

Shoulder Injuries (Separations, Dislocations, and Fractures)

Severe shoulder injuries are common in collision and throwing sports. In high school, these injuries are three times more likely to occur in competition than in practice and four times more likely in boys than in girls. The top three sports for these injuries are football, wrestling, and baseball, followed by girls' softball and volleyball (Bonza et al. 2009). The most common shoulder injuries are sprains or strains (40%), dislocations or separations (24%), contusions (12%), and fractures (7%). The most common mechanisms of injury are player-player contact (58%), playing surface contact (23%), improper rotation (10%), and overuse (5%). Overall, about 6% of all shoulder injuries required surgery and 23% were severe, keeping athletes out for 3 weeks or longer (Darrow et al. 2009; Hootman et al. 2007). The most common severe shoulder injuries are anterior subluxations or dislocations, acromioclavicular separations, rotator cuff and labral tears, and clavicular fractures. Each of these injuries is painful and may interfere with sleep during the acute injury or postsurgical periods. Prompt attention to range of motion is very important because prolonged immobilization of the shoulder can lead to reductions in the range of motion.

Case Study: My Doctor and Athletic Trainer Don't Think It Should Hurt This Much

A junior college football player sustained an anterior right shoulder subluxation during spring practices while attempting to tackle the returner with his arm out and up. He completed the afternoon practice but afterward noted throbbing pain and shoulder muscle spasm. On examination, he was very tender over the anterior shoulder and had much pain with partial abduction and external rotation. He was treated with icing, pain medication, and a muscle relaxant for the night but did not sleep. The next day, he was examined again and reported worsening pain even with his arm supported in a sling. Over the next week, he did not improve. He was seen by the sports psychiatrist in the training room while the other players were at practice.

Intervention: He reported a history of recurrent shoulder, hip, and knee injuries throughout his college career, although none required surgery. He often missed practices during the week but was able to play in games. He said he did not find pain medications very helpful and always worried that an injury would end his career. When asked about his early life, he became emotional when discussing his parents' separation while he was in middle school and having to go live with his maternal aunt while two of his older siblings went to another state to live with another relative. He excelled in football during high school but never felt emotionally secure when stressed, always fearing the worst would happen.

For the remainder of the spring and into the beginning of the season, the psychiatrist saw the player regularly and provided encouragement and support. Sleep became a main focus and was monitored. The player was eventually given an as-needed medicine in case he felt he would have difficulty falling asleep. He did well getting back to regular practice and play until he sustained another subluxation, causing him to miss several games. Whereas before he had minimal laxity on examination, this time laxity was more evident, so he wore a shoulder harness during practice and games. He made it through the season, making solid contributions to the team. In the off-season, he had his anterior shoulder repaired, and he returned for his final year with improved performance. He was identified as someone with a lower pain threshold and as stress sensitive and was seen regularly by the psychiatrist for as long as he remained with the team.

Emotions of Injury, Recovery, and Departure From Competition

Injury produces quick or reactive negative emotions and slower negative contemplative emotions that can interfere with injury management and recovery (see Table 6–2) (Galambos et al. 2005; Gobbi and Francisco 2006; Hamson-Utley et al. 2008; Kvist et al. 2005; Webster et al. 2007). The quick negative emotions are automatic responses that surface in tenths of seconds and include anxiety, confusion, fear, panic, annoyance, frustration, anger, tension, cautiousness, disappointment, sadness, hurt, distraction, embarrassment, and doubt. When these quick emotions arise, they are often intense and can lead to changes in thinking, behavior, and interpersonal interactions. Contemplative emotions occur after the athlete has time to process information and interact with teammates, staff, and family. The most common of these emotions are pressure, hostility, resentment, distrust, depression, shame, isolation, guilt, grief, indifference, apathy, jealousy, boredom, concern, apprehension, remorse, regret, distraction, contempt, and revenge. These emotions develop over time and are more common as the extent of the acute injury is processed and as the surgery and rehabilitation periods begin. The contemplative emotions that interfere are often magnified by the athlete's past life and injury experiences in the context of sudden change and social disconnection. In general, strategies to prevent injury emotions from interfering include the establishment of a support system, clarification of the injury, establishment of the injury treatment plan and timetable, and facilitation of positive emotions such as comfort, hope, relief, humor, pride, courage, grace, accomplishment, vitality, optimism, and confidence.

Acute Injury and Stabilization

Serious or minor injuries, especially if recurrent, can quickly trigger emotional changes that can interfere with pain control, sleep, energy, relaxation, information processing, and communication. The most common early emotions are hurt, anxiety, frustration, disappointment, sadness, and doubt. These reactive emotions should be identified and expressed; otherwise, they may evolve over the first week or two after the injury into complex pain, confusion, anger, fatigue, and tension. Interestingly, the presence of this latter group of contemplative emotions has been shown to correlate with increased injury risk and prolonged recovery time. To facilitate the release of emotions, sports psychiatrists should be available in the training room to interact with injured athletes within a few days of a new injury. Emotional release is facilitated by informal conversations about the circumstances of the injury; its impact on pain level, mood, and sleep; and the current understanding of the next step in assessment and stabilization. Repeated brief discussions with the athlete alone or with the athletic trainer and/or team physician present serve to continue a process of emotional release.

To help prevent complex, contemplative emotions from increasing during the acute injury stage, the clinician needs to target pain control and sleep immediately. Pain control is best achieved with more frequent dosing of lesser amounts rather than higher doses as needed during times of high pain. If muscle spasms accompany the injury, then a long-acting benzodiazepine, such as diazepam 5 mg, can be added several times a day or in the evening a few hours before bedtime. Sleep is usually addressed with a low dose (5 mg) or regular dose (10 mg) of zolpidem, depending on whether a benzodiazepine or another muscle relaxant is also being used.

Final early strategies are to ensure a clear understanding of the injury and to establish a support network. One of the best ways to ensure that a player understands the injury is to ask the athlete to explain it in detail and to describe the proposed surgery, if needed. Misconceptions or inaccuracies can then be corrected promptly. The support network typically consists of family, teammates, and the medical staff (athletic trainers, physicians, and chiropractors). A very helpful tactic is to encourage a contact between the injured player with another player who has had the same injury. In addition, to prevent the sense of isolation that can develop quickly, active involvement of the support network is useful.

Case Study: I Can't Play in the Tournament?

A senior lacrosse player scored the winning goal in the final minutes of the conference tournament, securing his team a bid to the NCAA tournament. Just as the game was winding down, however, he sprinted back on defense, and as he was turning to cut off a fast break, he heard something pop and knew he had torn his right ACL. He knew because he had torn his ACL before as a senior in high school, causing him to miss postseason play then as well. The swelling and instability evident during the team doctor's examination confirmed the injury. It wasn't so much the dread of another long rehabilitation period that consumed the player over the next week, but the deep disappointment and pain that he felt about missing postseason play as a senior and one of the team leaders. The situation was especially difficult for him because his team had never made it past the first round in the tournament, but this year they were expected to go far. He moped around the training room and practice field for 2 weeks while he waited for the swelling to subside. He had already decided to delay his surgery so that he could travel with his teammates.

Intervention: The player was seen by the psychiatrist in the training room at the beginning of the second week following his injury. When asked how he was doing, the athlete grimaced and then cried in anguish as he thought about his injury and the missed opportunity. He spontaneously mentioned how much this time reminded him of his senior year of high school and how helpless he felt back then when his team lost in the state finals. He seemed surprised when asked what positives had come from that injury, but quickly replied that it made him appreciate every moment in practice and competition and that he had worked harder to succeed. The psychiatrist told a story about another college team that made it to postseason play for the first time in 5 years, despite losing three upperclassmen to preseason ACL injuries. He explained that these three individuals were recruited to organize an intensive team building intervention before the tournament and to advise the coaches about the first two teams in their region because they had played them before. Over the course of the tournament, these three individuals sparked a rise in the team's confidence and unity. The team went on to an upset win in the second round to advance farther in their sport than any previous team from their college. The psychiatrist asked the player if he was willing to have a similar impact by activating his positive emotional circuitry rather than allowing his current negative emotions to dominate. After hearing the story, the athlete smiled and said, "Thanks, Doc."

Rehabilitation and Recovery

Due to the variability of injuries and time involved, the rehabilitation and recovery phase of injury management requires flexibility and adaptability by sports psychiatrists. Regular contact with rehabilitating athletes is recommended throughout this phase. This contact is especially important during long rehabilitation programs for more serious injuries, because negative emotions may disappear for a while and then reappear when return to practice is imminent. Clinicians should directly observe work on the training table, as well as the reconditioning and restrengthening efforts. Casual conversations with injured athletes can suffice to ensure that negative contemplative emotions are not interfering in recovery. To ensure that positive emotions are present and are influencing motivation and energy in the rehabilitative process, clinicians should begin with discussions of what is going well before discussing negatives. A prospective study of return to play after ACL tear and surgical repair confirms the importance of positive emotions, motivation, and optimism (Gobbi and Francisco 2006). High scores on a six-question psychovitality scale that asked about importance of return, speed of recovery, time commitment, doubts, and acceptance of lower functioning predicted return to play at the same competitive level.

Another strategy for the facilitation of injury rehabilitation is to teach athletes mental skills such as relaxation, imagery, visualization, positive self-talk, goal setting, and pain control through self-hypnosis. This phase offers an ideal time to expose athletes to these skills because they have free time and can combat the boredom and isolation with new reading, learning, and practice. An effective technique is to tell injured athletes success stories of other injured athletes from any sport and to describe how they benefited from emotional expression, use of a support network, and mental skills training. Athletic trainers and physical therapists can support these activities but are more inclined to do so if they have had some exposure or training or have worked collaboratively with an on-site sports psychiatrist or psychologist (Hamson-Utley et al. 2008).

Case Study: Recovery Is Boring and Takes Too Long

An early career professional football player tore his ACL in practice without contact early in the off-season. He knew immediately what the injury was, having heard other players describe that characteristic pop. He had little swelling and was able to go for surgery within a week of the injury. His surgery went well, and he began his rehabilitation program at the team's facility. Because it was the off-season, few players were around, and he was the only one with an ACL tear. As the first few weeks passed, he became sullen and more withdrawn, snapping at the athletic trainers and other team staff. He also reported being impatient, irritable, and bored at home, especially because his day was short. He said that he preferred to spend time in his basement away from his wife and daughter, even though he knew that he should take the opportunity to get better connected with them. Having had several serious injuries in college, he began to develop resentment toward his bad luck and to players that seemed to always stay healthy.

Intervention: The psychiatrist observed the athlete completing his rehabilitation protocol in the training room. The few players who were around came through the area on the way to complete their off-season strength and conditioning workouts. The injured player seemed annoyed when they would walk through without speaking. After his workout, he openly voiced his frustration and resentment and was beginning to have serious self-doubt about continuing his career. The discussion about the rest of his day clearly indicated that he did not feel productive about it either, and this feeling was further undermining his confidence. He agreed to bring back an old hobby of archery as a way to fill his time and to force himself into a parenting role by telling his wife that he would care for their daughter two afternoons per week. To deal with his sense of isolation at the facility, his rehabilitation time was changed to follow his upper-body workouts so he would have more contact with his teammates. These simple changes seemed to energize him, and after a few weeks the staff felt that he was over the hump and progressing well.

Return to Play

More pressure exists now than ever before for athletes to return to play quickly following minor or severe injuries. Athletes worry that if they stay away too long, they will get behind, someone else will take their spot, they will lose their competitive edge and confidence, or they will be forgotten by the coaching staff. Because reinjury and complications often result from premature return, athletes should be monitored when they return to play. Sports psychiatrists also should observe athletes for demonstrations of fear of reinjury (Kvist et al. 2005). This is a universal concern of any seriously injured athletes, and they must work through this fear by engaging in progressively intense training and open discussion of their thoughts and feelings. In a study that examined athletes' recovery from ACL repair, Webster et al. (2007) developed a 12-question psychological scale that inquired about their emotions of return to play (nervousness, frustration, relaxation, and fear), confidence (knee integrity, ability and performance level), and risk appraisal (likelihood of reinjury, concern about another surgery). Although the study did not identify correlates with successful return to play, this scale provides a good framework to guide clinical sports psychiatry and psychology. A reinforcement of the many small successes that occur during the return to play phase may boost confidence and counterbalance nervousness and fear.

Case Study: I Don't Think I Can Ever Vault Again

A college sophomore gymnast missed a difficult vault in an early season tournament and snapped her ACL. She had significant swelling and therefore had to wait 3 weeks before getting a patellar tendon reconstruction. She worked hard and returned to her sport after 8 months. With graduated activity, she was able to get back most of her routines on the beam, floor, and bars, but every time she went to do more difficult vaults, she balked in fear. She had begun to think that she might never overcome her fear and might always be haunted by the sound and feel of her ligament snapping when she badly underrotated on the vault during competition. Her athletic trainer referred her to a sports psychiatrist for evaluation.

Intervention: When seen in the psychiatrist's office after practice, the gymnast seemed confident about her progress except in vault. When asked to describe her injury and surgery, she was able to give a very clear description. She was not as clear, however, in describing the healing process of the knee and seemed uncertain that her reconstructed ACL would be strong and secure. The psychiatrist and gymnast had a joint meeting that day with the team orthopedist, who reviewed the recent MRI. The orthopedist was very encouraging after the review and examination, declaring that the athlete's injury was completely healed and the knee was stable enough for any challenging skill. The orthopedist said that in her experience, many ACL tears resulted from a one-time perfect storm of the wrong force and landing and that the gymnast should believe it would never happen again and commit to being so prepared that her confidence would be unshakable.

The athlete worked on a plan to replace her fear with confidence. She developed a graduated series of increasingly difficult vaults to be done over the next 6 weeks. She also began to visualize success each night and developed a mantra of "stick it" that meant both to stick the landing and to stick with the plan. Whenever she felt her anxiety or fear rise up, she would pause, clear out all her breath, and then do a single loud, prolonged exhale, ending with an "it." In her mind, this further reinforced her commitment to be adequately prepared to "stick it." Finally, she began to study the looks of confidence on various members of the men's and women's teams as well as athletes from other sports. She laughingly began to refer to herself as "the crook" for stealing everyone's confidence. As her practice intensity built, so did her confidence. She got very good at clearing out the fear and replacing it with her "C" (i.e., confidence). She returned to full competition the next season, successfully doing her injury vault and more difficult ones.

Transition Out of Sports

Some injuries prevent athletes from returning to competition or performance at the prior level, and they decide to leave their sport. Common reasons include loss of flexibility, speed, range of motion, and quickness; persistent pain and swelling; and fear of reinjury. Once the decision is made, the athlete must decide whether to give up sports completely or continue playing the same or another sport at a lower competitive level. In addition, if they choose not to return to competitive sports, they must decide on the type of lifestyle they will lead, addressing ongoing fitness and nutrition.

The departure from competitive sports is difficult, especially for an athlete who has been involved since youth. Just deciding how to fill available time can seem daunting at this juncture. A clinician can help the athlete to consider what else he or she is good at and interested in, and encourage a search for outlets in these areas. An athlete leaving a sport also has to deal with the losses of connection to teammates and coaches, his or her identity as a successful athlete, and the strict regimen of practice and play. The processing of this shift often provokes a grief reaction that may take months or a year or more to resolve. During this transitional period, athletes are at risk for depression, anxiety, low motivation, and excessive substance use.

The typical resolution of the loss comes with the development of a replacement activity or identity. Professional athletes leaving their sport often struggle with this transitional period longer than other athletes, because their sport may be all that they know. Some must go back to school or retrain to find a new career direction. Delay in doing this can result in chronic frustration, boredom, pain from injuries, and reduced self-efficacy and confidence. Sports psychiatrists can play an important role in facilitating a shift from one positive identity to another by meeting regularly with transitioning athletes and supporting their search and skill development. Involving a spouse or partner can be beneficial in this process to gain his or her perspective and to harness support. In addition, finding a mentor who can guide this shift and help an individual make new contacts is helpful.

Case Study: What Good Am I Now That I've Lost My Career?

A midcareer wide receiver and special teams player fractured his lower leg while attempting to tackle a player. He sustained compound fractures of his tibia and fibula that required internal and external fixation. Although he healed, he never returned to his former level of play and was not re-signed. Even though he had been paid well during his career, he overspent and struggled to pay the mortgages on his home and the home that he had bought for his parents. Although he looked for work, he could not find anything that was satisfying or paid as well. As his struggle to find a postcareer identity increased, he began to drink more. Being concerned about his downward spiral into alcoholism and depression, his wife drove him from another city for a psychiatric evaluation.

Intervention: At his initial evaluation, the player described intense frustration at the way his career had ended and deep disappointment that he had not taken better advantage of his opportunity for an education in college. He knew that a life of daily heavy drinking was leading him nowhere, but he felt trapped and hopeless. Several former teammates in his city had tried to get him to stop drinking and had offered him job opportunities, but he could not break his pattern. He felt particularly ashamed that he had slipped in his responsibilities to his wife and two children. He agreed to stop drinking and succeeded initially with outpatient detoxification, disulfiram, and weekly recovery counseling. He continued with the psychiatrist for eight sessions before abruptly stopping. A month later, he called to say that he had relapsed and that he wanted residential treatment. He was immediately sent to a residential program in his area for 30 days and again did well for a few months before he relapsed again. In his therapy sessions, he repeatedly criticized himself for his lack of determination and persistence. He continued his sessions, however, and eventually shifted into stable recovery, going back to college with the support of the player's union to find a new career.

Conclusion

Sports psychiatrists and other sports mental health clinicians need to know the types of, mechanisms of, interventions and surgeries for, and rehabilitative approaches to common athletic injuries so they can understand and help prevent emotional and behavioral issues that can interfere with athletes' return to play or increase their risk of reinjury. Whether sports clinicians work from a base of practice in the training room or an off-site office, they need to gain experience regulating the typical reactive and contemplative emotions and motivational fluctuations for each stage of injury and recovery. Establishing strategic linkages with athletic trainers, physicians, fitness staff, coaches, and family members helps to form the basis of integrated treatment, minimize complications, and facilitate successful outcomes. Athletes respond well to the presence of psychiatrists or other mental health professionals who can explain injury, surgery, and healing; manage pain and insomnia; and enhance motivation and confidence. Early preventive contact and regular monitoring throughout the rehabilitation and return-to-play phases are helpful. In cases where injury leads to an athlete's departure, especially retirement, from sports, psychiatric interventions can facilitate successful transitions while minimizing the disruptive effects of strong negative emotions and thoughts.

Key Clinical Points

- Sports injuries are common, and serious injury or reinjury often results in athletes' long absences from practice and competition or departure from sports. Dividing the injury process into four stages—acute injury, rehabilitation and recovery, return to play, and departure from sports—facilitates an intervention-oriented understanding of the common emotional, motivational, and attitudinal challenges that occur.

- A sports psychiatrist can actively work with athletic trainers and team physicians to facilitate athletes' acute injury management, rehabilitation, and return to play by being in the training room as a member of the medical staff. Critical early issues to address following injury are pain control, sleep, energy, information processing, decision making, and attitude.

- The rehabilitation of a serious injury requiring surgery can last from 6 to 12 months or longer. During this time, athletes often become disconnected from teammates and coaches, and struggle with boredom, pain, distrust, and apathy. Important roles for sports psychiatrists are the continuous monitoring for negative emotional interference or poor adherence to the recommended rehabilitation plan, as well as the creation of an encouraging support network.

- Serious injury can lead to a sudden departure from sports. These transitions are accompanied by grief, depression, chronic pain, insomnia, and loss of self-confidence. Psychiatrists and other mental health professionals can engage transitioning athletes in therapy to facilitate the identification of replacement activities.

- Retired professional athletes have typically suffered multiple injuries during a sports career. Injuries may lead to early traumatic arthritis, limited range of motion, chronic pain and insomnia, difficulty with anger control and depression, and substance misuse. These individuals can be successfully engaged in sports psychiatric treatment that is integrated with other medical and rehabilitative care.

References

Bonza JE, Fields SK, Yard EE, et al: Shoulder injuries among United States high school athletes during the 2005–2006 and 2006–2007 school years. J Athl Train 44:76–83, 2009

Boston University Center for the Study of Traumatic Encephalopathy: Case studies. Available at: http://www.bu.edu/cste/case-studies. Accessed January 25, 2012.

Chumbley EM, O'Connor FG, Nirschl RP: Evaluation of overuse elbow injuries. Am Fam Physician 61:691–700, 2000

Court-Brown CM, Wood AM, Aitken S: The epidemiology of acute sports-related fractures in adults. Injury 39:1365–1372, 2008

Darrow CJ, Collins CL, Yard EE, et al: Epidemiology of severe injuries among United States high school athletes: 2005–2007. Am J Sports Med 37:1798–1805, 2009

Galambos SA, Terry PC, Moyle GM, et al: Psychological predictors of injury among elite athletes. Br J Sports Med 39:351–354, 2005

Galbraith RM, Lavalee ME: Medial tibial stress syndrome: conservative treatment options. Curr Rev Musculoskelet Med 2:127–133, 2009

Gobbi A, Francisco R: Factors affecting return to sports after ACL reconstruction with patellar tendon and hamstring graft: a prospective clinical investigation. Knee Surg Sports Traumatol Arthrosc 14:1021–1028, 2006

Gordon MA: Psycholinguistic changes in athletes' grief response to injury after written emotional disclosure. J Sport Rehabil 19:328–342, 2010

Hamson-Utley JJ, Martin S, Walters J: Athletics trainers' and physical therapists' perceptions of the effectiveness of psychological skills within sport injury rehabilitation programs. J Athl Train 43:258–264, 2008

Heiderscheit BC, Sherry MA, Slider A, et al: Hamstring strain injuries: recommendations for diagnosis, rehabilitation, and injury prevention. J Orthop Sports Phys Ther 40:67–81, 2010

Hootman JM, Dick R, Agel J: Epidemiology of collegiate injuries for 15 sports: summary and recommendations for injury prevention initiatives. J Athl Train 42:311–319, 2007

Hoskins W, Pollard H, Daff C, et al: Low back pain status in elite and semi-elite Australian football codes: a cross-sectional survey of football (soccer) Australian rules, rugby league, rugby union, and non-athletic controls. BMC Musculoskeletal Disorders 10:1–9, 2009

Huffman EA, Yard EE, Fields SK, et al: Epidemiology of rare injuries and conditions among United States high school athletes during the 2005–2006 and 2006–2007 school years. J Athl Train 43:624–630, 2008

Ivarsson A: Psychological predictors of sport injuries among junior soccer players. Scand J Med Sci Sports 21:129–136, 2011

Kvist J, Ek A, Sporrstedt K, et al: Fear of re-injury: a hindrance for returning to sports after anterior cruciate ligament reconstruction. Knee Surg Sports Traumatol Arthrosc 13:393–397, 2005

Montgomery DL: Physiological profile of professional hockey players: a longitudinal comparison. Appl Physiol Nutr Metab 31:181–185, 2006

Mueller FO, Cantu RC: Annual Survey of Catastrophic Football Injuries 1977–2009. Chapel Hill, NC, National Center for Catastrophic Sports Injury Research, University of North Carolina, 2010

National Football League: NFL announces new sideline concussion assessment protocol. Posted February 25, 2011. Available at: http://www.nfl.com/news/story/09000d5d81e78cc4/article/nfl-announces-new-sideline-concussion-assessment-protocol. Accessed January 25, 2012.

National Football League: Safety rules & regulations. Available at: http://nflhealthandsafety.com/commitment/regulations. Accessed February 5, 2012.

Nelson AJ, Collins CL, Yard EE, et al: Ankle injuries among United States high school sports athletes, 2005–2006. J Athl Train 42:381–387, 2007

Rechel JA, Yard EE, Comstock RD: An epidemiologic comparison of high school sports injuries sustained in practice and competition. J Athl Train 43:197–204, 2008

Swenson DM, Yard EE, Collins CL, et al: Epidemiology of U.S. high school sports-related fractures, 2005–2009. Clin J Sport Med 20:293–299, 2010

Webster KE, Feller JA, Lambros C: Development and preliminary validation of a scale to measure the psychological impact of returning to sport following anterior cruciate ligament reconstruction surgery. Phys Ther Sport 9:9–15, 2007

Wood AM, Robertson GA, Rennie L, et al: The epidemiology of sports-related fractures in adolescents. Injury 41:834–838, 2010

Chapter 7

Common Mental Disorders

Psychiatrists, other mental health professionals, and sports medicine practitioners who treat adolescent and young adult athletes at any competitive level can expect to see the same disorders that are common in nonathletes of the same age in the general population. These include disorders of adjustment, anxiety, impulse and anger control, attention-deficit, learning, eating, mood, substance use, and sleep. Although athletes and nonathletes may have the same diagnoses, athletes' symptoms are often sports centered or sports aggravated. For example, although an athlete's anxiety may be generalized to sports, school, social networks, and family, it may be more specific to competition or conflicts with coaches or fitness staff. Although common and expected, performance anxiety can also manifest in extreme forms, such as panic, with strong physiological symptoms (e.g., vomiting, shaking, hyperventilation, fainting, muscle spasms) that require specialized psychiatric intervention. Depression in an athlete may be episodic and strongly linked to repeated mistakes, lack of playing time, or failure to perform to the expectations of the athlete, parents, or coaches. Depression in athletes can manifest in a typical way, but just as often manifests with frustration and anger, isolation from teammates, excessive alcohol use, or lack of intensity or enjoyment in practice (Glick and Horsfall 2005; Glick et al. 2009; Kamm 2005; McDuff et al. 2005).

Some of the disorders commonly seen in individuals ages 15–35 are more likely to be seen in athletes. For example, adjustment disorders with mixed disturbance of emotions and conduct are frequent following serious sports injuries or the death of a teammate or family member. In addition, somatoform disorders, such as pain disorder with psychological factors or somatoform disorder not otherwise specified (NOS), are more likely to be seen in athletes in whom serious injury leads to chronic functional impairment or pain, or in athletes who suffer from unusual problems such as chronic orthostatic intolerance or postural tachycardia syndrome. Also, eating disorders with or without compulsive overexercising are more common in athletes, especially in sports that are associated with lean body mass or endurance, including distance running, tennis, lacrosse, soccer, figure skating, gymnastics, and wrestling. In addition, eating disorders are more likely to be seen in athletes who are girls and young women than in those who are boys or young men and may be seen more often in women's sports that emphasize power and physicality, such as softball or rugby, than in men's collision or contact sports.

In this chapter, I discuss the typical manifestations and challenges of the most common mental disorders seen in sports. Because sleep and substance use disorders were discussed in Chapter 4, "Energy Regulation," and Chapter 5, "Substance Use and Abuse," respectively, those topics are not repeated in this chapter. Case studies highlight traditional and nontraditional treatment approaches and provide guidance on medication selection and dosage. The diagnoses for each case are presented using the DSM-IV-TR (American Psychiatric Association 2000) multiaxial format (i.e., Axis I—major mental disorders and other conditions that need clinical attention; Axis III—general medical illness or problems). In recommending medication selection, I address critical issues such as level of alertness, heat regulation, weight loss or gain, sleep disturbance, abnormal movements, motor quickness or rhythm.

Adjustment Disorders

Athletes are regularly exposed to stressors from practice, competition, and life that tax their adaptive capacities. Some athletes respond to events, such as injury, retirement, losing, role disappointment, academic ineligibility, failure to make a team, dismissal from a team, breakup of a relationship, serious illness, or deaths of others, with such strong emotions or behaviors that their functioning in and out of competition suffers. The most common emotions related to adjustment disorder are anxiety, depression, guilt, grief, and anger, and the most common related behaviors are aggression, arrests, insomnia, social isolation, substance misuse, conflicts in relationships, self-injury, poor performance, and quitting. Although many reactions are mild and self-limiting, others are more serious and require assistance from teammates, coaches, physicians, athletic trainers, or sports mental health professionals.

Injury is the most common stressor, affecting more than one-third of all athletes in a year. When serious injury occurs that necessitates discontinuation of training and competition, or immobilization or surgery, some athletes are devastated and react as if their dreams have been lost forever; this is especially true for an athlete who has had a previous serious injury that has caused significant missed time. Close monitoring of injured athletes that take them out of play is important to pick up distress in excess of that expected and to provide the needed support to work through the acute injury and rehabilitation phases. Although most athletes respond to team-based support, some need more formal therapy or short courses of medication for sleep, anxiety, or anger. Typically, therapy consists of gathering facts, developing perspective, instilling hope, reframing meaning, and identifying supportive persons. The most commonly used medications are either zolpidem for sleep or short-acting benzodiazepines for anxiety or anger. If symptoms persist, however, a trial of a selective serotonin reuptake inhibitor (SSRI) or a serotonin-norepinephrine reuptake inhibitor (SNRI) might be appropriate.

Athletes are not immune to the ongoing demands of life. In fact, some of life's more serious events, such as the death of a family member, coach, or teammate, can be particularly devastating because of the difficult decision between playing and attending to family needs or because of intense closeness to the deceased. Because teammates and coaches develop strong bonds during training, success, and defeat, the loss of a coach or a current or former teammate can be profound. Every year, the sudden deaths of athletes at all competitive levels—caused by suicide, murder, heat injury, automobile accidents, or even unknown heart pathology during competition—send ripples of emotion and grief through teams, departments, schools, and organizations for years. The presence of sports mental health professionals and clergy during these times can assist leaders, teams, and individuals in working through the loss while maintaining functioning.

Case Study: We Knew He Was Taking Stimulants and Trying to Lose Weight, But We Didn't Say or Do Anything

A talented young professional baseball player arrived at spring training with hopes of making the major league roster. He had an outstanding season the previous year and had been promoted when the roster expanded in September. He had a history of carrying more weight than ideal, and during the off-season he had been unable to reach his weight target. Therefore, he had started using high-dose ephedrine to suppress his appetite, speed up his metabolism, and boost his workouts. He collapsed while on the field after a few days of spring training, and he died some hours later of a severe heat injury, even though the day was neither hot nor humid. The team's leadership, coaching, and medical staff and players were stunned as he was taken off the field, during his brief hospitalization, after his death, and throughout the memorial service and funeral. His loss was made more difficult by the facts that the county coroner determined that the player's death was caused by ephedrine, which at the time was a legal supplement, and that his wife was pregnant with their first child.

Diagnosis: Axis I: Adjustment disorder with grief, depression, guilt, and anxiety (multiple individuals)

Intervention: The team's mental health staff was called to come to spring training early and asked to assist the organization in managing the response to the loss. Working with the general manager, field manager, and team chaplain, the mental health team established an assistance network. A constant presence on the field, in the clubhouse, and at the team hotel was maintained for the week following the death. Many individuals were seen for supportive counseling, and calls were taken through the day and night for individuals who wanted to talk through their perspective on the player's death. For the entire season, the mental health staff made additional site visits to the team's front office and to the major and minor league teams. That year, more players and staff used the team's assistance services than in any year before or since. The most common themes discussed were guilt about knowing the player's risk from using ephedrine and not intervening, and simply not being able to do something to prevent the tragic loss. (*Note:* This case was highly publicized in the national media because it involved the on-field death of an athlete. Neither the deceased player nor any of his family members were patients of the author.)

Case Study: I Don't Play Enough and I'm Thinking of Transferring

A second-year college soccer player was referred to a sports psychiatrist early in the season with assistance from a teammate for the evaluation of frustration and disappointment because of his limited role on his team. He had trained hard all summer and in fact had been told by his athletic trainers that he was good enough to play professionally. As preseason practices began, he noticed that the coach was favoring another player for the starting role as an outside midfielder. When the season began, he did not start and by his own admission started to sulk. While he was given opportunities to play in every game, he put so much pressure on himself to score that he made mistakes and in several games was pulled out after 10 minutes. The more time he spent as a bench player, the more bitter and self-critical he became. Eventually, his emotions started to affect his intensity in practices, and he could tell that the head coach had lost confidence in him. Every day after practice, he obsessively reviewed his situation and even started to think about transferring to another school in another conference so that he would not have to sit out a year without playing. During the week before his assessment, his sleep was poor and his class attendance and attention to required reading had slipped.

Diagnosis: Axis I: Adjustment disorder with mixed emotional features (frustration, anxiety, and depression)

Intervention: During the evaluation, the player revealed that his disappointment had actually started earlier in the summer when a fellow player in training received an invitation to try out for a developmental professional team. Because he thought he was better than the other player, he was hurt but did not say or do anything. As the season began he thought he was practicing well, but in retrospect he agreed that his internalized emotions and high expectations might have been noticeable to his coaches. He agreed to change his emotions by focusing on positive moments in the day and to spend more time with his nonsoccer friends. In addition, he agreed to spend more time playing piano, something else he had passion for and was good at. As his emotional patterns shifted, his practices improved. He began to get more playing time because he found a way to play in the moment rather than playing to score. His coach responded positively by giving him more minutes of playing time. He began to have an impact on the game, and by the end of the season, although he had never become a starter, he had more assists and goals based on time played than anyone else on the team. After the season, he met with his coaches and asked for feedback about what he needed to do to get better. They surprised him by saying that he needed to play with more ease and creativity and not with so much self-imposed pressure. They said they were sure he had the technical skills and tactical knowledge to succeed at this and the next level, but he needed to better manage his negative emotions. He seemed pleased with this feedback and felt that he had matured greatly as a player and person having gone through this period of adversity.

Anxiety Disorders

The pressure of athletic competition and the need to balance the demands of training, travel, family, finances, academics, and relationships can trigger performance, phobic, generalized, obsessive-compulsive, or panic anxiety. Performance anxiety most often manifests with heightened worrying and physiological arousal. Although common and expected, performance anxiety sometimes can become so persistent and intense that it interferes with consistency in practice and competition. Before a competition, athletes can present with mild or moderate racing or scattered thoughts, doubt, dread, fatigue, poor concentration, nausea, loss of appetite, rapid heart rate, tremulousness, dizziness, muscle tension, overbreathing, chest pain, numbness, sweating, or abdominal distress. These symptoms may start as early as the night before and result in inadequate rest, hydration, and nutrition. On the day of competition, athletes may be unable to relax or focus enough to quiet the mind, build intensity, and be ready to compete. Typical excessive performance anxiety results primarily in energy loss, muscle tightness, and inattention, which can lead to mistakes and subpar or inconsistent performance. Common strategies for reducing performance anxiety are improved preparation, positive self-talk, imagery and visualization, arousal, cognitive control, and relaxation amplification. Most of these strategies are organized into a structured precompetition routine that may be longer and more structured than before. In addition, work in practice must translate into confidence in competition. For example, an 800-meter track athlete may do interval training (alternating fast and slow runs) in the week before a meet to build confidence in his or her ability to race and recover. Sometimes, performance anxiety becomes extreme and evolves into recurrent panic attacks with or without hyperventilation. These are usually approached in the same way as precompetitive anxiety, but sometimes the short-term use of β-blockers such as propranolol or atenolol (if not banned in the sport) or short-acting benzodiazepines is helpful. If these strategies do not work and symptoms persist, and especially if the athlete has a background of generalized anxiety, then daily antianxiety medications can be started.

Phobic anxiety most often occurs following an injury or collapse in competition. This type of anxiety occurs most frequently in sports such as gymnastics, diving, rodeo, or cross-country running. When a gymnast falls from the balance beam, high bar, or vault and is seriously injured, he or she may develop a specific fear of the skill or apparatus. Phobic anxiety can also occur in divers who lose a dive, smack the water, and sustain a concussion, or in runners who push themselves so hard physiologically that they pass out in a race. Any of these competitors may not be able to regain their mastery of the requisite skill, or their phobic anxiety may generalize to all competition. The usual approach to treating specific phobia is to talk through the injury and make sure the athlete knows that he or she is healed enough to return to competition. Next, a graduated reintroduction to the lost skill is structured while enhanced calming and confidence-building techniques are taught. Collaboration with the athlete's coach or athletic trainers is critical at this stage. For example, if a gymnast sustains a fall doing a blind specific skill on the balance beam, then he or she practices the skill on the mat, low beam, high beam with mats, and high beam alone in succession, until confidence is restored. Each step in the succession is done with breathing-triggered calm, positive self-talk, and visualizations. As with preperformance anxiety, if these techniques do not work or if the injury is so catastrophic that posttraumatic anxiety develops, then a short course of the same medications mentioned in the previous paragraph may be tried.

Generalized and obsessive-compulsive anxiety affect athletic practice and competition, as well as social, academic, and leisure activities. Sleep disturbances are extremely common in athletes with these types of anxiety, because their overactive minds interfere with falling asleep or result in early awakening or interrupted sleep. Life balance is lost because anxiety, obsessions, or compulsions disrupt healthy interpersonal, nutritional, sleep, and energy-building routines, and then procrastination, inefficiency, and loss of confidence result. Because these disorders are typically not tied specifically to athletics and often date back to childhood, a combination of cognitive-behavioral or motivational enhancement therapy with longer-term medication is needed. For anxiety, response is usually good to typical or even low dosages of SSRIs. For sleep, daily or as-needed trazodone or zolpidem is used. Once the sleep pattern is improved, the sleep medication can be used only when the athlete senses that poor sleep is likely or a good night's sleep is critical. Occasionally, an SSRI response is not adequate, and a trial is needed of any of the following: another antianxiety agent (e.g., venlafaxine), adjunctive buspirone, an atypical neuroleptic such as aripiprazole (2 mg/day), or quetiapine (12.5 or 25 mg/day).

Case Study: I Get So Nervous That I Hyperventilate

A high school senior sprinter and her parents sought assistance from a sports psychiatrist because of performance anxiety that had progressively risen over the past 2 years after she had experienced some success in her sophomore year. Now before each meet, she would become so anxious that by the time the race began she would hyperventilate until she felt so light-headed that she could not run. In addition to feeling light-headed, she experienced blurred vision, shaking, and eventually muscle spasms in her hands. Six months earlier, she had gone to several physicians who had noted that she had a very reactive cardiovascular system, with an immediate pulse increase of 40 beats per minute with standing and then a rise to 170 beats per minute after just a few minutes of exercise. After undergoing extensive cardiac and pulmonary workup, she was diagnosed as having postural tachycardia syndrome and told that her total blood volume was too low. She was encouraged to stay well hydrated and was placed on salt tablets and birth control pills, but she continued to struggle with her breathing. In addition, a year before, she had been evaluated by an otolaryngologist who diagnosed her as having vocal cord dysfunction. Weekly sessions with a speech therapist had not improved her symptoms.

Diagnosis: Axis I: Anxiety NOS with hyperventilation; Axis III: Vocal cord dysfunction and postural tachycardia syndrome

Intervention: In the office, her pulse rose consistently by 38–42 beats per minute with simple standing, followed by a quick recovery when reseated. A short run around the office parking lot resulted in a rapid rise in her heart rate to 180 beats per minute and automatic gasping hyperventilation. Fortunately, she had a quick recovery, and her dizziness and blurred vision faded after a few minutes. Back in the office, she was instructed to reverse her breathing pattern while running to actively push the air out slowly with each stride and then to let air flow back in passively. She practiced this in the office and seemed ready to try a short run again. This time when she ran, she was easily able to slow her breathing down, and her heart rate did not activate as quickly and she did not automatically hyperventilate. After each lap, she was encouraged to recover by taking slow exhalations and passive inhalations, making sure she did not use her accessory chest or neck muscles to move the air in. She revealed toward the end of the interview that she had always been able to feel her heart beating too rapidly and had worried that she would either pass out on a run or even have a heart attack. When the physiology of exercise and respiratory drive were explained and the symptoms of hyperventilation were reviewed on the office computer, she seemed to relax. She was instructed to do 5–10 minutes of cardiovascular fitness work (running and stationary biking) daily at home, making sure that she was able to master this new way of breathing. In addition, she was instructed on patterned relaxation breathing (in through the nose for a count of four, hold for seven, and out for eight, repeated eight times) and encouraged to do this four to six times daily. Once she felt that she could breathe with a focus on exhalation, she went to an outdoor track on her own and tried to change her breathing pattern in this way while doing a slow distance run and then sprint intervals. After 2 weeks of running on her own, she returned to practice with her team and found that she could do the workouts with less distress. In consultation with her primary care physician, she was prescribed low-dose atenolol (25 mg/day) to suppress her cardiac hyperactivity.

Over the next 3 months, she continued to train with exhalation running, allowing her power to flow into each stride. Her confidence began to soar, and she entered her first competition in almost 6 months. She ran well, making sure she relaxed between events and stayed well hydrated. At a follow-up meeting before a bigger meet, she reviewed her prerace routines and made sure she kept her breath under control, with the idea that with relaxation breathing and a focus on music, she could reduce her heart rate activation and could easily recover after the race. She was also encouraged to visualize success each night and to do some interval runs at every practice, consisting of 200 yards fast then 200 yards slow, repeated first two, then four, then six times. She understood that this practice was intended to build her confidence with running race pace, as well as her confidence in her ability to recover and go again. At the next meet, she ran faster than ever before, posting two personal best times. She was more pleased, however, that she could practice and compete without such distress.

Case Study: I've Always Been a Worrier Like My Dad, But Now I Can't Stop Thinking or Get Rest

An early career professional football player was referred to a sports psychiatrist for an evaluation of insomnia early in the season by the head athletic trainer. The player had experienced difficulty falling asleep and staying asleep dating back to high school. He described being physically tired after practice and at bedtime, but being unable to turn off his thinking. After he got home and even when he got into bed, he would regularly review his football day, often dwelling on mistakes and worrying about his wife, newborn son, parents, and finances. He had never consulted a physician for sleep concerns and had never been evaluated for anxiety despite the fact that his father and two paternal uncles were being treated with medication for anxiety and insomnia. He had no history of excessive alcohol, tobacco, or stimulant use, and no history of illicit drug use, recent injury, or acute pain. He did, however, report fatigue and regular tension headaches two to three times per week at the end of the day, which were usually relieved by acetaminophen or ibuprofen.

Diagnosis: Axis I: Generalized anxiety disorder, insomnia; Axis III: Chronic muscle contraction headaches

Intervention: Initially, the main focus was on improving sleep to see what impact that change would have on his anxiety and fatigue. He started taking trazodone 50 mg 90 minutes before bedtime and developed a better unwinding routine. His sleep improved only modestly, however, so the dosage was increased to 100 mg. After 2 weeks of taking trazodone daily, he still needed 45–60 minutes to fall asleep, so escitalopram was added and raised to 15 mg at bedtime over 3 weeks. After a month, he reported that his day-to-day worrying had diminished and that with either 50 or 100 mg of trazodone, he was able to fall asleep easily and awaken refreshed the next day after 7–8 hours of continuous sleep. He continued on this combination through the end of the season. During the off-season, he reduced his use of trazodone to once a week, but continued taking escitalopram. During the following season, he continued escitalopram and used trazodone two to three times a week when he knew sleep would be difficult (e.g., pregame).

Impulse- and Anger-Control Disorders

The impulse-control problems that are most commonly seen in athletes at the professional level are overspending, substance misuse, aggression and fights, gambling, and risky sexual behaviors. These behaviors are usually present to some degree during the athletes' college years but often worsen with the sudden influx of money and lifestyle upgrade. Too often, professional athletes so substantially overspend for relatives and themselves that if their career changes or ends early, they face home foreclosure, automobile repossession, insurmountable credit card debt, or even bankruptcy. Binge drinking that does not meet the criteria for a substance use disorder occurs during the season on off-days and during the off-season, and sometimes leads to club or bar fights, partner aggression, and other risky behaviors, such as having unprotected sex with multiple partners. Athletes at the professional level sometimes feel that they work so hard that they deserve to party to escape or unwind. Although pathological gambling is not common, casino or online gambling is so readily available that some players occasionally spend more than is wise. Anger-control difficulties are the most common impulse problems seen and typically involve a wife or domestic partner. The conflicts usually center on finances, parenting, or lifestyle and occasionally result in a media event or an arrest (Burton 2005).

The typical approach to preventing or managing an impulse-control problem is to put it in the context of maturity and responsibility. Younger professional athletes should be informed that as late as age 25, the brain's cortical circuits are still being constructed, especially in those frontal areas that regulate executive functions such as judgment, critical review, error recognition and correction, organization, planning, and resisting temptation. Until the cortex is fully mature, the midbrain's impulsive pleasure- and thrill-seeking drive circuits may dominate. Discussion of the disciplinary consequences that can result from more serious impulsive behaviors can evolve into a dialogue about the pros and cons of such behaviors in the future and the impact that these behaviors have on the views of the coaching staff and the public. In the areas of responsibility, productive topic areas include achieving a consistent high level of play, and being a good teammate, son or daughter, and partner. A media event or arrest often presents an opportunity to work with the coaching staff and league administrators and clinicians who deal with disciplinary infractions to move athletes' behaviors in more positive directions. These discussions best occur soon after the event and in the training facility or clubhouse because the athlete can more directly experience the disappointment and support of his or her coaches and teammates. The most important goal is for the athlete to learn from his or her mistakes and make more contemplative and mature decisions the next time.

Case Study: I Take Out My Frustration With Lacrosse on My Girlfriend, Teammates, and Family

A fifth-year senior college lacrosse defenseman was referred for evaluation by the head athletic trainer after the player had an angry outburst in a meeting with his head coach. The athletic trainer had also noticed that this player had demonstrated a high level of frustration and irritability in the training room over the last few years when receiving treatment for injuries. The player described a long history of quick frustration, impulsivity, and anger dating back to middle school. He described himself as someone with a high energy level who needed to move constantly and greatly disliked sitting in meetings. In addition, he noted difficulty with verbal restraint if frustrated, and this difficulty often triggered conflicts with coaches and teammates, who viewed him as a "hothead." He preferred to take his intensity to the lacrosse field, where he was known as one of the hardest hitters on the team. In school, he described poor attention, restlessness, easy distractibility, disinterest in most subjects, and disrespect for his teachers. Consequently, he often got in trouble in class or just didn't go. His grades were far below his ability level because he did not read what was required or complete or turn in his assignments. He retained his academic eligibility in college by taking easier classes and using tutors. In relationships, he noted that conflicts with his girlfriend, parents, and teammates often resulted in intense arguments. In addition, while out with friends, he would get into fights with strangers whether or not he was intoxicated. He said that marijuana was one of the few things that calmed him down and helped him focus. He had never had a psychiatric or psychological evaluation and reported no depression, mania, hypomania, insomnia, or use of other illicit drugs. He had no history of tobacco or excessive stimulant use.

Diagnosis: Axis I: Impulse-control disorder NOS (anger control); attention-deficit disorder, combined type; marijuana and alcohol abuse

Intervention: The player agreed to weekly meetings in an office near the training room to develop anger-control strategies. He agreed to refrain from alcohol and marijuana and was interested in a trial of medication to improve his attention. A collateral contact with his girlfriend confirmed that he had a quick temper and sometimes would get so angry that he would scream in her face, throw things, or punch walls. Many times, she had left his apartment because of fear of being harmed even though he had never hit her. She did think he drank excessively and smoked too much weed and felt that both made him more likely to get into a confrontation. A trial of low-dose extended-release methylphenidate was started. After the dosage was raised to 36 mg/day, he began to note increased irritability and difficulty sleeping. Therefore, the methylphenidate was discontinued, and a trial of atomoxetine was started. The dosage was raised slowly to 60 mg/day, and he experienced improvement in focus and attention shifting, as well as reduced restlessness and impulsivity. The main behavioral strategy for anger control was to have increased awareness of the little things that frustrated him and to allow himself time and space to think before reacting. In addition, he shifted more attention to positive events in his day and to positive emotions. He also worked through some disappointments about his academic failures. When his parents visited town for a game, a family meeting was arranged to identify areas for change in communication style and emotional reactions. Through the combination of anger-control therapy, substance abstinence, improvement in his attention, reduction in impulsivity, and increase in success and positive emotions, the player experienced a gradual change in his interpersonal patterns and improvement in his athletic and academic performance.

Attention-Deficit and Learning Disorders

Problems with focus, concentration, learning, attention shifting, and sustained attention are common in athletes (Conant-Norville and Tofler 2005). These problems can be temporary, due to poor sleep, general stress, anxiety, injury and pain, performance slumps, or interpersonal conflict, or they can be more enduring and due to an attention-deficit disorder. Athletes are increasingly entering college and professional levels of competition already diagnosed with attention-deficit disorder and taking medications. Most of the evaluations done before or during college are of good quality, and if done by a neuropsychologist, have typically assessed intelligence, learning, attention, and personality. In these cases, athletes have already been diagnosed with attention-deficit disorder with or without hyperactivity and with executive functioning deficits and minor learning problems. Understanding of these athletes' learning styles is important, because instruction varies from sport to sport and can include a playbook, classroom talks, on-field skills building, film review and discussion, and home reading. In athletes of high school age and older, attention disorders might be the second most common psychiatric disorder, after performance anxiety.

Treatment of attention-deficit and learning disorders consists of medication and behavioral therapy. The most common starting medication is long-acting methylphenidate, beginning at the lowest dosage and increasing the dosage about every 2–3 weeks so that behavioral strategies can be incorporated into treatment as well. Rapid dosage escalations give the wrong message that the medication is the main solution and that the athlete can be passive in the process. For most athletes, two doses a day are needed. The first dose is taken upon awakening and the second in the middle to late afternoon depending on the medication's duration of action, which is unique to the individual. The beneficial effect of a single dose can vary from as little as 5–6 hours to as long as 8–10 hours. The clinician should emphasize that the medication will result in improvement in attention in a number of other areas besides sports, including academics, pleasure reading, hobbies, and relationships.

If long-acting methylphenidate is not effective, then a trial of long-acting amphetamine salts or the prodrug lisdexamfetamine, which also has a long duration of action, can be initiated. Again, starting with lower dosages and building up slowly works best in athletes, although they are often very impatient to improve their performance. With long-acting amphetamine salts, twice-daily dosing is necessary during the season, whereas once-daily dosing may suffice for the off-season depending on the individual's activity level. With lisdexamfetamine, once-daily dosing during the season may be sufficient, but for a sport like professional baseball, where days are often 12–14 hours long, overlapping two dosages, with the second dose being lower than the first, may be more effective. Although some athletes can take short-acting formulations, these medications often generate overstimulation if the dosage is too high or if the athlete is tired and takes more than prescribed. This stimulant effect is attractive to athletes in sports that are exhausting, such as baseball, and may become the main reason for a drug's use. In some individuals, the combination of a long-acting medication in the morning and a short-acting medication in the evening works best, because insomnia may be a problem with two long-acting doses.

The most common side effects of any of these medications are morning gastrointestinal nausea and irritation, appetite suppression, stimulation, irritability, headaches, sleep difficulties, and problems with heat regulation. Easy solutions to these side effects are available and include eating breakfast before the first dose, eating lunch before the second dose, taking the lowest effective dose, taking the last dose at least 6–8 hours before bedtime, and staying well hydrated on hot and humid days.

Combining behavioral therapy with medications is critical to long-term success for athletes with attention-deficit disorders. First, athletes need to understand the natural cycles of the brain's visual and attention circuits and the need for these to be given a break and refreshed. For example, the visual system usually needs refreshing every 10–15 seconds, so shifting to alternative visual targets or shifting from vision to kinesthetic (feel) and back to vision in an athletic routine can help. For longer attention tasks, such as meetings or studying films, the natural cycle is usually 30–60 minutes. Once this time boundary is crossed, attention fades quickly, even for individuals taking medication. Therefore, athletes can benefit from a quick resetting break involving simple standing or stretching with some activating or relaxation breathing. Coaches also need to be aware of the importance of breaks to attention maintenance.

Second, athletes need to refine their pregame and preaction routines to clear their mind and become ready to play. Pregame routines should involve a series of actions that repeatedly shift attention from out (visual) to in (kinesthetic) until the process is automatic. For example, alternating sprints and stretching before batting practice in baseball or drills in soccer. Preaction routines are the same as pregame routines, but on a shorter time cycle. For example, in baseball, a prepitch routine for an outfielder might involve a break in visual attention from the plate after a strike by looking blankly to the grass in front, adjusting the glove, and moving around in a circle or side to side. Then, when the pitcher steps back on the mound, the outfielder's attention shifts back to broad visual by looking lightly at the back of the pitcher until the pitch is thrown and then narrowing attention to the hitter and the pitch by zoning in.

Third, athletes need to learn the importance of relaxation to sustained attention. If competitive routines contain regular relaxation strategies, such as clearing breaths or stretches, then the athlete's mind and body can operate for long periods without mental or physical fatigue.

Finally, differences in learning styles, especially for athletes with learning disorders, must be identified and the teaching tailored to them.

For example, some athletes learn best through demonstrations or walk-throughs in which kinesthetic patterns can be felt and registered. Others may learn better through visual strategies, such as by looking at film or by seeing or drawing plays on a board. If verbal communication is to facilitate learning, then it should be slowed down, made simple, and repeated several times in different ways if possible to benefit all learners in the room. Using a combination of verbal, visual, and kinesthetic approaches will usually work for most learning styles. Interestingly, some athletes, especially those with attention disorder with hyperactivity, attend and learn best when standing or while moving rather than while seated on the ground or in a chair.

Case Study: I Knew I Wasn't Learning Like I Could so I Just Focused on Sports

A professional minor league baseball player was referred for evaluation by his manager because of difficulty focusing in the field. He was drafted as a center fielder out of high school 5 years earlier and quickly established himself as a solid hitter and base stealer. In the field, however, he seemed unfocused and distracted, often making errors by failing to get a proper read and jump on the ball even though he had good speed. In addition, he would make throws to the wrong bag or fail to hit the cutoff man. He had been diagnosed with attention-deficit disorder and a developmental reading disorder in late middle school. At that time, he was assigned a reading tutor and started taking short-acting methylphenidate, but he stopped taking the medication after a year because it made him irritable. In his first year of high school, he began taking extended-release amphetamine salts, which resulted in improved attention and reduced impulsivity. Even with the medication, however, he knew he was not learning at a maximal level and became less and less interested in studying, even though he found his high school classes interesting. As he moved through high school, he shifted his attention from academics to football and baseball. Reflecting back on that time, he commented that sports gave him the self-confidence that he lacked in the classroom. After he was drafted, he felt the pressure to achieve and began raising his amphetamine salts dosage, in part because the increase helped but also because he liked the intensity boost. Eventually, he got to a dosage that was actually disruptive to his attention because of overstimulation, so he stopped taking the medication. Although his hitting remained solid, he seemed distant from his teammates and was not improving in other aspects of his game.

Diagnosis: Axis I: Attention-deficit disorder, combined type; developmental reading disorder, mild; amphetamine medication misuse

Intervention: When asked about his focus and ability to shift his attention in the field, the player was defensive, saying that it wasn't that bad. Several of his past coaches, however, said that if he did not improve in his fielding, he was unlikely to advance beyond the AA class level. They also said that he definitely had the talent to rise to the major leagues, but they felt that he did not have the commitment. Given his tendency to misuse amphetamines, he did not want to try those again. When asked if he had read much about nonmedication strategies to improve focus and concentration, he said he did not read books but was open to hearing about mental preparation training. After a long discussion of options, including atomoxetine and long-acting methylphenidate, he decided on a trial of low-dose atomoxetine. He began taking 25 mg/day and after 2 weeks noted some improvement in his baseball focus and his ability to read a mental skills manual he was given. At that point, his dosage was increased to 40 mg/day, and his casual attitude toward his fielding and undeveloped prepitch routine was addressed. As suggested by the roving fielding instructor, the player committed to approach each pitch as an opportunity to make a great play. His prepitch routine was reworked to ensure that he gave his visual system a break between each pitch and that he did not focus on the batter too soon in the process. After each pitch, he would walk around looking at the ground and briefly glancing up until he saw the pitcher start his windup or stretch. As soon as the ball was released, he then zoned into the hitter in anticipation that the ball might be hit into his area. This routine, in combination with the atomoxetine, resulted in steady improvement in his fielding and further improvement in his hitting and base running. As a result of his improvement, he was sent to an AAA team during a late-season call-up.

Eating Disorders and Disordered Eating

Athletes at entry competitive levels repeatedly hear about the importance of nutrition to performance and to injury prevention and healing. At the highest competitive levels, an even stronger emphasis is placed on nutrition and weight, percentage of body fat, body shape, muscularity, strength, flexibility, power, and speed. Some sports that emphasize weight (low or high) and body shape seem to have a higher risk for disordered eating patterns or eating disorders. Sports that are more strongly associated with restrictive eating patterns and anorexia include those that are organized by weight categories, such as high school and collegiate wrestling and boxing; those that emphasize leanness, endurance, or small size, such as distance running or horse racing; and those that emphasize appearance and leanness, such as gymnastics, figure skating, and competitive cheerleading. Meanwhile, those sports that value larger size, weight, and power, such as football, rugby, softball, and professional and sumo wrestling, are more associated with binge eating and bulimia. In addition to placing an emphasis on nutrition, athletic competition requires regular cardiovascular training, making compulsive overexercising more likely, and weight training, making restrictive eating disorders harder to recognize early on because of the additional muscle mass.

The following are common clinical indications of restrictive eating patterns or disorders: reduced weight, muscularity, or body fat; distorted body image; injury proneness; amenorrhea; loss of energy or endurance; sudden drop in performance; social isolation; dental problems from self-induced vomiting; changes in emotions, including irritability, anxiety, and depression; and changes in behavioral patterns, such as dressing in baggy clothes, secretive eating, or disappearances after meals that may indicate purging. Binge eating patterns or disorders surface because of consumption of large quantities of high-calorie and high-fat foods; weight gain; facial puffiness; compensatory purging, fasting, or overexercising; and self-image that is based on weight or shape. Subthreshold or atypical syndromes, such as anorexia athletica, are characterized by fear of weight gain in lean persons, distorted body image, caloric restrictions with some bingeing, excessive exercising, menstrual dysfunction, and gastrointestinal complaints, whereas the female athlete triad comprises disordered eating, amenorrhea, and osteoporosis or osteopenia (Currie and Morse 2005).

Treatment of disordered eating patterns and eating disorders usually involves a team approach, with the selected involvement of the family, coach, athletic trainer, team physician, nutritionist, therapist, teammates, and sports psychiatrist, depending on the severity of the problem (Bonci et al. 2008). Initially, treatment focuses on improving nutrition, restoring general health, and treating comorbid mood, anxiety, sleep, substance use, personality, and somatoform disorders. Therapy can be done individually or in groups and usually addresses self-esteem, self-criticism, self-acceptance, self-destructive patterns, perfectionistic standards, stress, relationships, distorted beliefs and body image, and the typical emotions of fear, disappointment, rejection, and anxiety. Medications usually target anxiety, depression, and sleep, and sometimes emotional instability. They should be selected to ensure that weight gain or weight loss is unlikely and that the risk of abuse is low.

Case Study: I Began Binge Eating to Relieve Stress, and Then I Started Making Myself Vomit

A third-year college softball player was referred to a sports psychiatrist by the head coach at the end of fall ball because of concern about the player's low energy in practice, social isolation, and stress from grades. The player had been struggling to maintain her academic eligibility throughout college and was especially worried now that she was taking upper-level courses in her major of kinesiology. During the evaluation, the player revealed that she was recruited as a power-hitting first baseman, but she had been upset that she had no energy lately, and her hitting, defense, and base running had suffered. Over the summer, she had stayed on campus and had taken two difficult courses, barely passing each despite the assistance of a tutor. From the stress of the summer, she had activated a past pattern of binge eating of high-calorie, high-fat foods and consequently gained 15 pounds. Out of concern for the weight gain and for the first time ever, she started inducing vomiting using her fingers. She noted that she felt such stress relief from eating and vomiting that the practice seemed to quickly develop into a compulsive pattern. As she got into the fall semester, she became depressed and did not want to be around her coaches, athletic trainers, or teammates. Not long after the semester began, she began using laxatives excessively, and that is when her energy began to drop.

Diagnosis: Axis I: Bulimia nervosa; depression NOS; Axis III: Overweight

Intervention: The player was seen weekly, and cognitive-behavioral therapy was initiated. She was referred to a nutritionist, who helped her construct an adequate nutritional plan. In the early sessions, the main sources of stress (academics, strained romantic relationship with a teammate, and sexual identity) were identified and a plan for each was developed. She responded to the structure of weekly meetings and agreed to allow the head coach to be informed generally of her struggles. Her academic adviser took a more active role in course selection, assignment of tutors, and monitoring of weekly work. A joint meeting was arranged with her teammate, and most of the tension between them was diffused. At each session, the player was asked about her nutritional patterns and urges to binge or purge. She recorded small successes each day as a way to build her confidence. Over a few months, her disordered eating resolved as her stress became controlled. She was seen throughout the spring season and agreed to find a therapist and a nutritionist in her home town to continue her treatment during the summer.

Case Study: I Wanted to Run Faster, so I Reduced My Calories and Upped My Training

A high school sophomore distance runner was referred to a psychiatrist at the beginning of cross-country season because of overtraining and low energy. After an outstanding freshman year in cross-country and in indoor and outdoor track, the athlete looked forward to a summer of hard training and additional success. Due to developmental maturity, however, she had gained weight and her body shape had changed, with widened hips and additional body fat. She knew that she was running slower, so she began to up her miles, eventually running twice a day for an hour each. When her weight did not change, she began to restrict her food intake to three small meals a day, consisting mainly of salads and vegetables with little protein or fat. She started to drop weight and by the beginning of preseason workouts had lost so much weight that she had insufficient energy to complete her training runs and her menses had stopped.

Diagnosis: Axis I: Anorexia nervosa, restricting type; impulse-control disorder NOS (compulsive overexercising); Axis III: Amenorrhea, underweight (5'5", 103 lb)

Intervention: The athlete stopped running and was referred to an outpatient eating disorders program, where she began individual and group therapy with nutritional counseling. By the end of the fall, she had regained her weight and started to go on slow 20-minute runs three times a week. Her care was then transferred to an office sports psychiatrist, who saw her weekly. At the first visit with the athlete and her parents, the psychiatrist said the athlete was allowed to gradually increase her running as long as she kept runs under 30 minutes, adhered to a proper nutritional plan, maintained her weight, and had regular menses. At the second and subsequent meetings, discussions focused on her broadened hips and resultant mechanical changes that had slowed her down, and the need to develop additional core and upper-body strength to compensate. She understood that building body strength would require a balance between good nutrition, especially regular protein intake, and running and lifting. She gradually increased her training over the winter and was able to compete in several distance events in outdoor track. Although she did not best the times from her freshman year, she understood that persistence with her current training plan would eventually lead to positive results. She maintained good nutrition and training through the summer. By the start of cross-country season, she had much better core and upper-body strength and began to have stronger training runs. By the end of the season, she posted a personal best time on the very difficult state championship course.

Mood Disorders and Grief

Athletic competition is filled with opposing positive and negative emotions. Negative emotions include doubt, fear, frustration, disappointment, sadness, loneliness, isolation, pain, pessimism, embarrassment, shame, irritability, homesickness, and depression, whereas positive emotions include pride, ecstasy, joy, accomplishment, invincibility, entitlement, camaraderie, connection, mastery, optimism, and confidence. Within each athlete, an ongoing battle of competing emotions exists, along with positive and negative thought patterns and automatic actions (Figure 7–1). When negative emotions dominate over time, an athlete may develop depression and a sense of loss. As athletes move to higher competitive levels and practices become more intense and competition gets stronger, the athletes may experience low emotional periods during which mistakes may increase, performance may drop, playing time might be lost, and confidence may diminish or disappear. Depression in this situation is usually temporary and needs to be worked through with the support of the coaching staff, athletic trainers, team physicians, and teammates. Team captains and veteran players are expected to notice when players experience these low periods and to intervene with encouragement, hopefulness, and a message of persistence.

In addition to these expected episodes of depression during adjustment periods, athletes may experience more serious and complex episodes of depression, which are often triggered by a broader series of

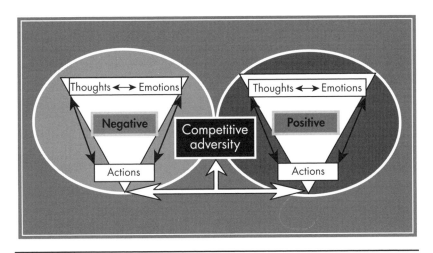

FIGURE 7–1. Positive and negative shifting in sports.
Competitive adversity=mistakes, poor performance, losing, injury, and the like.

events, such as serious injury, family loss, high sustained stress, or important transitions, including graduation, marriage, or retirement. These more persistent and serious episodes of depression are accompanied by poor concentration, indecisiveness, sleep and energy changes, loss of appetite, feelings of worthlessness, and diminished pleasure in sports and other areas. In these cases, an evaluation by the team physician or a sports psychiatrist or other mental health professional is warranted (Baum 2005). Although not common in sports among elite athletes, major depression does occur but may not be easily detected until it has substantially interfered with athletic performance and interpersonal functioning. The delay in noticing the change is often due to the athlete's determination to keep pushing through adversity to perform well. Usually, a family member, position coach, or the team's athletic trainer is the person who notices the distress.

When an episode of major depression is identified, the athlete and his or her support network should be involved in the assessment and treatment. Although collateral contact might not occur during the initial visit, such contact is important during follow-up visits. If possible, treatment should be delivered where training and competition occur to ensure adherence with appointments and connection with supports. Usually, combinations of typical antidepressant medications and therapy are used. First, an SSRI or SNRI should be tried, with consideration for sedation, weight gain, sexual effects, and activation. If a blood relative has been medically treated for a similar episode with good results, then that medication should be strongly considered. Therapy usually centers on addressing each precipitating stressor with a specific action plan. Because athletes are accustomed to practicing and competing as a team, creating a formal support network and involving these individuals in the solution are often helpful tactics. Sports psychiatrists should have comfort working with couples and families, as well as with strategic collateral contacts that may include coaches, parents, siblings, friends, and teammates. Information gained from these contacts is invaluable in understanding the development of an athlete's depression and working toward its solution.

Other serious mood disorders, such as bipolar disorder, substance-induced mania, and severe dysthymia, are not common among athletes at elite competitive levels because these disorders usually block success and promotion. However, because athletes at collegiate and professional levels are in the age ranges at risk for the onset of these disorders, new cases sometimes develop. When they do occur, they often result in missed playing time and more intense treatment. If a bipolar disorder develops, then the clinician must give special consideration in medication selection to acceptance and adherence and avoidance of certain side effects, such as electrolyte imbalance, sedation, slowed reaction time, impaired balance, and reduced mental quickness. Generally, if the current episode is mania or hypomania, then the clinician should consider treating the athlete with an atypical antipsychotic or with combination therapy with a low-dose antipsychotic, such as aripiprazole or quetiapine, and an anticonvulsant mood stabilizer, such as lamotrigine or oxcarbazepine, because blood level monitoring of these medications is not necessary. If the current episode is depression, then recommended treatment is either monotherapy with an atypical antipsychotic or lamotrigine, or combination therapy with either of these medications plus the cautious addition of a second-generation antidepressant. Therapy focuses heavily at first on sleep and safety, as well as the therapeutic alliance with the athlete and family. Severe mood disorders in athletes are difficult; of the four cases my practice group has seen in 15 years, only one athlete has returned to compete at the same level. Having a psychiatrist positioned at the team's practice facility is beneficial so that the athlete can be seen regularly during practice and injury treatment.

Case Study: I've Been Depressed My Whole Life, but My Divorce Tipped Me Into Deep Despair

A late-career baseball player was referred by the team physician to a sports psychiatrist during spring training. He had been married for 9 years and had two daughters, ages 7 and 5. According to the player, over the past year, increasing marital tension and a lack of love and communication led to an announcement in the off-season by his wife that she was moving out and filing for divorce. She took the children and moved in with her parents, who lived in the same city. This action devastated the player, who began to stay home and sleep excessively. The more he stayed home, the more depressed he became, with frequent crying spells, low energy, poor concentration, and feelings of worthlessness. A good friend and another athlete with whom the player trained convinced him to go to a therapist, who also referred him to a psychiatrist. When he arrived at spring training, he was much improved from weekly therapy, scheduled weekends with his daughters, and extended-release bupropion 150 mg/day. He described chronic low self-esteem, hypersomnia, fatigue, and difficulty making decisions, which he related to a dysfunctional family filled with criticism and fighting. In addition, his parents divorced when he was 12 and his dad quickly remarried and moved to another state. He expressed a desire to continue regular therapy with a team assistance provider during home stands.

Diagnosis: Axis I: Major depression, single episode, moderate, without psychotic features, in full remission; dysthymia; Axis III: Healthy, fit, no injuries or medications

Intervention: The player was seen twice weekly throughout the season during home stands and was maintained on extended-release bupropion. He hired a young adult to accompany his daughters to see him when he was on the road and at home on a monthly basis and communicated with them through Internet video regularly when they were not visiting. Therapy focused on improving his self-confidence and decision-making capacities. He successfully negotiated a separation agreement and visitation schedule with his wife and worked hard on improving his baseball. He used positive self-talk, visualizations, and relaxation to raise his baseball confidence, and this then spilled over to his personal life. He did well until the end of the season when his divorce was finalized and he learned that his wife had become serious with another man. Road trip phone sessions with the psychiatrist were added to the regular home-stand meetings, and the player successfully worked through this brief period of return of his prior symptoms. He left for the off-season and picked back up with the therapist he had seen earlier. He returned to training the following year with stable mood and improved self-confidence.

Case Study: I Can't Stay Awake and Sometimes I Zone Out at Practice and Games, but I Need My Meds

A 16-year-old high school junior soccer player and his parents were seen for a second opinion by a sports psychiatrist midseason because of concerns about periods of poor focus and sustained attention in sports and school. In addition, the player noted moderately severe midmorning (second period) and late-afternoon (prepractice) tiredness and sleepiness. He was diagnosed with rapid-cycling bipolar disorder at age 12 in sixth grade and had three prior hospitalizations, the last one 1 year earlier. He was currently being treated with a high dose of an atypical antipsychotic (aripiprazole 15 mg three times daily) and an anticonvulsant mood stabilizer (carbamazepine 400 mg twice daily), and had a therapeutic midrange blood level. He had been on this regimen since his last hospitalization. All three hospitalizations had been precipitated by uncontrollable aggression. A recent attempt to reduce his aripiprazole resulted in increased irritability and depression. No evidence suggested alcohol, marijuana, stimulant, or other illicit drug use. He did have prior neurological workup that was normal and neuropsychological testing that showed above average intelligence and no evidence of a specific learning disorder. In the interview, the player had constant conflict with his father over details of his history. His mother was passive and supportive. He described himself as a heavy sleeper who needed an alarm clock and his parents to awaken him. He usually slept for 9 hours a night. He tended to rush out of the house at 6:30 A.M. without breakfast and was extremely hungry by his 10:30 A.M. lunch break. Because of his hunger, he tended to overeat, consuming more than half his daily nutritional requirements at lunch. After school and before practice, he was very hungry again and tended to eat a high-calorie, high-fat meal before practice. He was overweight (5'10", 206 lb).

Diagnosis: Axis I: Bipolar II disorder, rapid cycling; impulse-control disorder NOS (anger control); parent-child problem; Axis III: Overweight; poor nutritional plan; medication sedation

Intervention: The initial focus of the consultation was on nutrition. Given the timing of his midmorning drop in energy and sleepiness, he was advised to begin eating breakfast that had a mix of simple sugars (fruit), complex carbohydrates (whole grains), and fats (nuts) to make sure he had energy to get him through his first two classes (90 minutes each) and to reduce his midmorning hunger. His lunch was modified to reduce the quantity and fat content, and a midafternoon nutritional bar was added. After school, he substituted a meal of complex carbohydrates and healthy fats for his former high-calorie, high-fat meal. After practice, he resupplied his carbohydrates with a nutritional drink. Next, his morning awakening routine and prepractice routines were revised to address the importance of actively raising his energy level for school and sports. He agreed to add in two 60-second cardiovascular exercise sets with controlled nasal hyperventilation for quicker and stronger awakening and to increase the structure and intensity of his preparation for practice and games. The sports psychiatrist suggested reducing his morning aripiprazole to 7.5 mg and adding 7.5 mg to his bedtime dose. Finally, because he was only being seen by his treating psychiatrist once a month for medication visits and he was having increasing conflicts and angry outbursts with his father and mother over studying and sports, he started meeting weekly with a therapist, who also met periodically with his parents. These changes gradually resulted in increased energy and alertness and reduced anxiety in school, reduced frustration and anger at home and practices, and improved focus and attention in competition.

Pain and Somatoform Disorders

Athletes pay constant attention to their bodies during endurance training, weight lifting, practice, medical evaluations, daily treatments, tapings, and long or short rehabilitation periods after surgery or serious injury. This constant body focus creates a high level of body awareness and routinely leads to continuous body scanning for imbalances or injuries. Some athletes seem injury prone, whereas others seem to practice and compete just as hard without incurring serious injuries. When injuries do occur, some athletes respond predictably to the treatment and return to play promptly, but others have slower and more complicated recoveries, causing the athletic trainers and medical staff to speculate about the presence of outside stress or the influence of emotional distress on the frequency and severity of the subjective symptoms of injury and the speed and character of the recovery.

When an athlete's emotional response to injury is substantial or unexpected or the recovery is not progressing well, his or her emotions may have magnified the intensity of the discomfort or disability and may have changed the athlete's experience of the injury. On every team and in every training room, there are certain athletes whose injury experiences are altered by past injury experiences, current stress reactions, or their particular emotional intensity and patterns. These athletes are baffling and frustrating to athletic trainers and the medical staff, and often require extra attention, more explanation and reassurance, or more diagnostic evaluation and second opinions. Sports psychiatrists can be helpful with these cases of somatoform disorders where quick and strong emotions, automatic thinking, and interpersonal patterns combine to complicate injury or illness recovery.

The clinician should begin the assessment of these athletes with a complete review of the circumstances of the injury or illness and the current treatment and prognosis. Any prior injuries or similar illnesses are also reviewed and understood, especially those with prolonged or complicated recovery. As the assessment proceeds, the clinician should conduct brief range-of-motion and strength testing or a simple examination to look for signs of guarding or unexpected distress. Problems with sleep, anxiety, frustration, and disappointment often co-occur with somatoform disorders and must be directly managed. These patients also have underlying pessimism and helplessness that accompany each interaction and that alter their view of the prognosis. After the injury and illness history is obtained, the clinician takes a sports history, allowing the athlete to share his or her life experiences in sports. Particular attention is paid to the presence or absence of key family members during the early competitive years and to the history of frequent moves, school failure, and early losses, separations, or trauma. In the context of an athlete's life story, his or her strong reaction to an injury or serious illness, as well as his or her need for more support during recovery, may make more sense.

Because the athletic trainers and team physicians likely do not have enough time to learn of these early life experiences or to talk extensively with the athletes about current stresses or concerns, the sports psychiatrist can perform this valuable function. What seems to help in the recovery process of athletes with somatoform disorders is for them to feel validated and secure that their needs will be met. When they have this feeling of reassurance, they will quietly and steadily improve and eventually return to full play, although sometimes after a longer than usual recovery period.

Case Study: This Pain Could Mean the End of My Career

A recently signed midcareer professional football player visited the sports psychiatrist in the training room complaining of right hip pain after practice during preseason camp. He seemed convinced that he had retorn his labrum, which had been surgically repaired 8 months earlier. He was anxious and despondent when seen in the training room. He described himself as an emotionally intense worrier all his life but said that over the past 4 years his worrying had gotten worse because a series of injuries had limited his play and because his marriage had dissolved. He said that his past team physician had encouraged him to see a psychiatrist and consider medications, but he had declined. He did go to a psychotherapist, who had helped him work through some past conflict with his parents and siblings. He described daily anxiety about small things and emotional lability, with anger and crying spells. His sleep, however, was normal, and although he had used alcohol to excess in the past, he had no current substance abuse or dependence. For a few days, he was held out of practice and given local heat and stimulation, along with anti-inflammatory medications and muscle relaxants. During this period, the team physician developed the impression that the intensity of the athlete's pain experience was being influenced by his anxiety and mood state.

Diagnosis: Axis I: Pain disorder with psychological factors; generalized anxiety disorder; depression NOS; Axis III: Degenerative traumatic hip disease with recent labral repair; chronic hamstring strains; high ankle sprain, healed

Intervention: The player saw the sports psychiatrist daily over the next week and agreed to assume that his hip was just inflamed and not reinjured. In addition, he agreed to counter any of his usual negative emotions with positive thoughts of optimism, calm, and confidence. After a few days, his hip improved and he returned to full practice. With continued encouragement, he began to more consistently find positive moments in his day and let these determine his emotional patterns. After a few weeks of rapport building, the psychiatrist more fully addressed the topic of the athlete's reluctance to take medications. The athlete stated that he had always viewed medications as an indication that he had a permanent disability, plus he had heard that all medications interfered with sex drive and caused withdrawal symptoms if stopped. After a complete review of the pros and cons of various medications, he agreed to a trial of extended-release venlafaxine. He started taking a low dosage (37.5 mg/day), and the dosage was raised slowly over the next month to 112.5 mg/day. Over the first half of the season, his constant worrying and anxiety diminished and his mood stabilized. He progressed nicely in his return to football and made excellent contributions on special teams and began to challenge for time as a backup linebacker.

General Approaches: Psychotherapy and Medication Management

The three time-limited types of therapy that work best in a busy sports psychiatric practice are stress control, motivational enhancement, and cognitive-behavioral therapy. Stress control therapy, which is described in detail in Chapter 3, "Stress Recognition and Control," involves 1) identification of the main stressors, the athlete's unique stress response, and any background factors that may have magnified or complicated his or her stress response; 2) identification of strategies for prioritizing, eliminating, managing, or changing the perspective of the current stressors; 3) use of strategies for changing or diminishing the patterned stress response (e.g., a support network; medications for sleep, anxiety, anger, depression, or mood instability; relaxation activities or breaks); and 4) review of background factors to place the current stress response into the context of past responses and to identify and work through past events such as childhood loss or trauma or major disappointments or failures.

Motivational enhancement therapy is based on the belief that the individual must find solutions to problems by using internal competencies and by actualizing self-efficacy. The clinician uses a range of interactive strategies to create an equal partnership and to maintain low resistance or defensiveness when discussing sensitive, personal, or emotional issues. The goal of the partnership is to facilitate a dialogue with enough exchange of information that the athlete discovers new perspectives and alters his or her readiness and capacity to change repetitive and unhelpful response patterns. Some of the main strategies used in this therapy are asking open-ended questions, providing affirmations, using reflective listening, rolling with resistance, and episodically summarizing the interaction through feedback.

Finally, cognitive-behavioral therapy is useful for athletes with adjustment or other mental disorders. This therapy identifies repetitive thinking patterns and more fundamental core beliefs that are associated with or even produce patterned emotional responses that interfere with performance, relationships, and quality of life. After identifying and challenging the validity of automatic thinking patterns and beliefs, the athlete can learn to create and substitute alternatives that produce different and more positive emotional patterns.

The use of medications in sports is common for insomnia, attention-deficit disorder, anxiety, and depression. Lower dosages can be used and side effects minimized if medication is combined with good therapist-patient rapport and brief therapy. Ideally, the clinician can be present on-site for two to three contacts with the athlete per week during the season and available for phone contacts if the team is away or out of season. Insomnia and attention-deficit disorder are two of the most common issues faced by athletes in college and professional sports. Insomnia most often occurs in individuals who are overactive thinkers or worriers or those who are so easily activated by competition that they cannot unwind. The most effective medications are trazodone or zolpidem, but their use may differ from sport to sport. For example, for baseball players who experience daily play and travel, trazodone is rarely used because it often takes 8–10 hours for its sedative effects to clear. In these baseball players, therefore, short-acting zolpidem is typically used. In contrast, football players get off earlier in the day and have time to go home and unwind during the week; therefore, they can take trazodone 60–90 minutes before bedtime, and its sedative effects will be completely cleared by morning. Football coaches with insomnia, however, have long days and short nights, so zolpidem in lower doses (5 mg) is preferred. Care must always be taken during sleep evaluations to make sure that alcohol or stimulants are not being used excessively or that another mental disorder is not present.

Athletes with attention-deficit disorder may already have tried methylphenidate and amphetamine salts and therefore may have a bias. The clinician needs to help them understand that stimulant medications should be started at a low dose and raised slowly to allow repeated exposure to important attention tasks in practice, competition, studies, and social interactions. If there are no contraindications, then long-acting methylphenidate is usually tried first and is often given twice daily if the period to be covered is 12 hours or more. With overlapping doses taken at 7–9 A.M. and 2–4 P.M., most essential daily tasks can be easily covered. If methylphenidate is not effective, then a trial of extended-release amphetamine salts can be instituted. Again, the starting dose is low because twice-daily use is necessary. Lowest effective dosing is facilitated by strategic shifting of the timing of the two doses to cover the highest period of attention demand.

For situational anxiety, typical agents are used. Short-acting benzodiazepines (e.g., alprazolam or lorazepam) that target specific symptoms or specific symptom time periods are helpful, and if used in low dosages, these agents do not typically produce sedation or motor impairment. Sometimes, a β-blocker such as propranolol or atenolol can be used for performance anxiety while relaxation or stress control skills are developing. For individuals with anxiety disorders, SSRIs or SNRIs are used, with the specific choice depending on prior experience, family history, and possible side effects. If started during the competitive season, then very low dosages (often half the typical starting amount) are recommended, with slow increases not more than every 7–10 days. The slower approach with regular therapy ensures that the lowest effective dose is used and side effects are minimized so that adherence rates are higher. Because anxiety often co-occurs with depression, medication should be chosen that is effective for both. The most common sports-compatible agents that are well tolerated are sertraline, escitalopram, venlafaxine, and duloxetine. As when treating other common problems, low dosages can be effective if concurrent therapy is provided. Because anxiety and depressive disorders are usually associated with sleep and energy disturbances, then a combination strategy is often necessary, with a quick-acting medication, such as a benzodiazepine or zolpidem, used first, followed by longer-term medication. If pain is an associated factor and the athlete is taking a narcotic analgesic, neuropathic agent (e.g., gabapentin or pregabalin), or muscle relaxant, then the choice of dosage of the antianxiety/antidepressant medication may be affected.

Conclusion

Sports psychiatrists need to be skilled brief therapists and able to prescribe medications that are effective and that address the unique requirements of athletic competition and training. Individual therapy often takes place in the training facility and addresses practical barriers to peak performance, such as confidence, stress, attention, and interpersonal conflict. The best approach involves a blend of stress control, motivational enhancement, and cognitive-behavioral therapies that promote self-efficacy and the ability to substitute positive thinking, emotional, and behavioral patterns for negative ones. In addition, clinicians can use mental preparation techniques to engage athletes to first work on performance directly and then eventually get at some underlying emotional or interpersonal barriers to long-term achievement. Skill in working with couples, families, and networks is also important. The lives of many professional athletes are filled with episodic conflicts with spouses, family members, agents, coaches, or teammates. The clinician's ability to gather information about the nature of these conflicts and then meet strategically with two or more individuals to quickly defuse heightened emotions and impulsive actions is critical. Clinicians can also help athletes learn parenting strategies, because athletes often live away from the support of family and friends and therefore benefit from practical advice about children's sleep, feedings, negative behaviors, habits, toilet training, learning, and emotional control.

Key Clinical Points

- Attention-deficit, learning, adjustment, anxiety, mood, impulse-control, eating, substance use, and sleep disorders are the most common mental disorders encountered in sports psychiatric practices. Eating, somatoform, impulse-control, sleep, and some substance use disorders are more common in athletes than in the general population.

- Performance anxiety is the most common problem in athletes and can usually be managed with the introduction of basic mental skills, especially breathing and relaxation, positive self-talk, and visualization, and a reworking of prepractice and precompetition routines and performance goals and expectations.

- For athletes with attention-deficit disorders who are facing long days of practice, travel, and competition, the best medication options are atomoxetine, the long-acting formulations of methylphenidate or amphetamine, or the prodrug lisdexamfetamine. Long-acting formulations are preferred over short-acting ones to prevent their misuse for stimulation effect during periods of low energy.

- Chronic insomnia is commonly encountered in athletes and often results from stress, overthinking, worrying, or injury and pain. Good sleep hygiene requires an earlier bedtime, the elimination of prebedtime excessive visual stimulation (e.g., TV, Internet) and heavy eating, and the regulation of noise and temperature. The introduction of improved unwinding, white noise, and relaxation breathing is also helpful. Medications that turn off active thinking and aid in unwinding, such as trazodone, or that induce sleep, such as zolpidem, are safe and have few side effects as long as alcohol use is minimal.

- Adjustment disorder, dysthymia, or more severe depression is encountered in athletes and usually is linked to poor performance, trauma, or loss. Therapy in combination with medications and team and family support is usually effective.

- Sports psychiatrists must be skilled at brief therapy for individuals, couples, and families, as well as have experience in developing support networks. The most common brief therapies are stress control (supportive), cognitive-behavioral, and motivational enhancement.

Adherence to treatment is more easily maintained if the therapy is provided at or proximate to the athlete's training site and integrated with the athletic trainers, team physicians, and coaching staff.

References

American Psychiatric Association: Diagnostic and Statistical Manual of Mental Disorders, 4th Edition, Text Revision. Washington, DC, American Psychiatric Association, 2000

Baum AL: Suicide in athletics: a review and commentary. Clin Sports Med 24:853–869, 2005

Bonci CM, Bonci LJ, Granger LR, et al: National Athletic Trainers' Association position statement: preventing, detecting, and managing disordered eating in athletes. J Athl Train 43:80–108, 2008

Burton RW: Aggression and sport. Clin Sports Med 24:845–852, 2005

Conant-Norville DO, Tofler IR: Attention deficit/hyperactivity disorder and pharmacologic treatments in the athlete. Clin Sports Med 24:829–843, 2005

Currie A, Morse E: Eating disorders in athletes: managing the risks. Clin Sports Med 24:871–883, 2005

Glick ID, Horsfall JL: Diagnosis and psychiatric treatment of athletes. Clin Sports Med 24:771–781, 2005

Glick ID, Kamm R, Morse E: The evolution of sport psychiatry, circa 2009. Sports Med 39:607–613, 2009

Kamm RL: Interviewing principles for the psychiatrically aware sports medicine physician. Clin Sports Med 24:745–769, 2005

McDuff DR, Morse E, White R: Professional and collegiate team assistance programs: services and utilization patterns. Clin Sports Med 24:943–958, 2005

Chapter 8

Teams, Medical Staff, and Sports Leadership

Experienced sports psychiatrists and psychologists can find opportunities to work with team owners, presidents, general managers, athletic directors, and coaches to improve team morale, cohesion, and performance; resolve conflicts between coaches and players; address a negative public relations event; or establish assistance services for athletes and team staff on an ongoing basis. Initial opportunities often arise during crises, such as unexpected or sustained poor performance, a serious incident or pattern of athlete misconduct, overt player-coach conflict, a tragedy like an accidental or unexpected death, or serious mental illness in an athlete or coach. Rarely will a team seek out sports psychiatric services with the intention of establishing a comprehensive set of preventive and intervention services for athletes and staff with performance or personal problems. Rather, comprehensive services typically evolve out of crisis services that are time limited but successful (Shapiro et al. 2001).

Interestingly, some professional sports organizations, such as Major League Baseball, require that every team establish and operate a team assistance program that provides free short-term evaluation, treatment, and coordinated referral services for stress, mental health, and substance abuse problems that affect performance or quality of life. Colleges and universities, on the other hand, usually rely on available campus resources, such as counseling or health centers, for general support or crisis services for athletes. Unfortunately, these services are often so busy that athletes cannot be seen promptly, or the services are not sensitive enough to the unique needs and time availability of athletes or to the culture of athletic training and competition. Some colleges have responded to this service gap by hiring full- or part-time sports mental health clinicians or consultants to work for certain teams or to provide general support to athletes from any team. Some of these services focus specifically on athletes with mental health or substance abuse problems, whereas others focus exclusively on performance enhancement (McDuff et al. 2005; Teleander 1994).

Most professional sports teams have access through the medical staff structure to an off-site psychiatric consultant who is available for routine or crisis evaluations and treatment. Although this model of service delivery is the most common, it leads to low service utilization because of logistical barriers to making or keeping appointments and stigma associated with receiving psychiatric care. Most referrals to off-site consultants occur late in the development of a crisis or mental disorder, when performance or relationships have already deteriorated. In addition, these consultant relationships are not usually established to address the more common needs of athletes, such as stress reactions, injury recovery, substance abuse prevention, family crises, or performance slumps.

Some team leaders, who appreciate the mental and emotional aspects of performance, hire on-site consultants with broad skills to establish regular contact with athletes and coaches and expand services over time. The organizations that invest in these on-site, year-round sports psychiatric services usually see utilization soar, satisfaction increase, misconduct decline, and treatment outcomes improve. Typically, off-site psychiatric or psychological consultants will see only 2%–5% of eligible individuals in a year, whereas on-site consultants see 25%–35% for a wide variety of concerns (McDuff et al. 2005). Although it is difficult to demonstrate a direct performance benefit with so many other relevant variables, the services will be valued and continued if utilization and satisfaction are high.

The best models of on-site services in professional sports use interprofessional, culturally competent staffs of psychiatrists, psychologists, employee assistance professionals, and substance abuse counselors who work collaboratively with medical, player development, and pastoral support staffs. Staffing should allow on-site services regularly each week during the competitive season and consistent availability and follow-up during off-season periods. Services can be offered in the training room or in a separate area of the training or competition facility. Although most athletes prefer to be seen at the team's facilities, some, especially if family members are involved, prefer off-site locations. The ideal situation is for one or more of the consulting staff to have off-site offices in the areas where the players and families live. In some cases, home visits are helpful, especially when the focus is on small children with behavioral or developmental concerns.

To work successfully with teams on-site, sports mental health practitioners must have broad diagnostic and therapeutic skills; comfort interacting with sports physicians, athletic trainers, and coaches; and most important, a superior ability to form quick therapeutic alliances in an intense, highly regimented, and unpredictable atmosphere. Practitioners also need to have extensive knowledge about the particular sport, sports culture, league rules and regulations, and the team's organizational structure and function. Another important skill is the ability to develop trust with players, coaches, and front-line medical staff. This trust develops over time with a visible, consistent presence and openness and honesty in work. Although confidentiality is important, trust develops more by word of mouth from one athlete to another or from an athletic trainer or team physician to an athlete. Interestingly, if athletes witness or overhear comfortable and helpful interactions with others in the training room or on the field, they will often seek assistance when the time is right. Therefore, it is essential for mental health practitioners to regularly walk around the key areas of the facility, such as the practice field, lunchroom, locker room, strength area, and training room, and talk with the athletes informally.

In this chapter, the focus is on sports psychiatric work at all levels of an organization using an on-site model. This model involves working with the following entities:

- Athletes, regarding goal setting and improving quality of life
- Team captains, about player concerns and morale
- Medical staff, regarding health promotion, stress control, and mental illness management
- Owners, about shaping corporate culture and policy development
- General managers and scouts, regarding player selection procedures and personnel decisions
- Coaches, regarding team morale, discipline, cohesion, and performance

Discussion and clinical examples for each of these entities are included to illustrate key points and strategies.

Working With Teams

Sports clinicians who provide services to entire teams rather than individual athletes are most active during a season but should be available during the entire calendar year. The focus is variable, depending on whether the work addresses crises, conflicts, or performance enhancement. The most common reasons for team interventions are problems with team morale, cohesion, discipline, or performance. The work opportunity usually starts with a call from a general manager, athletic director, or head coach, and the contact is usually made because of prior work, referral by a colleague, or connection through a practice's Web site (e.g., see www.mdsports.net). After an initial phone conversation, a face-to-face meeting is scheduled for the clinician to meet the coaching staff and learn about their concerns and goals. The clinician can prepare and distribute a set of handouts customized to the team and based on the phone conversation and provide an overview of the clinician's past experiences and capabilities. Even though the focus may be on a crisis or problem, the clinician should reframe it with a positive focus, such as mental skills training (Figure 8–1 provides an overview of these skills). Putting problems into a performance enhancement framework reduces defensiveness and resistance to an organized intervention that may be mandated (Anderson and Aberman 1999; Beswick 2001; DiCicco and Hacker 2002; Lynch 2001; Lynch and Scott 1999).

The next step of working with teams is to meet with the athletes, coaches, and athletic trainers. The purpose of this meeting is to outline the structure and timetable of the intervention, the approach, and the expected outcomes. Usually, the head coach or an assistant athletic director will present an overview, and then the sports psychiatric clinician provides a description of possible strategies for a successful intervention. Preferably, time should be allotted for discussion by team members. If the group is reluctant to talk or ask questions, then the captains or more experienced athletes can be called on directly. Once a few individuals make comments, then open dialogue usually develops. If the intervention originated because of tension between the coaching staff and players, then meeting separately with the athletes is necessary. Once the team meeting has clarified the general areas for improvement, then meeting individually with athletes is helpful. However, for large teams, such as football teams, individual meetings are impractical, and having small group meetings by position is a sensible alternative. Although these smaller meetings are time consuming, individual or position meetings facilitate acceptance of the process and provide critical information on the team's strengths and weaknesses. Additionally, any life- or performance-related issues that individual athletes identify serve as a basis for concurrent individual work.

After the individual meeting(s), the clinician holds a follow-up meeting with the coaches and the team captains to give feedback and clearly outline the goals and action steps in the process. This meeting provides an opportunity for modifying the plan to ensure that it is practical and

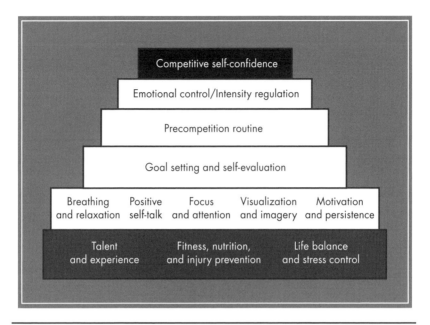

FIGURE 8-1. Pyramid of mental skills linking athletic fundamentals to competitive self-confidence.

has a likelihood of success. The meeting is also important for developing outcome goals, such as improved morale, compliance with team rules, or changes in performance, that are measured at the beginning, middle, and end of the intervention. When working with teams, the clinician needs to attend practices and games. Because practice is where the team becomes ready to play and builds confidence, the clinician's observations of practice length, organization, intensity, attitude, and energy are important. In addition, the time during practice provides an opportunity to briefly interact with resting or injured players, and the time after practice provides additional opportunity for in-depth talks with coaches or players. Attendance at games is important for the clinician to observe the pre-game routine; the team's reactions to success and adversity; the manner in which practice tactics and techniques are applied during competition; and the team's intensity level, communication, adjustments, and consistency. Riding on the team bus or plane or attending team meals provides an additional opportunity to assess team members' attitudes, values, interactive patterns, and confidence. In fact, road trips present the best opportunity for the clinician to do individual or small group work because of available time and fewer distractions.

Some teams benefit from learning formally about the characteristics of successful teams. In a simple and well-received model, Lencioni (2005) identifies five important characteristics (and supporting strategies):

1. Build trust (e.g., admit mistakes, offer feedback, accept apologies, ask for help)
2. Engage in conflict (e.g., have lively meetings, use everyone's ideas, minimize drama, examine mistakes, resolve core problems efficiently)
3. Commit fully to a common purpose (e.g., identify core values, find common goals, change direction, identify opportunities for group learning)
4. Hold one another accountable (e.g., put pressure on poor performers, hold everyone to the same standards, deal with rule violations decisively, question each other's approaches)
5. Focus on collective results (e.g., find success-oriented players and staff, reward group behavior, share the adversity and emotions of competition, emphasize team strategy and intensity)

By going over each of these characteristics and strategies as a blueprint for success, teams can learn to achieve and have fun along the way.

Case Study: This Team Has No Leadership

A new Division III college basketball coach became frustrated with her team's play during the first few games of the season after two disappointing losses to weaker opponents. She voiced her concern to the athletic director, who suggested that she contact the sports psychiatrist who had worked with a number of the college's other teams. In the meeting with the sports psychiatrist, the coach voiced concern about the team's laziness in practice and failure to execute the new offensive and defensive schemes that she and her new staff had installed. She was especially disappointed in the team's poor rebounding and point guard play. She had tried several players at point guard, but none had showed any leadership potential. She felt that the team was divided into subgroups that did not get along and that there were two players who did not respect her authority and were negatively influencing other players. She was getting numerous reports that team members were missing classes and study halls, and overall their grades were poor. Because she had not recruited any of the players, she had already written off the year and said she would need to recruit better players in the future. She had been hired to turn around a program that had been in decline for 5 years and was upset that she would need to wait a whole year to get that process going. When asked who the captains were, she said that none had been named because no one had impressed her.

Intervention: Because the athletic director had already agreed to fund the sports psychiatrist to work with the team for the remainder of the season, the coach was open to any assistance. Individual meetings were set up with the psychiatrist and each player, the assistant coaches, and the athletic trainer. Each individual was asked to name three strengths and three weaknesses of the team and to make suggestions for improvement. In addition, each player was asked to identify one aspect about her defensive and offensive play to improve during the year and to create three action steps for each. In addition, all players were asked who should be named team captain. Regarding the team's strengths, the most common responses were athleticism, good shooting, defensive intensity, and unity if the divisions in the team could be dissolved. For weaknesses, everyone agreed that there was no court leadership, too much dissension and disrespect, and poor rebounding. Because the team had only two seniors and one had been a starter last year, they were the logical captains. Reluctantly, the coach agreed and approached the two players. One, a point guard, was reluctant to be a captain because her minutes had been cut. The other, a center, was reluctant because her confidence was at an all-time low. They both agreed, however, to accept their new role, and weekly meetings with the sports psychiatrist were scheduled.

The sports psychiatrist began attending two practices each week and met regularly with individual players after practice to work on their individual goals. Out of several team discussions, two areas were selected for intense focus: 1) movement off the ball and 2) rebounding with heart. After a few weeks, the senior leadership felt more empowered to influence practice intensity. The confidence of both players soared, and their improved play began to spread to other players. The coach was able to relax at practice and let her assistants and the captains assume more responsibility. The half-time reviews became much more inclusive, and the players felt that their opinions were valued because each player was asked to make at least one observation. Over the next few games, the team was transformed. By the time conference play began, team members were playing with consistent intensity and their rebounding statistics had soared. Review of game film showed the players moving well off the ball and therefore getting easier, uncontested shots. The team finished the season with six conference wins and made it to the finals of the conference tournament, where they lost in overtime. Because of their good overall conference record and strong finish, they were selected for postseason play. They won their first two games, including an upset victory over a perennial elite program. They lost in the third round but felt proud of their hard work and success. This led to successful recruitment for the following year, and the team became the conference champion with three first-year players as starters.

Case Study: What Could Go Wrong Did Go Wrong

The athletic director of a medium-size Division I college asked for a sports psychiatric consultation for the baseball team after several members of the team complained to an assistant athletic director that the attitude and style of the coaching staff was so negative that they had lost the respect of the team. The sports psychiatrist met with the coaching staff as a group and asked what their sense of the situation was. They had lost many close games the previous year, and team members had more injuries than in recent memory. In addition, they had repeated problems with accessing their off-campus practice facility, which was undergoing renovation. They felt that these issues had taken a toll on the team's confidence and led to the adoption of a negative and defeatist attitude.

Intervention: The sports psychiatrist suggested that the coaching staff and athletic director create a positive focus by offering mental skills training for each player. In addition, the clinician, who had experience with professional teams, agreed to attend practices weekly and travel with the team to away games at least once a month. The head coach introduced the consultant to the team at a prearranged off-campus dinner. A brief presentation was given on team strategies for improving play and on basic and advanced mental skills. The team seemed excited by the addition of the psychiatrist, especially because several players hoped to be drafted and play professionally. An individual meeting was set up with each player to establish a team goal and individual goals with action steps. The team decided that its team goal should be to "prepare like champions" and to move on from last season's poor performance. Each player enthusiastically identified areas for individual improvement and developed written action steps to reach her goals. After each practice attended by the sports psychiatrist, a number of players would stay around asking questions about major league players' routines and approaches to the game. In addition, they were open to changing their commitment to academics, lifting, nutrition, and practice. After a month, the coaching staff noticed a marked change in team attitude, and problems with lateness and pessimism over the previous year's performance disappeared. The team started to believe that they could compete with any team in their conference, especially because they had several experienced pitchers who were having early success. Even though the team finished below .500 for conference play, they won more conference games than in any of the past three seasons, and most of their games with better teams had close scores, with losses occurring in late innings. The following season, a new enthusiastic assistant coach was added and several high-profile recruits were signed, making a young team even more confident and ready to play.

Case Study: We Have Too Many Personality Conflicts on Our Team

The head coach of a women's college lacrosse team asked for a sports psychiatric consultation for her team just before the beginning of the regular season. She wanted the team captains to meet and share their views about several players who were constantly introducing unhelpful drama into the team. The two captains identified two players whom they described as overly sensitive to criticism and perceived slights by others. When offended, they would lash out at after-practice gatherings or parties and send ripples of emotion and tension through the entire team. One of the players would also drink too much and then get angry and sometimes despondent. She had been unable to play for a few weeks because of postconcussive symptoms. A few times when drinking, she got so despondent that she took extra pain pills and once mentioned suicide. In these instances, she stayed with other team members who felt she needed constant watching.

Intervention: The team captains thought that individual meetings with all team members to talk about team goals and unity would be useful. They also suggested that barriers to team morale and cohesion be identified and presented at a players-only meeting. Thirty-minute individual meetings were scheduled over a 2-day period. The psychiatrist oriented each player to the purpose of the meeting by saying that the coaches and captains had asked for a team-building consultation. Each player was asked to cite two strengths of the team and to identify any current barriers to team unity. All players felt that the team had enough talent and commitment to compete at the highest level of their conference, but that players were distracted by too much off-campus team drama. A few said they were very worried about the injured player and felt that she needed mental health treatment. The two players identified as introducing tension and drama both felt that they were not liked by the coaches or most members of the team. The injured player opened up about past and current depression and insomnia that she linked to recurrent head injuries. She also acknowledged too many heavy drinking nights and was interested in assistance to change. At a players-only team meeting, the psychiatrist introduced Lencioni's model of successful teams (see the list presented earlier in this chapter). A lively 75-minute discussion occurred, and monthly follow-up meetings were suggested to the head coach and approved. The injured player was seen individually on a weekly basis for stress control therapy, and extended-release venlafaxine was started and the dosage ultimately raised to 150 mg/day. In addition, topiramate was added and raised to 100 mg/day for persistent headaches and mood stabilization. Although the injured player improved over the next month, she elected not to return to play out of concern for recurrent concussions. The team focused on building trust and communication and ensuring intense practices as preparation for competition. They played well all season and were able to avoid the interpersonal distractions that existed preseason.

Case Study: We Need Some Team Goals to Move to the Next Level

Members of an elite travel soccer team of girls under age 16 were frustrated that the team could not win tournaments or the state cup. The team had advanced to the semifinals or finals of large tournaments and had been state cup runners-up several times but just could not get to the next level. Several parents approached the head coach and asked if she thought that a team building process centered on goal setting might help the team improve and facilitate the integration of several new players. The team had been together for 8 years but seemed to have plateaued in the last two seasons. The coach readily agreed, and a sports psychiatric consultation was requested.

Intervention: The sports psychiatrist first met with the head coach and assistant coach and asked for areas for improvement. They identified the following as keys to more success: confidence in the attacking third of the field, consistent intensity and effort, defending by the midfielders, and stronger play in the air. Next, the psychiatrist met with the two captains, who echoed what the coaches had suggested but also added that the team needed to have more commitment and courage in the box, get more numbers in the attack, win more second balls, and play faster. The captains then called a brainstorming meeting with the team and listed the team's core values and additional process goals (Table 8–1). Then, an analysis of the team statistics was done for presentation at a second meeting. Based on these statistics, different specific outcome goals for the attack and defense were set (see Table 8–1). The sports psychiatrist was asked to take the input and come up with a final team document.

As a result of the goal-setting meetings and with the addition of some new players who brought additional depth and versatility, the practices became more competitive and intense. This intensity flowed over into fall league games and tournaments, and the team had much success. The team finished the highest ever (second) in their league and won a big tournament, upsetting a team they had never previously beaten. In the spring, they continued their commitment to steady improvement and again came in second in league play and for the first time ever won the state cup and went on to regional play. By focusing on the specific process goals that they had identified, the scoring and defending outcomes fell into place.

Working With Medical Staff and Athletic Trainers

A team's medical staff is the front line for injury and illness prevention and rehabilitation and for the identification of stress, risky behaviors, and early signs of problems with anxiety, depression, anger, insomnia, energy, attention, and confidence. The staff usually consists of physicians, dentists, chiropractors, podiatrists, dieticians, and athletic trainers. Physician groups for professional and college teams usually comprise team physicians (primary care sports medicine physicians and sports orthopedists) and consulting physicians. The team's physicians and athletic trainers have a regular presence at the training facility and usually travel with the team. The consulting physicians, who typically have off-site offices, include hand, foot and ankle, and spine surgeons; ophthalmologists; and neurologists. The chiropractors usually visit several times each week to deliver services to players in the training room and, depending on the sport, often travel with the team. The athletic trainers have the most contact with the athletes and, at professional and collegiate levels, are present all day at practices, games, and in the training room providing assessments and treatments.

The athletic trainers are usually the most aware of team members' stress, substance issues, and other personal problems and, because of the

TABLE 8–1. Soccer travel team goals

Main goal: Become state champions and compete well at tournaments and regionals

Core values	
Embrace the program	Championship mentality
Embrace each other	Create our opportunities
Industrious work ethic	Responsible
Trustworthy	Dependable

Process goals: how we play	
Attack: "Let the ball move"	**Defending: "Secure the ball"**
Work rate	Communication
Speed of play	Transition
Numbers in the attack	Physical play
Switch the point of attack	Pressure on the ball
Patterned attack	1 vs. 1 defending
Courage in the box	Maintain our shape
Ball movement	Possession
Win second balls	Cover/balance
Attacking half possession	Hard tackling
Play in the air	Disrupt opponent's flow
Pressure in the box	
Creativity	

Outcome goals: the results	
Attack: "Help each other"	**Defending: "Support and encourage"**
Goals (3 per game)	Goals allowed (1 per game)
Assists (2 per game)	Corner kicks allowed (4 per game)
Shots (15 per game)	Saves (8 per game)
Corner kicks (6 per game)	Shutouts (10 per season)
Opponent's saves (5 per game)	

trust they build with the athletes, are good facilitators of a connection to an on-site sports psychiatrist or other mental health provider. During the season, an active sports psychiatrist has near-daily contact with the head athletic trainer if the scope of psychiatric practice is broad and includes stress, substance issues, mental disorders, and pain management. Experienced athletic trainers usually ask sports psychiatrists to make contact

informally with athletes in the training room or at practice before sched-
uling formal, individual evaluations. Players typically trust athletic trainers more than any other provider, and players are more likely to use
psychiatric services if they see regular collaboration between psychiatry
and medical staff members. Contact between sports psychiatrists and
team physicians usually takes place in the training or examination room
and involves active dialogue in front of the athlete. If the issues are too
sensitive or personal to be addressed with a collaborative discussion, then
a separate evaluation is scheduled. In addition to after-practice interactions, team physicians and sports psychiatrists should have regular review
meetings of the entire team. In professional football, for example, a
weekly meeting might occur on Monday to review the entire roster, focusing on previously or newly injured players and those being followed for
psychiatric or performance concerns. This systematic review is needed in
football because of the large size of the team and the fact that 20–30 players are being followed throughout the season.

Documentation of sports psychiatric treatment in an athlete's medical record is another important way of integrating treatment with the
medical staff. Whether an electronic record or a standard paper chart is
used, a special section can usually be set aside for psychiatric evaluations,
medications, and follow-up meetings. Most importantly, psychiatric medications need to be documented in a way that all practitioners can easily
view all of an athlete's current medications. In addition to containing
evaluations and follow-up notes, records may also include mental health
screening tools (e.g., Appendix 8–1), as well as important letters related
to therapeutic use exemptions for banned substances or letters involving
legal matters. Usually, mental health screening is done during an athlete's preseason physical or right after a new player is signed. This screening allows for early detection of common problems like insomnia, stress,
or anxiety, and for an orientation to available support and services. Therapeutic use exemption letters are placed in the medical record, but communications to courts are kept in a separate mental health or substance
treatment record at the psychiatrist's office. Another good way for mental health clinicians to stay connected with the medical staff is to keep a
clinical database and produce regular (usually quarterly) and annual reports that detail the utilization rate, volume of service, and reasons for
interventions. These documents serve to educate the staff about the
broad scope of services and trends over time.

Case Study: Will I Ever Play Again?

A professional soccer player sustained a severe head injury in a car accident during the off-season. She was hospitalized and unconscious for

3 days because of a right temporal lobe contusion and skull fracture. She had no seizure or intracranial bleeding. She remained in the hospital for 2 weeks before being transferred to a rehabilitation facility to address her residual dizziness, poor balance, headaches, and difficulty hearing. She was prescribed topiramate 100 mg/day for her headaches, and for a while she took low-dose quetiapine for agitation and sleep. Her speech, gross motor functioning, and working memory were normal, but she did not remember anything before, during, or after the accident. While in the re-habilitation facility, she repeatedly asked the doctors and her parents if they thought she could play soccer again. After 2 weeks in the hospital, she returned to her apartment and rejoined the team for further assess-ment and treatment.

Intervention: The head team physician, head athletic trainer, team psychiatrist, and consulting neurologist met to review the acute care and rehabilitation hospital's discharge summaries and the recommended re-habilitation plan. The player then met individually with the team physi-cian, psychiatrist, and neurology consultant. Her main problems were balance while standing, which was made worse with her eyes closed or with rapid stepping and turning. The partial hearing loss in her right ear had resolved. Other coordinated movements were normal, but she had difficulty with convergent eye movements. A 3-day-a-week rehabilitation protocol at the local hospital was created, and she spent the other 2 days at the team's training facility working on regaining balance, strength, and cardiovascular fitness. In addition to the head injury, the player had a long history of attention-deficit disorder, inattentive type, which had been treated with long-acting methylphenidate. This drug had been stopped while she was in the hospital but was restarted and titrated back up from 18 mg/day to 36 mg/day over 2 weeks. Sleep was normal, but her overall energy was decreased. She was very discouraged and felt guilty about the accident when she learned that she had run a red light and was speeding. No alcohol or drugs were involved, however. Weekly meetings with the psychiatrist were held to address her concerns and facilitate her recovery.

Over the next 3 months, the team physician, psychiatrist, and athletic trainer met weekly to review the player's progress. Written progress re-ports were received twice monthly from the outpatient rehabilitation pro-gram. Although the player made steady progress, she was not ready to play when the season began. She attended practices and team meetings, but did not travel. She made steady progress and eventually returned to on-field training with the soccer ball, but was withheld from contact drills and scrimmages. Her balance steadily improved, and near the end of the sea-son, she was assessed for agility and speed by the strength and condition-ing coach and for soccer skills by the coaching staff. She received high marks on these assessments, and she was sent for a final neurological re-view before being cleared for full practice. The neurologist noted that the player had made a full recovery, and a repeat magnetic resonance imaging scan showed resolution of the cerebral contusion. She was sent for a sec-ond opinion to a specialist in sports head injuries, who agreed with the team neurologist that she could return to play but with a somewhat higher likelihood of concussion. The player discussed her injury and recovery with her parents and the team psychiatrist and decided to return to practice and competition if all went well. Although she had no prior sports or soccer concussions, she elected to wear head protection at first. After 3 weeks of full practice, she felt confident with her fitness and soccer skills and looked forward to her off-season training and play for next year.

Case Study: He May Be at the End of His Career if He Can't Get Over His Pain and Anxiety

A midcareer, recently signed free-agent professional football player had off-season surgery for a torn labrum on his right shoulder. The tear resulted from an anterior shoulder dislocation late in the preceding season. He returned to training camp fully rehabilitated and eager to compete. Two weeks into camp, he started to have right shoulder pain and tightness similar to what he had experienced the prior year. He became convinced that he had retorn his labrum or that he had loose bodies in the joint. Unfortunately, the player had experienced the same injury to the opposite shoulder in training camp for another team 2 years before and had missed an entire season.

The player was evaluated by the team's primary care sports medicine physician, team orthopedist, head athletic trainer, and chiropractor, who agreed that he had good shoulder stability, strength, sensation, and range of motion without catching, but that his shoulder muscles were tight and he consistently guarded with certain movements. Because he was convinced he had retorn his labrum, a magnetic resonance arthrogram (MRA) was done. When this test did not show any tears or loose bodies, the player was pulled from practice, administered anti-inflammatory medications and muscle relaxants, and given local treatments. Each time he attempted to return to practice, however, his pain levels and apprehension increased. The entire medical team felt that emotions and stress were affecting his pain experience, and they requested a psychiatric evaluation. The player described to the sports psychiatrist an injury-plagued career and indicated that he had grown weary of surgery and rehabilitation. He was frustrated that his talent had never been allowed to develop on the field, although when he did play, he was an impact player on offense. He became upset and tearful when describing his career. In addition, he noted chronic stress from a separation and divorce 2 years earlier and ongoing struggles with child support and visitation time. He became very sad when discussing the separation from his 4-year-old son. He had seen a therapist with the previous team but had not been open to any medication even though it had been suggested. When contacted, the prior therapist said he felt that the player had high levels of anxiety, resentment, and depression that were affecting his healing and that he had a very strong reluctance to take any psychiatric medications.

Intervention: A medical team meeting was held that included the team's primary care and orthopedic physicians, athletic trainer, and team psychiatrist. The player's anti-inflammatory medications were continued, but his muscle relaxant was changed from cyclobenzaprine 10 mg at bedtime to diazepam 5 mg twice daily to help with his worrying and apprehension. In addition, he was scheduled to see the chiropractor three times weekly to work on alignment and muscle release and reconditioning. The team physician agreed to go over his recent MRA and compare it to his postoperative one, and the athletic trainer worked with the athlete on muscle strength, flexibility, and soreness. After several long conversations with the team psychiatrist, the player reluctantly agreed to a trial of low-dose sertraline to target his anxiety, frustration, and obsessive thinking. The providers shared their weekly updates. Over the next few weeks, the player steadily improved. He seemed pleased with his multifaceted approach and appreciated that his providers were regularly communicating. He began to open up in his weekly psychiatric meetings about his off-the-field stressors, and some solutions for these were identified. By the end of training camp, he was at full speed and no longer complaining of pain or muscle tightness.

Working With Owners, General Managers, and Coaches

Some owners and general managers of professional teams and athletic directors of colleges have a visible presence at practices and games, but others do not. Over time in sports practice, psychiatrists will work with some leaders who want little involvement with mental health and substance services and others who seem more comfortable with regular contact. Most sports team leaders understand that regular involvement with sports psychiatry could introduce in them a bias for personnel decisions or create the perception among athletes that confidentiality for mental health meetings is variable or absent. Whether leaders are on one end of the involvement spectrum or the other, they need to get written or verbal summaries from the director of medical services (usually the head team physician or athletic trainer) on utilization rates, range of services, athlete satisfaction, and return-to-play and performance effects. Occasionally, athletes or coaches with good outcomes will directly let an owner or general manager know of the helpfulness of on-site sports psychiatric services. These types of testimonials should not be solicited by mental health providers but do have tremendous impact on a leader's view of the value of these services.

Coaches vary in their experiences and interactions with sports psychiatric or mental skills services. Some coaches may have a view that too much emphasis on personal problems can detract from a needed focus on training and competition. Many coaches have worked with athletes who, for example, have gotten into trouble, struggled with anxiety or depression, or developed a performance slump; however, few coaches have had prior involvement with on-site psychiatric services that are integrated with medical staff services and training. At first, coaches may view the services as a distraction, but over time and with the support of key medical staff, the coaches will come to appreciate the value-added impact of sports psychiatry.

With the athlete's permission, direct work between a sports psychiatrist and assistant or position coaches can be extremely helpful. For example, when a player is struggling with return from an injury or has a learning style that makes mastering plays or strategy more difficult, he or she may ask the sports psychiatrist to explain the nature of the struggle to the coach so that collaborative and expanded approaches can be developed.

Interacting with a head coach about individual players is more difficult, however. Because head coaches are involved in personnel decisions and playing time, they may develop subtle biases against players with emotional or behavioral problems. Even if a bias does not develop, athletes are more sensitive to information being shared with the head coach than they are with their position coach or an assistant coach in whom they have usually confided. Because each organization and coach has a specific culture and style, information sharing must be considered on a case-by-case basis. Generally, an effective approach is for a sports psychiatrist to share information with the lead medical staff, who then relay it to the head coach. Direct communication with the head coach is often warranted, however, in complicated cases that involve 1) legal trouble or mental illness that affects practice or game availability, or 2) medications that temporarily affect alertness or movements. This communication will often take place in a special meeting involving the team psychiatrist, general manager, athletic director, head coach, and head team physician.

Case Study: He Can't Keep Getting in Trouble Like This

Over three seasons, a veteran professional basketball player had repeated alcohol-related incidents that seemed to be getting more frequent and serious. After two additional incidents in a 3-week period, a meeting was called involving the owner, general manager, manager, head team physician, and team psychiatrist to develop a strategy to get the player the assistance he needed. Over the past 2 years, the player had several evaluations and outpatient treatment plans but was only partially compliant. The league's collective bargaining agreement did not specifically address problems with alcohol, so the team had to determine the appropriate action. Before the meeting, the team psychiatrist reviewed the protected health information release that was signed by the player and searched the player's contract for clauses that might provide some leverage for getting him to be more serious about change and treatment. Finally, with the player's permission, the psychiatrist contacted his agent, baseball mentor, and family and recorded their perspectives; all of them expressed concern about the player's heavy drinking, impulsiveness, and aggression, and agreed to have their views shared with the player and the organization.

Intervention: At the meeting, the general manager and manager presented an overview of the case to the owner. The team psychiatrist, within the limits of the player's signed release, discussed past treatment and current assessment and recommendations. The contract review did reveal several specific references to patterns of misconduct and a requirement to maintain good fitness and health, and the group decided to discuss these points with the player and take progressive disciplinary action if needed. The following day, the psychiatrist visited the player in the locker room to discuss the player's version of the last two incidents. The player agreed that his drinking had become a problem and was open to doing more about it. He seemed surprised, however, to learn that his father, aunt, sister, agent, and long-time mentor had all been concerned about his drinking and aggression since his college days. He was also informed about and shown the specific clauses in his contract that addressed his pattern of behavior and was told that the team was prepared to fine him or suspend him if he did not follow through with a revised treatment plan. With this leverage and with the encouragement of his agent and mentor, he agreed to begin intensive outpatient treatment 3 days a week and to see the team's substance abuse counselor once weekly and speak by phone an additional time each week. He also agreed to abstain completely from all alcohol, improve his health and fitness, and begin taking disulfiram daily. Over the next 3 months, he complied with all the requirements of his treatment plan and remained abstinent. His fitness and nutrition improved dramatically, and he lost 20 pounds. These changes led to a dramatic increase in his performance and self-confidence. By the end of the season, he continued to do well and agreed to stay in town during the off-season to train and continue his treatment. A year later, he and his agent expressed thanks to the organization that he had been forced to do the right thing.

Case Study: He May Need to Be Suspended for the Rest of the Season

A fifth-year starting college football defensive player was called to the head coach's office in the summer before his final year after another player reported seeing him pull out a pistol at an off-campus party. The player told the head coach that he had gone to the party and shortly after his arrival was confronted by several nonstudents who accused him of hitting their car and cracking their windshield. Even when he told them he had not done this, they followed him and his girlfriend to his car and would not let them leave. At that point, he felt threatened and showed them an unloaded pistol so they would leave. This player had a history of repeated off-campus incidents that seemed to correlate with periods of injury that prevented him from practicing or playing. He was a good student and did not drink, but always seemed to be either angry or depressed. The head coach knew that the player had grown up without a father figure and seemed to carry much resentment because his mother had to raise him and his two siblings without assistance. The head coach called the team psychiatrist and asked for an evaluation.

Intervention: The player told the psychiatrist the same story he had related to the head coach, and collateral contact with the player's girlfriend confirmed this. He expressed disappointment with his college career, feeling that injuries had blocked him from achieving athletically as he thought he might. He began having recurrent right knee pain with the start of preseason practice and was worried that he might miss the opportunity to start during his senior year. When asked about the weapon, he said it was not his and he knew that what he had done was risky and serious. He agreed to return the weapon to his friend. He also agreed with the head coach's assessment that he was carrying resentment from his youth and that his anger and moodiness were related to that and his frustrations with his injuries. He agreed to meet with the psychiatrist weekly through the remainder of the season to develop alternative strategies to manage his emotions and to improve his mental toughness. He also agreed that given the seriousness of the incident, the psychiatrist could give feedback to the head coach and athletic director. The next morning, the psychiatrist met with the athletic director alone to discuss the plan to see the player regularly and for the player to return the weapon. The psychiatrist assured the athletic director that the player was not at risk for self-harm or a risk to others. After thinking it over for a day, the athletic director approved the plan and did not feel that the player needed to be disciplined as long as he continued his treatment. The player saw the psychiatrist weekly for the rest of the season. He won a starting job but late in the season suffered a serious concussion that did not allow him to return to play. He felt proud of his accomplishments, however, and ended up graduating on time with a 3.5 grade-point average.

Conclusion

If on-site sports psychiatric services are provided to teams at practices or before games, utilization rates by players and coaches rise over time. The regular availability of sports practitioners at team facilities helps build trust with players and accelerates the development of functional working relationships with team leadership and medical staff. As a result, most player-clinician contacts result from the clinician walking around team training rooms and practices or from referrals by the athletic trainer or team physician. Because many of the interactions take place in open areas, other players may overhear or even become involved in discussions, especially when the topics are injury, pain control, sleep, or performance. Making services available in the athletes' training and treatment home appears to increase their comfort with personal discussions.

Most of the time, strong boundaries are kept between the sports psychiatrist and the team owner, general manager, and head coach. The head team physician is usually designated as the one member of the medical staff to relay all pertinent medical and psychiatric information to team leaders. This arrangement allows the team psychiatrist to focus mainly on services to players and coaches while providing confidentiality and privacy, to the extent possible.

Key Clinical Points

- Typical team interventions are designed to 1) improve team morale, cohesion, and performance; 2) resolve conflicts between coaches and players; 3) address a negative public relations event; or 4) establish assistance services for athletes and team staff on an ongoing basis.

- Initial opportunities for team consultation arise during crises, such as 1) an unexpected or sustained poor performance, 2) a serious incident or pattern of athlete misconduct, 3) an overt player-coach conflict, 4) a tragedy such as an accidental or unexpected death, or 5) a serious mental illness in an athlete or coach.

- According to Lencioni's (2005) model, a successful team 1) builds trust, 2) engages in conflict, 3) commits fully to a common purpose, 4) holds one another accountable, and 5) focuses on collective results. This model is simple, is well received, and can be used to create initial dialogue with team members (see the list in the section "Working With Teams").

- The team physician and athletic trainers are the front line for injury and illness prevention and rehabilitation and for the identification of stress, risky behaviors, and early signs of problems with anxiety, depression, anger, insomnia, energy, attention, self-harm, and confidence. The sports psychiatrist's on-site presence in the training room facilitates integrated treatment. Symptom screening can be formally done during an athlete's preseason physical (e.g., using a form similar to that presented in Appendix 8–1).

- The head team physician is usually designated as the one member of the medical staff to relay all pertinent medical and psychiatric information to owners and other team leaders. This allows the team psychiatrist to focus mainly on services to players and coaches while providing confidentiality and privacy. An on-site model for services results in increased utilization rates after a few years.

References

Anderson J, Aberman R: Why Good Coaches Quit and How You Can Stay in the Game. Minneapolis, MN, Fairview Press, 1999

Beswick B: Focused for Soccer: Develop a Winning Mental Approach. Champaign, IL, Human Kinetics, 2001

DiCicco T, Hacker C: Catch Them Being Good. New York, Penguin, 2002

Lencioni PL: Overcoming the Five Dysfunctions of a Team: A Field Guide for Leaders, Managers, and Facilitators. San Francisco, CA, Jossey-Bass, 2005

Lynch J: Creative Coaching: New Ways to Maximize Athlete and Team Potential in All Sports. Champaign, IL, Human Kinetics, 2001

Lynch J, Scott W: Running Within: A Guide to Mastering the Body-Mind-Spirit Connection for Ultimate Training and Racing. Champaign, IL, Human Kinetics, 1999

McDuff DR, Morse E, White R: Professional and collegiate team assistance programs: services and utilization patterns. Clin Sports Med 24:943–958, 2005

Shapiro RM, Jankowski MA, Dale J: The Power of Nice: How to Negotiate so That Everyone Wins—Especially You. New York, Wiley, 2001

Teleander R: From Red Ink to Roses: The Transformation of a Big Ten Program. New York, Simon & Schuster, 1994

Symptom Screening Form

Name:_____

Date:_____

Date of birth:_____

Many players on our team have symptoms or concerns that have interfered or will interfere with sports, relationships, or happiness. Place a mark (X) in the box to the right of each question to show how much each question has bothered or has been bothering you in the past 12 months.

	0 Not at all	1 Some- times	2 Often	3 A lot
Depression				
1. Have you been feeling sad, disappointed, or upset?				
2. Does your future seem bleak or hopeless?				
3. Do you feel worthless or inferior to others?				
4. Have you lost interest in activities you used to enjoy?				
5. Do you feel that life is not worth living?				
Anxiety				
6. Do you feel nervous or shaky inside?				
7. Do you feel tense, keyed up, or restless?				
8. Do you worry a lot or feel afraid?				
9. Do you have physical stress such as tense muscles, headaches, shortness of breath, or upset stomach?				

	0 Not at all	1 Some-times	2 Often	3 A lot
Sleep				
10. Do you have trouble falling asleep or staying asleep?				
11. Do you have excessive daytime sleepiness?				
12. Do you snore loudly or have pauses in your breathing?				
Anger				
13. Do you get easily frustrated or irritated?				
14. Do you lose your temper?				
15. Do you worry that you may break things or fight?				
Eating				
16. Do you need a special diet?				
17. Do you skip meals?				
18. Do you binge eat and later regret it?				
19. Do you struggle to lose weight?				
20. Do you use energy drinks, liquids, or supplements?				
21. Do you struggle to maintain weight?				
Mood				
22. Do you have mood swings?				
23. Do your thoughts race, or is your mind too active?				
24. Does anyone tell you that you talk too quickly or loudly?				
25. Do you do things that others think are risky or foolish?				
26. Are there times when you don't sleep but don't need it?				

	0 Not at all	1 Some- times	2 Often	3 A lot
Pain				
27. Do you have chronic pain that interferes with your sport, sleep, relaxation, or relationships?				
28. Do you take medications for chronic pain that worry you?				
Substances				
29. Have you thought you needed to cut down on alcohol?				
30. Have you thought you needed to cut down on tobacco?				
31. Have you used medications not prescribed for you or in ways not prescribed (e.g., pain meds for energy)?				
32. Have you thought you needed help for drug use?				
Attention				
33. Do you have trouble paying attention or with distractions?				
34. Do you have problems getting organized or finishing tasks?				
35. Do you feel overly active or compelled to move around like you were driven by a motor?				
36. Do you have problems learning or remembering?				

Chapter 9

Developmental and Cultural Competence

Sports mental health providers who work with individuals and teams need comfort and skill in dealing with athletes across broad age ranges. In a typical office practice, a clinician might be asked to see, for example, 1) middle school gymnasts, wrestlers, and swimmers; 2) high school swimmers, runners, and soccer, lacrosse, and basketball players; 3) college soccer, football, lacrosse, and basketball players; and 4) professional golfers, tennis players, and triathletes. Therefore, knowledge of key developmental issues in the context of sports across a life span from early adolescence to midlife is critical.

In addition to being comfortable working with athletes of different ages and developmental levels, sports clinicians need cultural competence in diverse areas. If a clinician's work spans the full range of competitive levels from youth club to professional, then comfort and skill in working with people of different genders, ethnicities, sexual orientations, geographic regions, religions, values, philosophies, and politics are important. For example, clinicians working with college and professional team sports will see athletes born both in the United States and in foreign countries, representing diverse cultures from Australia, Canada, Eastern and Western Europe, the Middle East, the Pacific Islands, Continental Africa, Latin America, and Asia. A typical professional sports team in the United States will have players representing rural, suburban, and urban locations, as well as multiple regions and states of the country. Athletes affiliate with a variety of religions, including Christianity, Judaism, Islam, Buddhism, Hinduism, Mormonism, and atheism. Athletes also represent all sexual orientations, including gay, lesbian, straight, bisexual, and transgender. Any of these differences has the potential to create tension or division within a team, between a coach and his or her players, or between the clinician and the athlete. Clinicians who have lived, traveled, or been exposed in other ways to the diverse dimensions of various cultures and clinicians who speak or understand other languages typically have greater cultural competence than those with less varied cultural experiences.

One good way to understand and bridge the differences that naturally occur among the players, coaches, and staff of any team is to have a definition and model of culture that incorporates and explains these differences. A practical definition of *culture* for use in sports suggests that each group of people can be described or characterized by a set of beliefs, attitudes, and values; formal expressions, such as art, religion, or literature; and popular expressions, such as music, food, dance, and traditions. Individual athletes should be viewed in the broader context of their cultural group and life story rather than according to obvious differences, such as language, race, skin color, religion, or sexual orientation. Even generational differences can represent subcultural or cultural differences and may affect lack of team unity or a sense of disconnection with a particular athlete. Descriptive terms, such as the Baby Boomers (Me Generation), Generation X, Generation Y (Millennials), and the Cyber Generation, are used to characterize the distinct cultural differences that develop across generations. The critical task for sports clinicians, therefore, is to be curious and outgoing, with a specific intent to become more informed about the different cultural groups represented on a team or the specific cultural set of an individual athlete. This effort requires active solicitation of unknown aspects of cultural groups that are encountered in different clinical or consultative settings.

In this chapter, I focus on the competencies needed by sports mental health clinicians to work effectively with athletes in youth sports, athletes of different genders and sexual identities, and athletes from various cultural groups. I discuss the common and critical issues encountered in clinical practice and present case studies to serve as a foundation for attitude formation and skill development in this area.

Youth Sports

As mentioned in the introduction to this book, youth sports participation rates have risen steadily since the 1990s. Surprisingly, childhood obesity rates and sedentary lifestyles have also increased over roughly the same time period. Although the increased participation in sports seems to logically flow from America's endorsement of sports branding, athletic competition and notoriety, and the importance of winning as a central part of the culture, Americans have an equally strong fascination with fast foods and the digital worlds of fiber-optic and satellite television, gaming, the Internet, texting, and cyber networking, which are characterized by low activity, high-calorie consumption, late nights, and reduced sleep, energy, and productivity. Too often by age 12 or 13, American boys and girls have dropped sports or regular fitness routines in favor of digital marathons. In addition, many U.S. schools have replaced physical educa-tion with academic enrichment in the curriculum. Although these two polar-opposite lifestyle choices are certainly not mutually exclusive, they do seem to be battling for supremacy in American culture.

In addition to childhood obesity and inactivity as problems in Amer-ican society, sports injury and burnout are issues of concern. Although sports participation is generally viewed more positively for its ability to promote socialization, commitment, responsibility, teamwork, organiza-tion, goal achievement, leadership, independence, efficiency, mental and physical health, and positive self-esteem and confidence (Bortoli et al. 2011), participation is also associated with a growing set of negatives. These negatives include overtraining, disordered eating, social isolation, immaturity, entitlement, aggression, early sexual activity, high stress, competitive failure, parent-coach and parent-child conflict, and damage to self-esteem and confidence (Brink et al. 2010; Fields et al. 2010; Habel et al. 2010). These negatives often result from a trend in the United States toward early single-sport specialization (Malina 2010), early expo-sure to ultracompetitive teams that emphasize winning, year-round train-ing, parental achievement by proxy (Tofler et al. 2005), and a lack of recognition of the importance of children's developmental stages (Mur-phy 2008).

To ensure that the positives of sports participation for young athletes outweigh the negatives, sports programs should recognize the phases of youth sports development, the importance of parental and coaching influ-ences, and the need for training breaks and life balance. Youth sports de-velopment should be divided into stages or phases that emphasize different tasks or skills that are appropriate to the child stages of emotional and behavioral maturity. A model developed by Jon Hellstedt and recently updated by Shane Murphy (2008) includes three phases: 1) exploration (ages 4–12)—trying different sports; 2) commitment (ages 12–15)—move-ment to a specific sport; and 3) proficiency (ages 15–18)—incorporating and pursuing a sports-centered lifestyle. In the exploration stage, parents allow their children to try as many different sports as possible to find the ones that they enjoy and are good at. In this phase, the emphasis is on va-riety, skill development, and enjoyment. Parents should carefully monitor for too strong an emphasis on winning and choose coaches who know how to motivate and raise a child's skills, interest, and confidence. In the commitment phase, athletes narrow their focus to one particular sport and begin to find internal reasons for training and competing apart from those of coaches or parents. At this phase, athletes need to feel that they are in control of their participation rather than that their sport or the expectations of others are in control of them. If not, then burnout and dropout are inevitable, and the child may be turned off from sports forever. In the proficiency phase, the sport becomes the central focus, and goal setting for improvement becomes a lifestyle. At this stage, selecting the proper competitive level is important, because too high a level may result in too little playing time and a sense of failure.

Another model, described by McCormick (2005), is used routinely in England and also consists of three stages: 1) fundamentals, 2) training to train, and 3) training to compete. In the fundamentals stage, athletes ages 4–8 years master general motor development, fitness, and sports enjoyment. Emphasis is on running, jumping, balance, and hand-eye coordination rather than sports-specific skill acquisition. The training-to-train stage, which is for athletes ages 9–13, emphasizes basic sports skills and fitness, with about 75% of the time spent in training and only 25% spent in competition. The training replicates the intensity of competition but in an encouraging and enjoyable environment. In the training-to-compete stage, for athletes ages 14–18, the focus shifts to sports-specific training, technical skills, fitness, game strategy, and mental toughness. By this point, the sport becomes central and the full dedication of the athletes shifts to increasingly intense training and the development of competitive self-confidence through quality preparation.

Throughout these stage models of youth sports development, the role of the parents and coaches is critical (Bois et al. 2009; Gould et al. 2006). Rushing young athletes too early into intense competition, without adequate exploration of other sports or inadequate time to develop an inner love of the sport, leads to conflict, negativity, dread, declining motivation and performance, and eventually dropout. Parents err in the early stages by pushing a child into a specific sport that the parents have chosen or played, emphasizing winning over skill development and fun, and living their sports dreams through a child rather than letting the child find his or her own path. Good coaches seem to instinctively know the importance of these stages and recognize that athletic development takes time and care. For younger children, developing basic motor skills through constant movement and mastery of balance and motor repetition is critical. Coaches err early by placing too much emphasis on sport-specific skill development that is accompanied by idle time, or by promoting competition before athletes are emotionally ready for success or failure. In later stages, good coaches know how to keep all athletes involved in fitness and training so that they truly become self-motivated. A coaching style that acknowledges the positives of play and emphasizes skill achievement and improvement in the long run leads to athletes who appreciate the artistry and creativity of sport and therefore are able to genuinely play for the love of the game.

Case Study: My Daughter Seems Overwhelmed, and Her Grades Are Dropping

A 13-year-old seventh-grade soccer player was seen by a sports psychiatrist in the spring of the year after she moved up from a high-level community recreational team to a travel team. With this shift came a year-round commitment to soccer, including three practices per week with a 1-hour commute, two games each weekend that were often 1–2 hours away, indoor winter soccer and fitness training, out-of-town tournaments on holiday weekends and school breaks, and an expectation for additional daily technical work. Although her child had not said anything, the mother was beginning to feel that this commitment was too much and noted that her daughter was constantly fatigued and her academics were slipping. The athlete confirmed that the shift to a travel team had indeed been difficult and that she was tired all the time. Even though she had not been injured, her legs always ached and she just wanted to nap or sleep in her spare time. She had stopped socializing with her school peers and was not socializing with the members of her soccer team because most went to private schools in another county. She liked her coach and teammates, felt satisfied about her improved soccer skills, and was playing regularly and having an impact. She was growing very weary, however, of the additional running and training that her coach expected on off-days.

Intervention: Several key issues were addressed in the initial meeting with the athlete. The first was the need to take physical and mental breaks from soccer for recovery to prevent injury, fatigue, and burnout. She agreed to stop the additional training between practices and use that time to catch up on her schoolwork. The second issue was her disconnection from her school social group and therefore an absence of fun. She agreed to reconnect with them and in fact noted that they had kept asking her to hang out even though she had been too busy with soccer. The third issue was the intense culture of this team and whether it provided her with enough life balance. She and her parents agreed that she would finish out this season but also look into other travel teams that were not as far away and that might allow involvement in other activities or cross-training in other sports. She was seen monthly through the end of the school year, and she felt better after resting physically on her nonpractice days. She was able to reconnect with her community friends, and this break from soccer seemed to free up energy for school and soccer. She also approached her coach for feedback about her development. He was very pleased with her improvement and seemed open to her taking a summer and winter break. She therefore decided to stay with this team for another year.

Gender and Sexual Identity

Participation rates of girls and women in sports have increased dramatically since the passage of Title IX in 1972. The rate of hiring of female coaches, however, has lagged behind this rise, and the coaching culture in high school and college sports is still quite patriarchal. When the sources of stress for female athletes and coaches are compared with those of their male counterparts, some differences are apparent. Female athletes identified coaching-related conflicts as the primary source of stress and identified using approach-behavioral and avoidance-cognitive coping styles more than did males (Anshel et al. 2009). Interestingly, white women reported higher stress levels than African Americans or Hispanics. In another study, women were more likely than men to use problem-focused strategies, such as planning or direct communication, for dealing with stressful events (Nicholls et al. 2007). Kamphoff (2010) surveyed 121 women who had left coaching about their experiences; the most common reasons for leaving were family commitments and desire for free time. In a smaller sample that was interviewed, women coaches identified important cultural concerns, such as gender discrimination, dominance by male coaches, and destructive homophobia. In another study, female coaches reported feeling much pressure to constantly prove themselves in a hostile male-dominated culture (Norman 2010). In addition, issues of equity in hiring, pay, and promotions were identified. Both female athletes and coaches also spend considerable time responding to the influence and perspectives of others and cultural norms. Therefore, it is important to monitor the female coach–athlete relationships and female coach–male coach/administrator relationships when working with college or professional women's teams.

Before the increase in women's teams, not much was written about gay male athletes except in occasional media reports about diving and figure skating (Anderson and McCormick 2010). As women's visibility in sports has increased, so have awareness and discussion of the existence of differences in sexual identity, including lesbian, gay, bisexual, and transgender male and female athletes and coaches (Sartore and Cunningham 2007). Some countries, such as the United States and Canada (Canadian Association for the Advancement of Women in Sport and Physical Activity 2006), and some athletic departments (Maurer-Starks et al. 2008) are attempting to create sports cultures that are more accepting of sexual orientation differences as a way to combat homophobia and homonegativity as possible sources of ongoing hostility, harassment, rejection, degradation, employment discrimination, and even negative recruiting (e.g., by making negative comments about another team's lesbian coach or players). Even though these are difficult cultural issues, they must be addressed openly with messages of acceptance and respect. Because sports psychiatrists are usually experienced with these issues from general practice, they can facilitate resolution to conflicts that develop and perhaps contribute to progressive cultural change.

Case Study: My Players Seem to Shut Down When I Push the Intensity in Practice and Games

A newly hired male coach for a private high school girls' basketball team consulted a sports psychiatrist early in the season to discuss his feelings that his players were not responding to his coaching style. He said that he had been hired by the athletic director specifically to upgrade the level of the team's play. For 10 years, he had coached high school boys at a nearby private school with much success. In addition, he had played Division III basketball as a starting point guard for 4 years. He felt that he knew the game and how to win, but acknowledged that coaching girls was different and challenging. He described his personality style as intense and did say he was prone to frustration and confrontation. Even though he had money in his budget, he had not yet selected an assistant coach.

Intervention: He was open to all suggestions and agreed to provide the names and numbers of the two captains and to allow the psychiatrist to attend a practice and a game before meeting again. The captains were called, and both confided that at times the coach was often too intense and critical and that some of the girls were intimidated by him. They were very pleased, however, with his basketball knowledge and felt already that his stressing of fitness and fundamentals, as well as good defense and communication, would pay off. At the practice and a game, the coach was clearly emotionally reactive and passionate about the game. When his emotions intensified, however, he would raise his voice and single out players regarding poor effort or mistakes. When he did this, his players tended to get quiet, drop their energy level and communication, and begin playing more cautiously.

At the second meeting with the coach, the psychiatrist provided some feedback and made several suggestions. The coach seemed surprised about the reaction of his players to his intensity, stating emphatically that his behavior was not meant as a personal attack but only to help the team get better. He understood, after discussing the girls' reactions, that calling out individuals in the presence of a group might embarrass or humiliate them and that they might carry these emotions for a while. He agreed to try to regulate his emotional intensity by controlling his vocal intensity and rate of speech. In addition, he agreed to promptly hire an assistant and to ask the individual to help him better regulate his emotions. He also agreed to two other things: First, he would shift his attention to positive play and try to first give a compliment about things done well before reviewing mistakes. Second, he would insert some "fun breaks" into practice by challenging the girls to short games of bounced shots and backward shots in which he participated. They responded instantly to these changes with a noticeable shift in facial expression, body language, enthusiasm, and intensity. After 2 weeks, he found two women, a graduate student and a former college player, who became his assistants. Both developed instant rapport with the girls and also agreed to keep his passion and vocal intensity in check. The team improved steadily throughout the season and was playing its best at the time of the conference tournament. After upsetting two teams that the school had never previously beaten, the team lost a close game in the semi-finals. Follow-up with the captains revealed that they and their teammates were proud of the season and knew they had all improved. They also noted that the coach had modified his style and moderated his intensity, and the girls had responded and put effort into practices and games.

Case Study: Two Girls on the Team Are in a Relationship, and It's Causing Tension and Division

A second-year college softball coach asked to meet with a sports psychiatrist out of concern about a breakdown in the cohesion on her team. Even though she had learned in her first year that a number of lesbian players were on her team, she did not consider that a problem and had no issues during her first season. The team members played well together and had exceeded her expectations. Going into her second year, she was concerned about team unity after losing eight seniors, including both captains. Because this was her first recruited group of players, she decided to expand the roster and brought in a more diverse group of players, some of whom were junior college transfer players from other states, including several African Americans from urban areas. This strategy was a first for this school's program but had brought consistent success at the coach's prior school. On a road trip shortly after the season began, she learned that one of the captains had allowed two players to change rooms and that two of the resulting roommates were known by most of the team to be in a relationship. The coach was infuriated by the captain's actions and addressed it directly, saying that all future room assignments were her decision. Over the next 2 weeks, the coach noted that divisions between the old and new players were widening and that more confrontations and less unity were apparent at practice.

Intervention: After the initial meeting with the psychiatrist, the coach met with her two assistants and the two captains to discuss the situation. They all agreed that this incident and its implications needed to be addressed directly during a team meeting and that the coach's views about player-player relationships should be shared. They asked the sports psychiatrist to meet with them to think through the best way to frame the presentation to the team. A consensus was reached that the coach and one of the captains would colead the meeting with the theme of creating team unity.

Both spoke to the team about their sense that more cultural differences were represented on this year's team than ever before and that this would make team unity and cohesion more challenging. They also stressed that the talent level and potential of this team were strong and that if these differences were embraced, then the team could surpass last year's success. Each team member was then asked to share something about herself that others in the room did not know. The coaches and the captains started the process, and this seemed to reduce the tension level and even introduced some humor and laughter. Because of the team's size, the process took 75 minutes. The coach summarized what she had

heard about members' differences and similarities and committed herself to learn more about her players as the season went on. She stated that
she also knew that some differences in the group included sexual preference and that those too were understandable and acceptable. She then
sensitively stated her position about teammates in relationships, saying
that she thought it could complicate the team's ability to come together
just as a relationship between coworkers in the workplace might. The
meeting concluded on an upbeat note. Later that week, the coach called
in the players who had developed a relationship and explained her position to them individually and allowed them to discuss their views. Both
understood the coach's position and said that they would respect it by
breaking off their relationship. Over the next few weeks, the team practiced hard and the natural divisions and subgroupings that could have
formed did not. Instead, the team developed into a strong performer in
the conference and finished with the first 20-win season in school history.

Common Cultural Groups

Sports psychiatrists who work with teams in high school, college, or professional sports will be exposed to many different cultural groups. In professional sports in the United States, common groups currently include
African Americans in football, basketball, and track; Latinos in baseball
and soccer; and Asians in golf, tennis, and baseball. Generalizations
about these groups, however, need to be considered carefully. For example, African Americans originate from various African or Latin countries
or from different parts of the United States that have considerable cultural diversity. Similarly, a Latino from Argentina with Western European
influence is quite different from a Dominican or Venezuelan with African and native ancestry heritage. Also, although Chinese, Japanese, and
Korean athletes are all Asian, they likely have quite different beliefs, values, traditions, music, languages, and food. Using the concepts of culture
outlined earlier in the chapter makes it clear that none of these major
groups are homogeneous or similar; instead, each athlete comes from a
unique cultural place that can only be learned about by hearing a detailed narrative of his or her life and family.

Sports mental health clinicians must appreciate cultural differences
and be curious and respectful enough to help each athlete to understand
them. The strategies that facilitate steady cultural exchange come from
asking each athlete something about his or her early life and exploring
how it influenced his or her path to sports and current beliefs and values.
In addition, discovering the most influential persons in his or her life
and learning the details of their influence can be useful. Having individuals from the same culture as part of the medical team—to answer questions or create a referral bridge—is beneficial but not essential. Prior

experiences living in other cultures and even prolonged or frequent travels can create a cultural sensitivity that guides all interactions. Most important, a clinician working with diverse populations can learn from every interaction and ask openly and regularly for feedback about the services provided. If asked, athletes are typically glad to help educate sports clinicians about the fundamental elements of their culture.

Case Study: Latino Players and Front Office Personnel Are Not Using Available Mental Health Services

At a mid-year review of professional team assistance service utilization patterns, it became clear that Latino players and front office staff were not as likely to use the services as other groups. The Latino players tended to sit together in the clubhouse, conversed only in Spanish, and did not seem as approachable in the training room. In addition, the non-Latino staff did not have as much comfort approaching them as did a Latino provider in the mental health services group. In addition, Latino music and food were notably absent in the clubhouse. When consulted for information about the front office staff, the director of human resources said that she believed that many of the staff resented the amount of attention that the player side of the organization received and that overall they felt devalued and neglected.

Intervention: To reach out to the Latino players, our Latino provider agreed to begin making regular visits to the clubhouse, joining the regular staff member who had been assigned there for years. During his first few visits, he and the primary provider spoke informally with each Latino player in Spanish and in English. Because many new players were on the team, formal introductions were made and basic information about country of origin, family status, and playing history was shared. After a few visits, one of the veteran Latino players asked to meet about a difficult family situation. Both providers met with him, and several helpful solutions were identified. This one connection seemed to break the ice, and the Latino utilization rate soared over the course of the next two seasons, with most of the referrals coming from the veteran player who was seen first.

To reach out to the front office staff, a mental health counselor visited the front office for a half-day each week to mirror the regular visits to the clubhouse. The human resources director identified space and informed the front office employees by e-mail that assistance time was now available weekly. In addition, monthly lunchtime topic discussions (e.g., fitness and nutrition, stress control, parenting, caregiver stress and responsibility) were held; after each one, several new referrals occurred. The utilization rate rose after a full year of on-site services from 3% to 5%, and later to 12%.

Conclusion

Sports psychiatric practice occurs in a multicultural society with important differences in age, stage of development, gender, sexual orientation, and primary cultural affiliation. Attention to these issues is an essential part of practice to promote engagement and active participation in treatment. In addition, utilization of services from player-to-player referrals will increase if a culturally sensitive approach is adopted. In working with young athletes, clinicians need awareness of structured developmental approaches that avoid 1) early exposure to a single sport or intense competition, 2) sports-specific training, and 3) winning as a primary objective. These strategies can prevent burnout and sports dropout and assist athletes in developing their own reasons and motivations for sports training and competition.

Key Clinical Points

- A practical definition of *culture* for sports suggests that each group of people can be described or characterized by 1) a set of beliefs, attitudes, and values; 2) formal expressions, such as art, religion, or literature; and 3) popular expressions, such as music, food, dance, and traditions. Individual athletes should be viewed in the broader context of their cultural group and life story rather than according to obvious differences, such as language, race, skin color, religion, or sexual orientation.

- Sports mental health clinicians need developmental and cultural competencies that address differences in gender, ethnicity, sexual orientation, geographic region, religion, values, philosophy, and politics. They can help athletes and coaches understand the potential strengths of these differences by discovering and revealing the common struggles and values within the detailed narrative of each athlete's life and unique family history.

- Even though youth sports participation rates have risen steadily since the 1990s, childhood obesity and sedentary lifestyles have also increased, due in part to the obsession with the Internet, gaming, video music, and television, as well as increasing sport dropout rates.

- Youth sports participation is positive for its ability to promote socialization, commitment, responsibility, teamwork, organization, goal achievement, leadership, independence, efficiency, mental and physical health, and positive self-esteem and confidence. Negatives, however, include overtraining, disordered eating, social isolation, immaturity, entitlement, aggression, early sexual activity, high stress, competitive failure, parent-coach and parent-child conflict, and damage to self-esteem and confidence.

- The negatives of youth sports often result from a trend in the United States toward early single-sport specialization, early exposure to ultra-competitive teams that overemphasize winning, year-round training, parental achievement by proxy, and a lack of recognition of the developmental stage of the child.

- Female athletes have identified coaching-related conflicts as the primary source of stress and noted that coaches who constantly criticize, focus only on mistakes, or call out athletes in front of the team are the least accepted and effective even if technically competent.

- Female coaches' hiring rates have lagged behind the dramatic increase in the number of women's teams since the 1970s. Even more distressing are the high quit rates that link to the following concerns: 1) family commitment; 2) lack of free time; 3) gender discrimination in hiring, pay, and promotion; 4) destructive homophobia; and 5) performance pressure in a hostile male-dominated culture.

- By modeling tolerance, respect, and open discussion, sports mental health clinicians can play critical roles in combating cultural homophobia and homonegativity as possible sources of ongoing hostility, harassment, rejection, degradation, employment discrimination, and even negative recruiting.

References

Anderson E, McCormick M: Intersectionality, critical race theory, and American sporting oppression: examining black and gay male athletes. J Homosex 57:949–967, 2010

Anshel MH, Sutarso T, Jubenville C: Racial and gender differences on sources of acute stress and coping style among competitive athletes. J Soc Psychol 149:159–177, 2009

Bois JE, Lalanne J, Delforge C: The influence of parenting practices and parental presence on children's and adolescents' pre-competitive anxiety. J Sports Sci 27:995–1005, 2009

Bortoli L, Bertollo M, Comani S, et al: Competence, achievement goals, motivational climate, and pleasant psychobiosocial states in youth sport. J Sports Sci 29:171–180, 2011

Brink MS, Visscher C, Coutts AJ, et al: Changes in perceived stress and recovery in overreached young elite soccer players. Scand J Med Sci Sports Oct 2010 [Epub ahead of print]

Canadian Association for the Advancement of Women in Sport and Physical Activity: Seeing the Invisible, Speaking About the Unspoken: A Position Paper on Homophobia in Sport. Scarborough, ON, Canada, Glisa International, 2006. Available at: http://www.caaws.ca/pdfs/CAAWS_Homophobia_Discussion_Paper_E.pdf. Accessed March 30, 2011.

Fields SK, Collins CL, Comstock RD: Violence in youth sports: hazing, brawling, and foul play. Br J Sports Med 44:32–37, 2010

Gould D, Lauer C, Rolo D, et al: Understanding the role parents play in tennis success: a national survey of junior tennis coaches. Br J Sports Med 40:632–636, 2006

Habel MA, Dittus PJ, DeRosa CL, et al: Daily participation in sports and student sexual activity. Perspect Sex Reprod Health 42:244–250, 2010

Kamphoff CS: Bargaining with patriarchy: former female coaches' experiences and their decision to leave collegiate coaching. Res Q Exerc Sport 81:360–372, 2010

Malina RM: Early sports specialization: roots, effectiveness, risks. Curr Sports Med Rep 9:364–371, 2010

Maurer-Starks SS, Clemons HL, Whalen SL: Managing heteronormativity and homonegativity in athletic training: in and beyond the classroom. J Athl Train 43:326–336, 2008

McCormick B: Stages of youth athletic development: an informed approach to sports training. Associated Content, Oct 16, 2005. Available at: http://www.associatedcontent.com/article/9840/stages_of_youth-athletic_development.html. Accessed March 30, 2011.

Murphy S: Three phases of development in youth sports. MomsTeam, May 16, 2008. Available at: http://www.momsteam.com/print/484. Accessed March 30, 2011.

Nicholls AR, Polman R, Levy AR, et al: Stressors, coping, and coping effectiveness: gender, type of sports, and skill differences. J Sports Sci 25:1521–1530, 2007

Norman L: Bearing the burden of doubt: female coaches' experiences of gender relations. Res Q Exerc Sport 81:506–517, 2010

Sartore ML, Cunningham GB: Gay and lesbian coaches' teams: differences in liking by male and female former sports participants. Psychol Rep 101:270–272, 2007

Tofler IR, Knapp PK, Larden M: Achievement by proxy distortion in sports: a distorted mentoring of high-achieving youth: historical perspectives and clinical intervention with children, adolescents and their families. Clin Sports Med 24:805–828, 2005

Chapter 10

Evidence Base and Future Directions

Because sports psychiatry is a relatively new specialty, its evidence base is not well established. Through evidence-based medicine, clinicians are encouraged and allowed to introduce useful clinical findings from studies and recommendations stratified by quality. In the evidence base for practice in sports psychiatry, surprisingly more information is available about professional athletes than about high school and college athletes, who make up much larger groups. In addition, because serious injuries requiring surgery and especially head injuries (e.g., concussion) are high-profile areas, more studies and data sets exist about these medical issues in sports. The most studied areas in sports psychiatry are 1) participation rates in high school and college sports, 2) expansion of women's sports, 3) injury surveillance and return-to-play rates, 4) mental preparation training effectiveness, and 5) substance misuse and dependence rates. Not surprisingly, the least studied areas are those that require random assignment, control or comparison groups, or large-scale epidemiological methods. These include patterns and prevalence of mental disorders by competitive level and gender, mental disorder treatment effectiveness, serious injury treatment outcomes, injury prevention strategies, youth single-sports specialization effects, and gender and cultural differences in mental disorder prevalence and engagement and retention in treatment.

In this chapter, I review the evidence for different aspects of some of the eight core competencies for sports psychiatry described in this book. Emphasis is given to areas within each competency for which the evidence base is strong and to areas that are important but for which the evidence base is weak. Some evidence is presented from my own data sets about service utilization rates, activity levels, and types of problems by sport. This review is provided for the purpose of identifying areas in which enough consensus exists to guide service design and standards of care. Additionally, future directions for the field, specific to the core competencies reviewed, are presented as possible road maps for the growth and development of this exciting and interesting specialty. What should be clear from reading earlier chapters is how intertwined sports psychiatry is with sports medicine, orthopedics and neurology, sports and organizational psychology, sports nutrition, general and addiction psychiatry, and exercise science. Given the popularity and growth of sports globally and in the United States, tremendous opportunity exists for psychiatrists and other mental health specialists to develop specialized clinical or consulting practices for work with sports organizations, teams, or individual athletes. Just as in psychiatric, mental health, and addiction treatment, factors such as stigma, priority, technology, and funding limit the acceptance, importance, and effectiveness of sports psychiatry.

Injury

Evidence Base

Sufficient evidence to guide future practice and research has been found in three areas related to sports injuries: 1) clinical outcomes following surgery for serious injuries; 2) differences in emotional responses by injury type and the relevance of these emotional responses to return to play; and 3) the effectiveness of prevention training programs for reducing serious injury and reinjury rates, such as from anterior cruciate ligament (ACL) tears or hamstring strains. Outcome data following surgery have come primarily from case-controlled studies of professional athletes collected by active sports orthopedic clinical centers. The two most interesting aspects of these studies are comparisons of performance before and after the surgery using sports performance data sets and comparisons of return-to-play rates and functioning between those receiving surgery and control groups of similarly competitive noninjured players. Regarding studies of emotional responses to injury, the most interesting aspects are the methods used to track emotion response and models for using this information during acute injury, rehabilitation, and return-to-play phases. From studies of injury prevention programs comes awareness of the difficulty of developing standardized prevention programs across enough teams and time with consistency and a comparison group to demonstrate a preventive effect. In the following subsections, I review these three areas and discuss the implications for sports psychiatric practice.

Return to Play Following Surgery

Return-to-play rates following various surgeries for serious injuries in professional and other competitive levels range from 68% to 83%, depending on the injury and the type of surgery (Table 10–1) (Anakwenze et al. 2010; Busfield et al. 2009; Cain et al. 2010; Carey et al. 2006; Cerynik et al. 2009; Gibson et al. 2007; Mithoefer et al. 2009; Namdari et al. 2011; Parekh et al. 2009; Richetti et al. 2010; Savage and Hsu 2010). Although most athletes return to the same level of play as before their injuries, some experience a decrement in performance and playing time. As shown in Table 10–1, the injury with surgical repair that results in the greatest likelihood of an athlete's return to the prior level of play is an ulnar collateral ligament tear of the elbow (83%), whereas an Achilles tendon rupture repair results in the lowest rate of return overall and also the lowest likelihood of returning to the prior playing level. Surprisingly, overall return-to-play rates at the prior level are good for lumbar disc ruptures for men and ACL tears for both men and women in basketball. Even though the return-to-play rate following ACL tear repair was good for football, the postsurgery level of play was reduced significantly. Any sports psychiatrist working with injured athletes requiring surgery and lengthy rehabilitation should be aware that 17%–32% will not return to any play and that some with certain injuries and in certain sports will not return to a prior level of play. This knowledge, along with prognosis predictors, allows for better management of the emotions of injury and potential transition out of sports.

Emotions Related to Injury and Return to Play

A recent area of active investigation in sports involves athletes' emotional reactions to serious injury. Some studies using a longitudinal cohort design have identified variable emotional response patterns to different common injuries. For example, differences have been identified between the emotional responses to concussion, ACL injuries, and musculoskeletal injuries using the short form of the Profile of Mood States (POMS). POMS scores are provided for six mood states—tension, depression, anger, vigor, fatigue, and confusion—and total mood disturbance. In one study, athletes with concussion developed fatigue and decreased vigor, whereas athletes with musculoskeletal injury developed short-lived anger (Hutchison et al. 2009). In contrast, another study documented that athletes with concussion developed significant changes from baseline in depression and total mood disturbance, whereas athletes with ACL injuries reported significant changes in depression only (Mainwaring et al. 2010). The POMS appears to be a useful tool for systematically screening and monitoring athletes' emotional responses from injury throughout rehabilitation.

TABLE 10–1. Return-to-play rates following serious injury and surgery

Injury surgery	Professional league	Return-to-play rate	Return-to-preinjury-play level	Comparison control group	Average time to return (months)
Achilles tendon rupture	National Football League (*N*=31)	68%	Poor	No	?
Knee articular cartilage damage	Professional and college (*N*=1,363)	73%	68%	No	7–18
Glenoid labral repair	Major League Baseball (*N*=51)	72.5%	72.5%	No	13.1 Mean
Lumbar discectomy	National Football League (*N*=23)	74%	74%	No	?
Lumbar discectomy	National Basketball Association (*N*=24)	75%	75%	Yes (88% returned)	?
Anterior cruciate ligament tear	Women's National Basketball Association (*N*=18)	78%	78%	Yes	?
Anterior cruciate ligament tear	National Basketball Association (*N*=27)	78%	Good	Yes	?
Knee articular cartilage damage	National Basketball Association (*N*=24)	79%	Poor	Yes	7.5 Mean
Anterior cruciate ligament tear	National Football League (*N*=64)	80%	33% Reduction	Yes	13.8 Mean

TABLE 10–1. Return-to-play rates following serious injury and surgery *(continued)*

Injury surgery	Professional league	Return-to-play rate	Return-to-preinjury-play level	Comparison control group	Average time to return (months)
Ulnar collateral ligament repair	Major League Baseball (N=68)	82%	82%	Yes	18.5 Mean
Ulnar collateral ligament repair	All levels (N=743)	83%	83%	No	11.6 Mean

Note. ?=not reported.
Source. Anakwenze et al. 2010; Busfield et al. 2009; Cain et al. 2010; Carey et al. 2006; Cerynik et al. 2009; Gibson et al. 2007; Mithoefer et al. 2009; Namdari et al. 2011; Parekh et al. 2009; Richetti et al. 2010; Savage and Hsu 2010.

Other researchers have attempted to develop methods for assisting with rehabilitation activities, return-to-play decisions, and injury prevention. In one study, Hamson-Utley et al. (2008) surveyed athletic trainers' and physical therapists' attitudes about the use of mental imagery, goal setting, positive self-talk, and pain control to enhance injury recovery speed. Both athletic trainers and physical therapists had generally positive attitudes to these mental approaches but were even more likely to be positive if they had prior training. In another study, Mankad and Gordon (2010) investigated the use of longitudinal therapeutic writing to reduce the negative emotions of serious injury. The authors reported that therapeutic writing about the injury and its emotional impact several times during the rehabilitation period helped athletes to feel less devastated, dispirited, and restless while maintaining positive attitudes for eventual recovery. Sports psychiatrists with expertise in mental preparation techniques can use these strategies formally or informally to facilitate injury recovery motivation and protocol adherence. In addition, athletes who like to write should be encouraged to create an injury journal or document their rehabilitation process through e-mails to family or friends.

Finally, other researchers have attempted to identify the emotional and behavioral readiness of athletes to return to play following serious injury. One study validated the usefulness of the six-item Injury-Psychological Readiness to Return to Sport (I-PRRS) scale, for use by athletic trainers (Glazer 2009), whereas another validated a three-category, 12-item ACL-Return to Sport After Injury (ACL-RSI) scale (Webster et al. 2008), for use by athletes. The first study positively correlated the I-PRRS with the POMS total mood disturbance score, whereas the second study identified the ACL-RSI scale's 12 items and three response areas (emotion, confidence, and risk appraisal) to be highly interrelated, internally consistent, and response diverse. These are examples of validated rating scales that are short enough that they could easily be used by athletic trainers or sports mental health clinicians to monitor athletes' injury emotions and return-to-play readiness.

Injury Prevention Programs

Good agreement exists on the mechanisms of injury and the underlying risk factors for common injuries, such as hamstring strains, and serious injuries, such as ACL tears (Alentorn-Geli et al. 2009a). No agreement, however, has been reached regarding what the best specific protocols are for preventing such injuries or when and how they should be organized into team practices and pregame routines. Because hamstring strains are common across a number of different sports and are highly likely to recur, prevention protocols based on risk factors have been developed that target hamstring stretching, eccentric hamstring strengthening, lower-extremity neuromuscular control exercising, and running with varying trunk movements. All of these except simple hamstring stretching show promise in reducing strains (Heiderscheit et al. 2010).

Although not as common as hamstring strains, ACL tears are also the focus of active investigation because of the significant amount of lost playing time and because they are three to eight times more likely (depending on the sport) to occur in women than in men. Most ACL prevention protocols have multiple elements, including lower-extremity plyometrics; core training; dynamic balancing, strengthening, and stretching; body position awareness; and competitive decision making (Alentorn-Geli et al. 2009b). Such protocols need to be tested on teams over time, however, to determine which elements are most important, the practicality of their implementation, and how consistently individuals and teams will follow them.

Surprisingly, two randomized controlled trials of noncontact ACL prevention protocols have been reported. The first study randomly assigned 61 participating National Collegiate Athletic Association (NCAA) Division I women's soccer teams during the fall 2002 season to a neuromuscular and proprioceptive training protocol 3 days a week or to a control group (Gilchrist et al. 2008). Overall, the prevention protocol athletes (N=583) were 41% less likely than the control athletes (N=852) to experience an ACL injury, and those prevention protocol athletes with a history of a prior ACL injury were also significantly less likely to have another one. A second randomized study did not look at injury prevention but rather sought to determine whether a pregame ACL injury prevention protocol had a positive impact on adolescent female soccer players' linear sprint speed, countermovement jumping, and agility (Vescovi and VanHeest 2010). Over the 12-week study period, the prevention protocol teams did not develop enhanced athletic performance over controls. Because an ideal protocol could both prevent injury and improve sports-specific fitness, these results were disappointing. Sports psychiatrists need to be aware that the success of injury prevention protocols may depend on how well the team can adhere to them. Monitoring or supporting motivational levels and consistency is a role that can easily be assumed by on-site sports mental health clinicians.

Future Directions

Sports mental health clinicians should develop active roles in serious injury recovery monitoring and injury prevention. Monitoring emotional responses and motivation from initial injury through return to play is important because some injuries requiring surgery develop complications, whereas other injuries prevent return to play or reduce the level of play and playing time. In addition, some researchers and clinicians are arguing for an expanded paradigm of injury management and prevention that goes beyond neuromuscular, environmental, and anatomical factors and includes lifestyle modeling that addresses early sport specialization, chronic stress, insomnia and fatigue, poor nutrition or disordered eating, substance misuse, and psychological distress. Athletes who do not return to play because of a serious injury may be another group to target for sports mental health intervention, because up to half of this group may have an emotional barrier for returning, such as fear (Elliott et al. 2010; Lee et al. 2008). Future studies need to more fully define the emotional patterns of the entire injury and return-to-play process and consider how they vary by age, sport, gender, and culture. In addition, agreement about the technical, emotional, and behavioral components of injury prevention programs needs to occur, and more long-term randomized trials across sports need to be carried out.

Mental Disorders

Evidence Base

According to Reardon and Factor (2010), no large-scale epidemiological studies have been done on the pattern and prevalence of the most common mental disorders of athletes at any competitive level. However, targeted prevalence studies have been reported on specific areas, including eating, gambling, sleep, and substance use disorders. In addition, no reports have been published on randomized trials of medications or psychotherapy that address the most effective approaches for athletes of different ages who have the most common disorders (i.e., attention-deficit, anxiety, and mood disorders). In the absence of well-designed prevalence or effectiveness studies, clinicians are left to rely on case series or clinical experience. Presuming that the most common mental disorders are just as likely to develop in athletes of the same age, race, and gender as nonathletes, then service design strategies for identifying and treating illness-impaired and suffering athletes becomes even more important.

Throughout this book, I recommend an on-site model for sports psychiatry because utilization rates are dramatically higher than if the same services are available from an office base. In addition, retention in treatment approaches 100% at collegiate and professional levels when a sports program offers free, frequent, on-site, and year-round services. An earlier study, reported in McDuff et al. (2005), demonstrated a progressive rise in the utilization rate for two professional sports organizations that had on-site services. In one organization, the utilization rate rose from a mean of 16% of all athletes per year in the first 3 years (1996–1998) to 40% per year over the next 6 years (1999–2004). In the other organization, where fewer resources were available, the utilization rate rose from a mean of 13% in the first 3 years (1997–1999) to 20% over the next 5 years (2000–2004). More recent utilization rates for these same professional teams reveal the same impressive utilization patterns, as well as rising rates of services for mental disorders in the last 5 years (Tables 10–2 and 10–3). The team with interprofessional sports mental health staffing had utilization rates for athletes that ranged from 23% to 43% over 10 years (Table 10–2), for an average athlete utilization rate of 33%. In comparison, the team that was staffed with a sports psychiatrist with a more substantial on-site presence (i.e., 2–3 half-days per week) had utilization rates for athletes that ranged from 18% to 59% over 8 years. Notably, the mean athlete utilization rate for this team rose from an average of 23% per year to an average of 55% per year beginning in 2008, when the role was expanded to include more injury monitoring and management (Table 10–3). The most common psychiatric diagnoses for the two teams were attention-deficit, sleep, anxiety, substance use, and mood disorders. Attention-deficit disorders were far more common among baseball players, and sleep disorders were more common among football players.

Eating disorders (and subclinical disordered eating) and postconcussive depression are two specific mental disorders that have been receiving recent research attention because of their high profile in the media, rising prevalence rates in athletes, and potentially serious outcomes. One prevalence study of 204 female college athletes representing 17 different sports from three universities was completed using the Questionnaire for Eating Disorder Diagnoses and the Bulimia Test—Revised (Greenleaf et al. 2009). Although only 2% of the subjects met criteria for a current eating disorder, an additional 25.5% had subclinical symptoms that were interfering with functioning and performance. A more detailed study, however, of elite female Norwegian soccer, handball, and endurance athletes ages 13–39 years, which included a clinical interview of screened positives using a detailed questionnaire and an age-matched control group randomly selected from the population, revealed very high rates of eating disorders in the athletes (Sundgot-Borgen and Torstveit 2007). Specifically, 32% of all athletes (N=244) met diagnostic criteria for anorexia nervosa, bulimia nervosa, or eating disorder not otherwise specified. The prevalence rates varied by sport: soccer, 24%; handball players, 29%; and endurance athletes, 44%. Across all athletes, 11% met criteria

TABLE 10–2. Intake and utilization data for professional team with interprofessional sports mental health and performance training services: 2001–2010

	2010	2009	2008	2007	2006	2005	2004	2003	2002	2001
Intake										
Total	95	97	75	116	147	115	84	142	100	92
Players	59	60	56	91	97	74	51	95	66	69
Team staff	8	14	13	11	31	23	13	28	16	7
Front office	24	16	4	10	8	8	12	8	10	3
Family	4	7	0	4	7	7	8	6	6	8
Other	0	0	2	0	4	3	0	5	2	5
Athlete utilization rate	29%	27%	33%	40%	43%	33%	23%	42%	29%	31%
Organization utilization rate	24%	24%	19%	29%	37%	29%	21%	36%	25%	23%
Primary problem										
Mental health	50 (52%)	32 (34%)	49 (65%)	41 (35%)	36 (25%)	21 (18%)	20 (24%)	28 (20%)	16 (16%)	8 (9%)
Relationship	14	18	4	16	27	15	17	13	22	14
Substance prevention	18	21	14	35	48	46	34	38	32	43
Stress	11	16	3	17	36	29	10	41	30	27
Performance	4	8	5	7	0	4	3	22	0	0

TABLE 10–3. Intake and utilization data for professional team with frequent on-site sports psychiatric and performance training services: 2003–2010

	2010	2009	2008ᵃ	2007	2006	2005	2004	2003
Intake								
Total	77	73	70	50	32	29	27	30
Players	50	43	48	30	18	20	16	15
Team staff	12	13	11	7	5	4	5	9
Front office	8	8	5	7	3	2	1	0
Family	7	9	6	6	6	3	5	6
Athlete utilization rate	59%	51%	56%	35%	21%	24%	19%	18%
Organization utilization rate	39%	37%	35%	25%	16%	15%	14%	15%
Primary problem								
Mental health	29 (38%)	35 (48%)	34 (49%)	29 (58%)	17 (53%)	13 (45%)	8 (30%)	6 (20%)
Injury/pain	25 (32%)	20 (27%)	16 (23%)	1	1	4	2	2
Substance prevention	4	3	3	7	2	5	4	2
Stress	15	10	12	9	8	6	6	11
Performance	4	5	6	4	4	1	7	9

ᵃInjury recovery and pain control services were expanded in 2008.

for low bone mass and 17% reported current menstrual dysfunction, although the rate for menstrual dysfunction was not statistically different from that for controls (15%). The growing recognition of higher prevalence rates of eating disorders in athletes has led many organizations, such as the American College of Sports Medicine and the National Athletic Trainers' Association, to recommend routine screening because eating disorders are so easily missed. The preseason/participation and annual health examinations offer ideal opportunities to screen, evaluate, and refer an athlete to a sports mental health clinician and nutritionist if needed (Bonci et al. 2008; Nattiv et al. 2007; Rauh et al. 2010).

The second psychiatric condition receiving recent research attention is postconcussive depression (Chen et al. 2008). Concussion rates in sports are rising and more concern is being expressed about the short- and long-term consequences of repeated or severe head injury. Although depression is not a core symptom of postconcussive syndrome (PCS), which is characterized by headache, irritability, dizziness, visual problems, poor concentration, and memory difficulties, the presence of depression can signal more serious functional impairment and a prolonged clinical course. In a study to determine whether depression associated with concussion represents current pathophysiological change, 56 male athletes with or without concussion were administered a concussion checklist and a depression rating scale, and were subjected to T1- and T2-weighted magnetic resonance imaging (MRI) and functional magnetic resonance imaging (fMRI) during a functional memory test (Chen et al. 2008). Although the four groups—concussion–no depression, concussion–mild depression, concussion–moderate depression, and normal controls—had no memory performance differences, fMRI revealed that those with PCS and depression had reduced activation in the dorsolateral prefrontal cortex and striatum, attenuated deactivation in the medial frontal and temporal regions, and actual gray matter loss in these regions. These findings suggest that depression following head injury is more serious than previously known and likely represents underlying and ongoing limbic-frontal pathophysiological change.

Because concussion is serious and its symptoms and diagnosis have historically often been missed, immediate return to play in competition is now routinely blocked when concussion is recognized, and return to play subsequently is more systematically and objectively determined. To make return-to-play decisions more objective, the combined use of a PCS checklist and computerized cognitive testing is now the standard protocol at some high schools and for most college and professional teams. (A baseline evaluation is obtained for subsequent comparison with postconcussive scores.) In addition, exercise provocation testing and a clinical examination are used to make the final decision. To validate the Post Concussion Symptom Scale for use in concussion recovery monitoring, Chen et al. (2007) grouped 28 male athletes with and without concussion according to their scores and then administered an eight-task computerized cognitive test (CogSport) and fMRI. Higher self-reported PCS scores correlated well with poorer performance on several cognitive subtests and with activation patterns on the fMRI.

Future Directions

Sports psychiatrists should be familiar with the treatment of common mental disorders in athletes, but need to have special skill with attention-deficit, eating, substance use, sleep, impulse-control, performance anxiety, and postconcussive cognitive and mood disorders. Effective care for many of these disorders requires collaboration with other health professionals, including sports neurologists and primary care physicians, sleep specialists, neuropsychologists, dietitians, and substance abuse counselors. In some cases, linkages with higher levels of care, such as intensive outpatient programs, are also needed. Family involvement is also an essential part of working with athletes with mental disorders, as is skill in working with couples. Future research in this area must include large-scale epidemiological studies of athletes of all ages and competitive levels to find out whether prevalence rates differ from those in the general population. In addition, medication effectiveness and psychotherapy trials need to be instituted to determine whether age, gender, and cultural groups have unique safety, acceptance, engagement, retention, and treatment response issues. Research on the most cost-effective and successful ways of getting untreated athletes the care that they need is also critical.

Working With Sports Teams

Evidence Base

One of the most interesting aspects of working with sports teams is collaborating with coaches to improve team and individual play, as well as players' personal development and quality of life. Several studies point to the impact that coaching style can have on player self-image, emotions, motivation, and satisfaction, as well as team performance. One study examined fear-of-failure levels of youth swimmers over a season and found that these levels related to three factors: affiliation, control, and self-blame. Specifically, perceived positive affiliation from coaches predicted autonomy and satisfaction and reduced the development of failure internalization (Conroy and Coatsworth 2007). Blame from coaches, on the other hand, predicted negative self-talk and fear of failure. Another study of youth swimmers documented the positive impact of coaches' autonomy support and process-focused praise on athlete satisfaction, self-esteem, competence, initiative, and identity (Coatsworth and Conroy 2009). Finally, a study of female adolescent soccer players examined the relationship of coaching performance feedback and motivational climate to perceived competence, motivation, and enjoyment (Weiss et al. 2009). Not surprisingly, more positive and informational feedback and an atmosphere of sport mastery rather than performance were significantly related to positive perceptions in all areas. Perhaps early experiences with coaches who notice and praise positives in practice and competition and who emphasize mastery and improvement rather than performance and winning may shape athletes' emotional response patterns and self-image into their adult competitive life.

Future Directions

Sports psychiatrists and other clinicians can work with coaches and parents to create a climate of praise, constructive correction, and mastery. This positive foundation of competence and confidence can serve athletes, especially young ones, throughout their athletic careers and even cross over to positively impact other important areas, including academics and social development. Future studies need to address coaching styles and team culture at higher competitive levels, where mistake-based learning and repetitive criticism, intimidation, and threats of lost playing time are often used as motivational tools.

Sleep and Jet Lag

Evidence Base

Sports psychiatrists encounter insomnia and fatigue in athletes who play professional sports such as baseball and basketball, which have long seasons, late night games, and much travel, and collision sports such as football, which are played less frequently but with high intensity and injury rates. Choosing a sleep medication that fits the athlete, sport, practice and playing schedule, sleep-awake times, and likelihood of episodic heavy alcohol use can be challenging. Some athletes need medications that act quickly and last for 6–8 hours, but then clear out fully the next day without interfering with alertness, reaction time, or motor coordination. Other athletes need medications after a game or practice to unwind and turn off overactive thinking and analysis. Still other athletes need medications to reset their circadian rhythm due to changing time zones and jet lag. Possible choices for quick-acting medications include zolpidem and eszopiclone. Unwinding medications include benzodiazepines, such as lorazepam or alprazolam; sedative antidepressants, such as trazodone or mirtazapine; or very low doses of atypical neuroleptics, such as quetiapine. Circadian rhythm–resetting agents include over-the-counter melatonin or prescription melatonin agonists, such as ramelteon. None of these medications have been systematically studied in athletes, so clinical experience or case series are used as guides.

A few studies have examined the effects of short-acting sleep medications on next-day alertness and motor performance. One study was a small double-blind placebo-controlled study of zolpidem (10 mg) with a cross-over design (Ito et al. 2007). Over 2 consecutive nights, seven athletes were given either zolpidem or placebo and then assessed for alertness or fatigue using rating scales and for psychomotor and physical performance using vertical jump, 50-meter sprint, and finger dexterity and critical flicker fusion tests. In this study, zolpidem shortened self-reported sleep latency and increased total sleep time but did not reduce next-day alertness or increase fatigue. Of interest, next-day subjective well-being was slightly worsened. The fact that no adverse effects were found on any motor performance testing suggests that this medication is a good match for those athletes who need a fast-acting, short-duration sleep medication. An older French study was similar in design to the Ito et al. (2007) study but evaluated zopiclone (7.5 mg) versus placebo for 2 nights using similar measures of daytime alertness and psychomotor and physical skills in eight athletes (Tafti et al. 1992). Although zopiclone is not available in the United States, its active stereoisomer, eszopiclone, is available. The findings were identical to the study for zolpidem, making this agent an alternative for athletes needing a fast-acting, short-duration sleep medication.

Another area of active investigation is the study of biological rhythms in sports. This area of sports chronobiology examines biological rhythms associated with wakefulness, fatigue, sleep, energy, and focus (Reilly and Waterhouse 2009). Much of this area has already been covered in detail in Chapter 4, "Energy Regulation," but the active development of protocols for teams and individual athletes to combat chronic fatigue or reduced alertness from game times and travel is worth mentioning. These protocols start with individual profiling (chronotyping) of athletes as either morning persons, night owls, or neither. Then they examine and profile individual napping patterns, environmental barriers to sleep, sleep debt, and personal discipline and behaviors. For teams, the times of competition, sleeping facilities, travel demands, time zone changes, and training, practice, and meal schedules are reviewed and documented. A draft protocol for teams and individuals is then created that incorporates the natural peaks and valleys of energy, alertness, and focus. The final protocol recommends ideal times for training, breaks, meals, naps, and sleeping (Postolache et al. 2005; Samuels 2009). These protocols have been developed in response to recent studies of college basketball, professional baseball, and professional football that demonstrate a strong disadvantage to athletes and teams that travel three or more time zones and compete immediately. No systematic study of the effectiveness of a comprehensive chronobiological protocol has been conducted.

Future Directions

Sports psychiatrists must be able to conduct a thorough evaluation of insomnia to determine whether it is due to stress, environmental problems, poor sleep habits, acute or chronic pain, substance misuse, obstructive or central sleep apnea, or an anxiety or mood disorder. In addition, clinicians need clinical knowledge and skill in the following areas: 1) behavioral strategies for improving sleep; 2) changes in patterns of stimulant and sedative use; 3) stress control therapy; 4) pain control; 5) medication strategy; and 6) mechanical soft tissue devices, positive pressure machines, and surgical options for airway obstruction. Research is needed to determine which medications are best suited for various individuals in different sports. Long-term studies on sleep effectiveness, next-day alertness, and motor performance are also needed for chronic daily use of short-acting medications, such as zolpidem, and short- and long-term studies are needed for the other agents mentioned above in the "Evidence Base" section, especially trazodone and benzodiazepines. For chronobiological protocols, studies need to be done to determine their adherence rates and effectiveness with control or comparison groups.

Substance Misuse

Areas of Study

Two areas of study related to substance use and sports are of particular interest. The first concerns the reliability of urine testing methods for performance and illicit substances, and the second is whether caffeine and other weak stimulants have performance-enhancing effects. As mentioned in Chapter 5, "Substance Use and Abuse," all college and professional sports have urine testing programs to detect banned substances. The frequency of testing and the specific substances tested, however, are highly variable from one sport to the next and from one competitive level to another. In addition, few U.S. professional sports perform postgame testing, in which short-acting stimulants are most likely to be detected. One interesting study examined the accuracy of urine drug testing for performance enhancers and illicit drugs in junior members of all German national teams (Striegel et al. 2010). In this study, athletes either completed an anonymous standardized questionnaire (*N*=1,394) or were interviewed using a randomized response technique (*N*=480). Interestingly, in contrast to official doping tests, which indicated an overall 0.81% positive urine test rate for performance enhancers, both study methods revealed a prevalence rate of approximately 7% for illicit drug use; however, the randomized response technique revealed that 6.8% of the athletes confessed to having practiced doping, but the standardized questionnaire did not indicate a realistic prevalence of doping (0.2%). This study shows that urine testing with its current frequency and timing dramatically underestimates the true prevalence of doping and illicit drug use by elite athletes.

Athletes widely use caffeine in coffee, tea, sodas, energy drinks, or pills. The NCAA bans caffeine in some sports, but no U.S. professional sport bans it. Several recent studies have examined whether caffeine is performance enhancing at certain dosages and therefore should be banned during competition. In one study that sought to address caffeine's effect on performance in a simulated soccer match (Foskett et al. 2009), 12 trained athletes completed two 90-minute soccer running trials, along with periodic tests of soccer skills. In the randomized crossover design, the players received either caffeine (6 mg/kg body mass) or placebo 60 minutes before exercise. Movement time, accrued penalty time, jumping ability, and total time for the soccer skills testing were recorded for both trials. When taking caffeine, the athletes had greater passing accuracy and jump performance, without any negative effects.

Another study investigated adding caffeine to a carbohydrate solution during two 90-minute intermittent shuttle running exercises alternating with measures of soccer skill (Gant et al. 2010). The caffeine-infused carbohydrate solution or the carbohydrate solution only was ingested 60 minutes before the trial and every 15 minutes during the trial in a double-blind crossover design. After ingesting moderate amounts of caffeine in the carbohydrate solution, the soccer players demonstrated improvements in sprinting performance, countermovement jumping, and subjective well-being. Caffeine seemed to specifically offset the fatigue-induced decline often seen in skills requiring self-motivation.

Finally, a comprehensive review of caffeine and sports performance by the International Society of Sports Nutrition confirmed that caffeine in low to moderate dosages (3–6 mg/kg) enhances performance in trained athletes (Goldstein et al. 2010). In addition, the society determined that caffeine is a more effective performance enhancer when consumed in a capsule, tablet, or powder than in a liquid and that it enhances vigilance during sustained endurance exercising and after prolonged sleep deprivation. Caffeine was specifically noted to be effective in sports with time trials, such as cycling, sprinting, or swimming, and those requiring a mix of endurance and sprinting, such as soccer, lacrosse, and rugby. These studies have very interesting implications for other, even stronger stimulants like amphetamines, and in sports like baseball, in which sleep disruption and chronic fatigue are common.

Future Directions

Sports psychiatrists need to be knowledgeable about oral and urine testing methods for performance-enhancing and illicit substances and the limitations of these methods in detecting substance use because of technical barriers, such as adulteration, dilution, and designer drugs, or the frequency and timing of the testing. More studies need to be done comparing one testing protocol to another and especially comparing large numbers of frequently obtained postgame stimulant test results with pregame test results. The complex issue of stimulants as performance enhancers needs to be regularly reviewed as new studies document the specific benefits in specific sports.

Conclusion

Sports psychiatry is a new specialty that overlaps significantly with sports primary care, neurology, orthopedics, chiropractics, nutrition, fitness and exercise science, chronobiology, physical therapy, athletic training, and sports psychology. As a new interprofessional sports specialty, its evidence base therefore comes from diverse areas. In this chapter and book, I have described an expanded role for sports psychiatrists and emphasized eight specific core competencies. Although sports-involved clinicians may not develop expertise in all eight areas, those who work on site with teams or in training rooms will need very broad skills. Even if a clinician's sports psychiatric practice is limited to the treatment of athletes with mental disorders, he or she needs substantial knowledge beyond the usual treatments of common disorders in this age group. Engagement, retention, and success in treatment come not only from technical clinical competence but also from awareness of athletes' lifestyles, pressures, identities, vulnerabilities, injury risks, and changing self-confidence. In addition, knowledge of the specific mental, emotional, and physical requirements of the sports, as well as sports culture and media coverage strategies, is critical.

Although the current evidence base for sports psychiatry is not strong, current and proposed research can guide practice in the coming years. Individual clinicians can contribute to this evidence base by creating clinical databases that collect demographic, diagnostic, and simple outcomes information over time. If data are systematically collected over 5 or 10 years in different sports at the same competitive level or in the same sports at different competitive levels, then a contribution to the specialty can be made. Because youth sports touch the lives of so many boys and girls in the United States and are so fundamental to the development of their self-image, self-esteem, emotional patterns, and sense of competence and confidence, greater involvement by sports-aware mental health clinicians is needed. My hope is that the information and cases contained in this book will inspire other clinicians to see more athletes and to reach out to teams and coaches and offer assistance. In doing this work, however, the clinician needs to remember that athletes, even elite ones, are just people struggling to adjust and adapt to challenging circumstances, hoping to realize their potential, and striving to build lasting and affirming relationships while developing pride in their hard work and accomplishments.

Key Clinical Points

- Return-to-play rates following various surgeries for serious injuries in professional and other competitive levels range from 68% to 83% depending on the injury and the type of surgery (see Table 10–1). Although most athletes return to the same level of play as before the injury, some experience a decrement in performance and playing time.

- The Profile of Mood States rating scale assesses tension, depression, anger, vigor, fatigue, and confusion, as well as total mood disturbance, and appears to be a useful tool for systematically screening and monitoring emotional responses from injury through rehabilitation.

- Therapeutic writing about an injury and its emotional impact several times during the rehabilitation period helps athletes to feel less devastated, dispirited, and restless while maintaining positive attitudes for eventual recovery. Sports psychiatrists, therefore, can encourage athletes who like to write to create an injury journal or document their rehabilitation process through e-mails to family or friends.

- Office- or team-based sports mental health clinicians should develop active roles in serious injury recovery monitoring and injury prevention. Because emotional barriers, such as fear, are common in athletes who do not return to play, some clinical researchers are arguing for expanded paradigms of injury management that address lifestyle, early sport specialization, chronic stress, insomnia and fatigue, poor nutrition or disordered eating, substance misuse, and psychological distress.

- Sports psychiatrists should have special skills for diagnosing and treating attention-deficit, eating, substance use, sleep, impulse-control, performance anxiety, and postconcussive cognitive and mood disorders. In athletes, the prevalence rate of each is sufficiently high to justify annual universal screening.

- Because studies highlight the impact that coaching style can have on player self-image, emotions, motivation, and satisfaction, as well as team performance, consultative work in this area is indicated. Positive and informational feedback and sports mastery–oriented training, rather than performance emphasis, significantly relate to positive perceptions. In addition, positive affiliation from coaches predicts autonomy and reduces the development of failure internalization.

- Few studies have examined insomnia medication effectiveness or the effect of jet lag on fatigue, next-day alertness, and motor performance. Some studies indicate that zolpidem and eszopiclone are good choices for athletes who need fast-acting, short-duration sleep medications with few side effects.

- Studies show that the current frequency and timing (i.e., primarily pregame) of urine testing dramatically underestimates the true prevalence of doping and illicit drug use in elite athletes.

- Caffeine appears to offset the fatigue-induced decline often seen in athletic skills requiring self-motivation and enhances vigilance during sustained endurance exercising and after prolonged sleep deprivation. Caffeine is most likely to be effective in sports with time trials, such as cycling, sprinting, or swimming, and those requiring a mix of endurance and sprinting, such as soccer, lacrosse, and rugby. In addition, caffeine is a more effective performance enhancer when consumed in a capsule, tablet, or powder than in a liquid.

References

Alentorn-Geli E, Myer GD, Silvers HJ, et al: Prevention of non-contact anterior cruciate ligament injuries in soccer players, part 1: mechanisms of injury and underlying risk factors. Knee Surg Sports Traumatol Arthrosc 17:705–729, 2009a

Alentorn-Geli E, Myer GD, Silvers HJ, et al: Prevention of non-contact anterior cruciate ligament injuries in soccer players, part 2: a review of prevention programs aimed to modify risk factors and to reduce injury rates. Knee Surg Sports Traumatol Arthrosc 17:859–879, 2009b

Anakwenze OA, Namdari S, Auerbach JD, et al: Athletic performance outcomes following lumbar discectomy in professional basketball players. Spine 35:825–828, 2010

Bonci CM, Bonci LJ, Granger LR, et al: National Athletic Trainers' Association position statement: preventing, detecting, and managing disordered eating in athletes. J Athl Train 43:80–108, 2008

Busfield BT, Kharrazi FD, Starkey C, et al: Performance outcomes of anterior cruciate ligament reconstruction in the National Basketball Association. Arthroscopy 25:825–830, 2009

Cain EL Jr, Andrews JR, Dugas JR, et al: Outcome of ulnar collateral ligament reconstruction of the elbow in 1281 athletes: results in 743 athletes with minimum 2-year follow-up. Am J Sports Med 38:2426–2434, 2010

Carey JL, Huffman GR, Parekh SG, et al: Outcomes of anterior cruciate ligament injuries to running backs and wide receivers in the National Football League. Am J Sports Med 34:1911–1917, 2006

Cerynik DL, Lewullis GE, Jones BC, et al: Outcomes of microfracture in professional basketball players. Knee Surg Traumatol Arthrosc 17:1135–1139, 2009

Chen JK, Johnston KM, Collie A, et al: A validation of the post concussion symptom scale in the assessment of complex concussion using cognitive testing and functional MRI. J Neurol Neurosurg Psychiatry 78:1231–1238, 2007

Chen JK, Johnston KM, Petrides M, et al: Neural substrates of symptoms of depression following concussions in male athletes with persisting postconcussion symptoms. Arch Gen Psychiatry 65:81–89, 2008

Coatsworth JD, Conroy DE: The effects of autonomy-supportive coaching, need satisfaction, and self-perceptions on initiative and identity in youth swimmers. Dev Psychol 45:320–328, 2009

Conroy DE, Coatsworth JD: Coaching behaviors associated with changes in fear of failure: changes in self-talk and need satisfaction as potential mechanisms. J Pers 75:383–419, 2007

Elliot DL, Goldberg L, Kuehl KS: Young women's anterior cruciate ligament injuries: an expanded model and prevention paradigm. Sports Med 40:367–376, 2010

Foskett A, Ali A, Gant N: Caffeine enhances cognitive function and skill performance during simulated soccer activity. Int J Sport Nutr Exerc Metab 19:410–423, 2009

Gant N, Ali A, Foskett A: The influence of caffeine and carbohydrate coingestion on simulated soccer performance. Int J Sport Nutr Exerc Metab 20:191–197, 2010

Gibson BW, Wedner D, Huffman GR, et al: Ulnar collateral ligament reconstruction in Major League Baseball pitchers. Am J Sports Med 35:575–581, 2007

Gilchrist J, Mandelbaum BR, Melancon H, et al: A randomized controlled trial to prevent noncontact anterior cruciate ligament injury in female collegiate soccer players. Am J Sports Med 36:1476–1483, 2008

Glazer DD: Development and preliminary validation of the Injury-Psychological Readiness to Return to Sport (I-PRRS) scale. J Athl Train 44:185–189, 2009

Goldstein ER, Ziegenfuss T, Kalman D, et al: International Society of Sports Nutrition position stand: caffeine and performance. J Int Soc Sports Nutr 7:5, 2010

Greenleaf C, Petrie TA, Carter J, et al: Female collegiate athletes: prevalence of eating disorders and disordered eating behaviors. J Am Coll Health 57:489–495, 2009

Hamson-Utley JJ, Martin S, Walters J: Athletic trainers' and physical therapists' perceptions of the effectiveness of psychological skills within sport injury rehabilitation programs. J Athl Train 43:258–264, 2008

Heiderscheit PT, Sherry MA, Silder A, et al: Hamstring strain injuries: recommendations for diagnosis, rehabilitation and injury prevention. J Orthop Sports Phys Ther 40:67–81, 2010

Hutchison M, Mainwaring LM, Comper P, et al: Differential emotional responses of varsity athletes to concussion and musculoskeletal injuries. Clin J Sport Med 19:13–19, 2009

Ito SU, Kanbayashi T, Takemura T, et al: Acute effects of zolpidem on daytime alertness, psychomotor and physical performance. Neurosci Res 59:309–313, 2007

Lee D, Karim SA, Chang HC: Return to sports after anterior cruciate ligament reconstruction: a review of patients with minimum 5-year follow-up. Ann Acad Med Singapore 37:273–278, 2008

Mainwaring LM, Hutchison M, Bisschop SM, et al: Emotional response to sport concussion compared to ACL injury. Brain Inj 24:589–597, 2010

Mankad A, Gordon S: Psycholinguistic changes in athletes' grief response to injury after written emotional disclosure. J Sport Rehabil 19:328–342, 2010

McDuff DR, Morse ED, White RK: Professional and collegiate team assistance programs: services and utilization patterns. Clin Sports Med 24:943–958, 2005

Mithoefer K, Hambly K, Della Villa S, et al: Return to sports participation after articular cartilage repair in the knee: scientific evidence. An J Sports Med 37:167S–176S, 2009

Namdari S, Scott K Ba, Milby A, et al: Athletic performance after ACL reconstruction in the Women's National Basketball Association. Phys Sportsmed 39:36–41, 2011

Nattiv A, Loucks AB, Manore MM, et al: American College of Sports Medicine position stand: the female athlete triad. Med Sci Sports Exerc 39:1867–1882, 2007

Parekh SG, Wray WH 3rd, Brimmo O, et al: Epidemiology and outcomes of Achilles tendon ruptures in the National Football League. Foot Ankle Spec 2:283–286, 2009

Postolache TT, Ming Hung T, Rosenthal RN, et al: Sports chronobiology consultation: from the lab to the arena. Clin Sports Med 24:415–456, 2005

Rauh MJ, Nichols JF, Barrack MT: Relationships among injury and disordered eating, menstrual dysfunction, and low bone mineral density in high school athletes: a prospective study. J Athl Train 45:243–252, 2010

Reardon CL, Factor RM: Sport psychiatry: a systematic review of diagnosis and medical treatment of mental illness in athletes. Sports Med 40:961–980, 2010

Reilly T, Waterhouse J: Sports performance: is there evidence that the body clock plays a role? Eur J Appl Physiol 106:321–332, 2009

Richetti ET, Weidner Z, Lawrence JT, et al: Glenoid labral repair in Major League Baseball pitchers. Int J Sports Med 31:265–270, 2010

Samuels C: Sleep, recovery, and performance: the new frontier in high-performance athletics. Phys Med Rehabil Clin N Am 20:149–159, 2009

Savage JW, Hsu WK: Statistical performance in National Football League athletes after lumbar discectomy. Clin J Sport Med 20:350–354, 2010

Striegel H, Ulrich R, Simon P: Randomized response estimates for doping and illicit drug use in elite athletes. Drug Alcohol Depend 106:230–232, 2010

Sundgot-Borgen J, Torstveit MK: The female football player, disordered eating, menstrual function and bone health. Br J Sports Med 41 (suppl 1):i68–i72, 2007

Tafti M, Besset A, Billiard M: Effects of zopiclone on subjective evaluation of sleep and daytime alertness and on psychomotor and physical performance tests in athletes. Prog Neuropsychopharmacol Biol Psychiatry 15:55–63, 1992

Vescovi JD, VanHeest JL: Effects of an anterior cruciate ligament injury prevention program on performance in adolescent female soccer players. Scand J Med Sci Sports 20:394–402, 2010

Webster KE, Feller JA, Lambros C: Development and preliminary validation of a scale to measure the psychological impact of returning to sport following anterior cruciate ligament reconstruction surgery. Phys Ther 9:9–15, 2008

Weiss MR, Amorose AJ, Wilko AM: Coaching behaviors, motivational climate, and psychosocial outcomes among female adolescent athletes. Pediatr Exerc Sci 21:475–492, 2009

Index

*Page numbers printed in **boldface** type refer to tables or figures.*

Achievement pressure, and case study, 24–25
ACL. *See* Anterior cruciate ligament
ACL-Return to Sport After Injury (ACL-RSI) scale, 238
Activation breathing, 11
Addiction, and anabolic steroids, 108
Adenosine triphosphate (ATP), 69, 70
Adjustment disorders, 166–169
Adrenaline, 81
Aerobic metabolic system, 69–70
African Americans, and cultural issues, 227
Age. *See also* Development
    alcohol use and, **116**
    anabolic steroids and, 107
Alcohol use
    banned substances by sport and, **88**
    case study of, 14
    common mental disorders and, 18
    effects of on athletic performance, **116–118**
    issues in use and misuse of, 92–97
    reasons for use and misuse of, 13–14, **116**
    stress control and, 64
    zolpidem and, 76
Allergic rhinitis, 79
Alprazolam, 76, 247

American College of Sports Medicine, 244
Amphetamines, 15, 81, 82–83, 86, 104–105, 106, **122, 124,** 176, 178–179, 190, 250
Anabolic steroids, 86, **88,** 106–110, **126**
Anaerobic glycolysis system, 69
Androstenediol, **126**
Androstenedione, **126**
Anger
    attention shifting and control of, 40
    common mental disorders and, 173–175
    stress reaction patterns and, 8
    symptom screening form and, 216
Ankle injuries, 133–134, 147
Anorexia athletica, 180
Anorexia nervosa, 181. *See also* Eating disorders
Anterior cruciate ligament (ACL), 150–152, 235, 239
Antidoping policies, 87, **88–89,** 91, 106–107
Antiestrogenic agents, **88**
Anxiety and anxiety disorders. *See also* Generalized anxiety disorder
    common forms of in sports, 165, 169–173
    medication management for, 19, 190–191

257

Anxiety and anxiety disorders
(*continued*)
stress reaction patterns and, 8
symptom screening form and, 215
working with medical staff and,
208–209
Aripiprazole, 171, 184, 186
Armodafinil, 105
Aromatase inhibitors, **127**
Asian Americans, and cultural issues,
24–25, 227–228
Asthma medications, **122**
Atenolol, 170, 191
Athletic trainers, role in. *See also* Case
studies; Teams, medical staff,
and sports leadership
detection and treatment of mental
disorders, 166, 170, 180, 182,
183, 187, 188
detection and treatment of
substance use, 14, 85, 92, **122**
injury prevention and recovery,
16, 130, 136, 154, 155, 156,
238
Atomoxetine, 19, 81, 175, 179
ATP (adenosine triphosphate), 69,
70
Attendance at games, by clinicians
working with teams, 199
Attention, and symptom screening
form, 217
Attention cues, and precompetition
routine, 48
Attention-deficit disorder, 19, 21–22,
175–179, 190
Attention shifting, and mental
preparation, 38–41
Atypical antipsychotics, 184, 247
Awakening routine
energy management and, 10–11
stress control and, 66–67

Background factors, in stress, 55
Back pain, 149–150
Badminton, 41

Baseball. *See also* Major League
Baseball; Softball
common mental disorders and,
167–168, 177, 178–179, 184–
185, 190
cultural issues and, 25–26
employee assistance programs
and, 22
energy regulation and, 76–77, 82–
83
injury recovery and, 140, 146–147
insomnia and, 75
mental preparation and, 35–36, 48
positive self-talk and, 37
precompetition routine and, 6
psychiatric consultation for team
and, 201–202
repetitions of athletic movements
and, 41
stress control and, 58, 66–67
substance use and, 13, 14, 15, **88–
90,** 95–100, 101–102, 103, 106
wakefulness cycle and energy
regulation for, 74
Basic mental skills, and mental
preparation, 2, **3,** 4–5, 29, 33–44,
199
Basketball. *See also* National
Basketball Association; Women's
National Basketball Association
energy regulation and, 78–79
gender issues and, 225–226
injury recovery and, 133, 138–139
issues in working with coach, 22–
23
mental preparation and, 40–41
repetitions and performance
under pressure, 41
substance use and, **88–90,** 98–100
team leadership and, 200–201
working with coaches and, 210–211
Behavioral therapy, for attention-
deficit disorders, 177
BELIEVE IT (acronym), and mental
preparation, 31–32

Benzodiazepines, 19, 76, 154, 170, 190, 191, 247, 248

Beta-adrenergic agonists, **88,** 108, **127**

Beta-blockers, **88,** 170, 191

Biceps femoris, and hamstring strains, 136

Binge drinking, 173

Binge eating, 180

Biofeedback, 32

Biological rhythms, and sleep, 74, 247–248

Bipolar disorder, 184, 185–186

Blood doping, **88,** 249

Body awareness, and somatoform disorders, 187

Body building, 107, 108–109

Body temperature, and energy regulation, 80

Boldenone, **126**

Brain. *See also* Brain imaging
development of cortical circuits in and impulse control, 174
ideal levels of energy, alertness, and focus and, 73
injuries to, 141–146

Brain imaging, and research on mental preparation, 36, 37–38, 41, 43, 49

Breaks
energy management and, 11, 81
stress control and, 61–62

Breathing
basic mental skills and, 33–36
energy management and, 11
stress control and, 58–59

Broad external focus, 39

Broad internal focus, 38

Bulimia nervosa, 181. *See also* Eating disorders

Bulimia Test—Revised, 241

Bupropion, 19, 185

Burnout, energy regulation and prevention of, 77–80

Buspirone, 171

Caffeine
awakening routine and, 11
case studies of substance use and, 14, 15, 101–102
effects of on athletic performance, **121**
energy management and, 81
stress control and, 64
substance use and, 101–102, 104, **123,** 249–250

Carbamazepine, 185

Carbohydrates
alcohol use and, 94
energy maintenance and, 11, 70, 71

Cardiovascular system, and anabolic steroids, 108

Case studies
of common mental disorders, 20–22, 167–169, 171–175, 178–182, 184–186, 188–189
of cultural issues, 24–26, 228
of development, 24–25, 223
of energy regulation, 71–73, 76–83
of gender issues, 225–227
of injury recovery, 17–18, 133–140, 144–153, 155–160
of mental preparation, 4–8, 35–37, 40–42, 44, 47–50
of pain management, 17
of sleep issues, 11–12
of stress control, 9–10, 56–57, 58, 59–67
of substance use, 14, 15, 95–100, 103–106, 108–110
of working with coaches, 22–23, 210–212
of working with medical staff and athletic trainers, 206–209
of working with teams, 200–204, **205**

Catastrophic injuries, 141

Chiropractors, 204

Choking
focus and attention shifting in, 39
stress control and, 59–60

Chorionic gonadotropin, **127**
Chronic traumatic encephalopathy
    (CTE), 142
Circadian rhythm, of sleep, 74
Clearing breath, 35
Clenbuterol, **126**
Coaches. *See also* Teams, medical
    staff, and sports leadership
    case study of resistance to
        psychiatry by, 22–23
    gender issues and, 224, 225–226
    issues in working with, 198, 209–
        212, 246
    scope of sports psychiatry and, 22–
        23
    treatment of common mental
        disorders and, 19
Cocaine, **122, 124**
Cognitive-behavioral therapy, 189–190
Cognitive profiling, 32
Cognitive issues
    stressors and, **54**
    symptoms of concussion and, **143**
Colleges and universities, and
    available resources for athletes,
    195–196. *See also* National
    Collegiate Athletic Association
Commitment, and youth sports
    development, 221, 222
Competitive adversity, **183**
Complex concussions, 142
Complex mental skills, 5–8, 29, 44–50
Computerized cognitive test
    (CogSport), 245
Concentration meditation, 36
Concussion, 17–18, 141–146, 244–245
Confidence, and injury recovery, 130.
    See also Self-confidence
Consciousness, altered states of, 38
Contemplative emotions, and injury
    recovery, **132,** 153–154
Core competencies, in sports
    psychiatry, 2, **3**
Corticotropins, **127**
Crack cocaine, **122**

CTE (chronic traumatic
    encephalopathy), 142
Culture
    competence, and key clinical
        points, 229–230
    definition of in context, 220
    overview of issues in, 219–220,
        227–228
    scope of sports psychiatry and, 23,
        24–26
Cyclobenzaprine, 208

Danazol, **126**
Dehydration, and heat illnesses, 144–
    146
Dehydroepiandrosterone, **126**
Delta-9-tetrahydrocannabinol (THC),
    97, 98
Dental injuries, 144–146
Depression
    common mental disorders in
        sports and, 165, 182–186, 188
    medication management and, 19
    research on postconcussive, 241,
        244
    symptom screening form and, 215
    stress reaction patterns and, 8
Development. *See also* Age
    competence, and key clinical
        points, 229–230
    overview of issues in, 219–220
    scope of sports psychiatry and, 23,
        24–25
    youth sports and, 220–223
Diazepam, 154, 209
Diet. *See* Nutrition
Dihydrotestosterone, 107, **126**
Diphenhydramine, 12, 150
Disappointment, and stress, 8, 9–10
Disulfiram, 160
Diuretics, 94, 106, **128**
Diving, and anxiety, 170
Documentation, of sports psychiatric
    treatment, 206
Dopamine, 81

DSM-IV-TR, 166
Duloxetine, 191
Dysthymia, 21–22, 184, 185

EAPs (employee assistance
    programs), 22
Eating disorders, 18, 166, 179–182,
    216, 241. *See also* Anorexia
    nervosa; Bulimia nervosa
Elbow injuries, 139–140, 148
Electrolytes, and energy regulation,
    71
Emotion(s). *See also* Anger; Negative
    emotions; Reactive emotions
    concussion and, **143**
    injury recovery and, 16, 130, **132,**
        234, 235
    mental preparation and
        competencies in, 30–31
    stress and, 8, **54**
Emotional control, 30, 49–50
Empathy, and emotional
    competencies, 31
Employee assistance programs
    (EAPs), 22
End-of-day routine, and stress
    control, 66
Energy management
    alcohol use and, 94
    alertness, fatigue, and sleep issues
        in, 73–77, 247–248
    basic physiology of energy and,
        69–70
    key clinical points, 83–84
    nutrition and hydration, 70–73
    prevention of chronic fatigue and
        burnout, 77–80
    scope of practice in sports
        psychiatry and, 10–12
    stimulants and, 80–83
Environment, and types of stressors,
    54
Ephedrine, 81, 104, **124**
Epi-dihydrotestosterone, **126**
Epinephrine, 81, **121**

Epitestosterone, **126, 128**
Erythropoiesis-stimulating agents,
    127
Erythropoietin, 108
Escitalopram, 20, 191
Evaluation, of goals, 45. *See also* Self-
    evaluation
Exercise, and awakening routine, 11
Exploration, and youth sports
    development, 221–222
Eye injuries, 144–146

Family
    history of alcohol use in, 93
    involvement of in treatment of
        common mental disorders,
        19, 245
    parent-child conflict and
        achievement pressure in, 24–
        25
Fatigue, and energy regulation, 73,
    75, 77–80, 247–248
Fats, and aerobic metabolic system,
    69–70
FDA (Food and Drug
    Administration), 97, 104
Fear, and injury recovery, 17–18, 157
Focus, and attention shifting, 38–41
Food and Drug Administration
    (FDA), 97, 104
Football. *See also* National Football
    League
    common mental disorders and,
        172–173, 188–189, 190
    energy regulation and, 72–73, 81–
        82
    goal setting and, 5–6
    injury recovery and, 17, 131, 136,
        137, 151–152, 152–153, 156–
        157, 159–160
    insomnia and, 11–12
    mental preparation and, 4–5, 35,
        42
    physicians and medical staff in,
        206

Football *(continued)*
    sleep interference and, 75
    stress control and, 56–57, 61–62,
        63–65
    substance use and, 13, 86, **88–90,**
        100, 103–105
    working with coaches and, 211–
        212
    working with medical staff and,
        208–209
Fractures, and injury recovery, 146–
    147
Frustration, and stress, 8
Fundamentals stage, of youth sports
    development, 222
Furosemide, **128**

Gambling, and impulse control, 173
Gender
    blood alcohol content and, **94**
    eating disorders and, 166
    injury rates and, **131,** 151
    overview of issues in, 224–227
    rates of participation in sports
        and, 224
    scope of sports psychiatry and, 23–
        24
    substance use and, 91, 107
Gene doping, **89**, 107
Generalized anxiety disorder, 20–21,
    170, 188
General managers, of sports teams,
    209
Gestrinone, **126**
Ginseng, **123**
Glucose, 69
Goals and goal setting
    complex mental skills and, 5–6,
        44–45
    soccer and examples of, **46, 205**
Golf, 37, 39, 40, 41, 43, 48–49, 149–150
Golfer's elbow, 140
Grief. *See also* Loss
    mood disorders and, 182–186
    stress and, 58

Growth factors, **89, 127**
Growth hormone, **127**
Gymnastics, 17–18, 158, 170

Hamstring strains, 136–137
Hangovers, and alcohol use, 94
Health. *See also* Injury recovery;
        Medication management; Pain
        control; Physicians; Somatic
        symptoms
    alcohol use and, 95
    anabolic steroids and, 108
    stress and, 55
Heat illnesses, 144–146
Hepatic system, and anabolic
        steroids, 108
Herbal alternatives, to marijuana, 98
Hobbies, and stress control, 65–66
Homophobia, 224
Hormones, and substance use, **89,**
        107, 108, **127**
Hydration, and energy regulation,
        70–73
Hydrocodone, 17, 150, 152
Hypnotic susceptibility/subliminal
        attention, and personality
        profile, 33
Hypomania, 184

Ice hockey, 40, **88–90,** 131, 133
Illegal substances, 91, **122**
Imagery, and visualization, 41–43
Immediate Post-Concussion
        Assessment and Cognitive
        Testing (ImPACT), 142
Impulse control
    anabolic steroids and, 108
    common mental disorders and,
        173–175
Injury-Psychological Readiness to
        Return to Sport (I-PRRS) scale,
        238
Injury recovery. *See also* Pain control
    adjustment disorders and, 166–
        167

common and less severe types of
injuries and, 131–140
emotions and, 16, 130, **132, 153–**
160
evidence for practice and
research, 234–239
future directions in, 239–240
key clinical points, 161
overview of issues in, 129–131
scope of sports psychiatry and, 15–
18
serious, rare, and catastrophic
types of injuries and, 140–153
somatoform disorders and, 187
substance use and, 86
Insomnia. *See also* Sleep
case studies of, 11–12, 17
medications for, 75–76, 190
Insulin and insulin-like growth factor,
127
Intensity regulation, and emotional
control, 49–50
Internalization, of goals, 45
Internal motivation, and emotional
competencies, 30–31
International Society of Sports
Nutrition, 249
International Society for Sports
Psychiatry, 1
I-PRRS (Injury-Psychological
Readiness to Return to Sport),
238
Irritability, and substance use, 100

Jet lag, 247

Key clinical points
developmental and cultural
competence, 229–230
energy regulation, 83–84
evidence base and future
directions, 251–252
injury recovery and pain control,
161
mental disorders, 192–193

mental preparation, 50–51
scope of practice, 26–27
stress recognition and control, 67–
68
substance use and misuse, 110–
111
teams, medical staff, and sports
leadership, 213
Knee injuries, 137–139, 150–152
K2, 98

Lacrosse, 21–22, 59–61, 155–156,
174–175, 202–203
Lactic acid, 69
Lamotrigine, 184
Lateral collateral ligament (LCL),
150–152
Latino culture, 25–26, 227, 228
LCL (lateral collateral ligament),
150–152
Leadership. *See* Teams, medical staff,
and sports leadership
Learning disorders, 175–179
Legal substances, 91
Lesbian, gay, bisexual, and
transgender individuals, 224–
225, 226–227
Lidocaine patch, 138
Life balance
high athletic achievement and, 31
stress control and, 8–9
Life events, and common mental
disorders, 167, 187–188
Life goals, 45
Light therapy, 11, 81
Lisdexamfetamine, 176
Lorazepam, 76, 247
Loss, and transition out of sports
after injury, 159. *See also* Grief
Luteinizing hormone, **127**

Major League Baseball (MLB), 87,
88–90, 195, **236, 237**
Mania, 184
Marijuana, 13–14, 97–100, **119–120**

Masking agents, and banned
    substances, **89**
Medial collateral ligament (MCL),
    138, 150–152
Medial tibial stress syndrome
    (MTSS), 134–136
Medical staff. *See* Teams, medical
    staff, and sports leadership
Medication management. *See also*
    Pain control; Side effects;
    Stimulants
    common mental disorders and,
        19–20, 190–191
    documentation of, 206
    insomnia and sleep disorders, 19,
        75–76, 246–247
Meditation, 36
Melatonin, 247
Mental disorders, common forms of
    in sports. *See also* Adjustment
    disorders; Anxiety and anxiety
    disorders; Attention-deficit
    disorders; Depression; Eating
    disorders; Impulse- and anger-
    control disorders; Mood
    disorders; Obsessive-compulsive
    personality disorder;
    Somatoform disorders
    evidence base for, 240–245
    future directions in, 245
    key clinical points, 192–193
    medication management for, 19–
        20, 190–191
    overview of issues in, 165–166
    psychotherapy for, 189–190
    scope of sports psychiatry and, 18–
        22
Mental health services, and
    utilization rates, 240–241, **242–
    243**
Mental health screening, and
    documentation, 206
Mental preparation
    basic mental skills and, 2, **3,** 4–5,
        29, 33–44

BELIEVE IT acronym and, 31–32
    complex mental skills and, 5–8,
        29, 44–50
    emotional competencies and, 30–
        31
    evidence-based techniques for,
        32–33
    key clinical points, 50–51
Mental stressors, **54**
Methamphetamine, **122, 124**
Methandrostenolone, **126**
Methylphenidate, 19, 21, 81, 86, 105,
    122, 125, 175, 176, 179, 190, 207
Mirtazapine, 247
MLB. *See* Major League Baseball
Modafinil, 81, 105, **122, 125**
Mood disorders, 182–186, 216. *See
    also* Depression
Mood disturbances, and anabolic
    steroids, 108
Mood stabilizers, 184
Motivation
    injury recovery and, 130
    mental preparation and, 43–44
    substance use and, 100
Motivational enhancement therapy,
    189
Motor planning, and brain imaging
    research, 41
MTSS (medial tibial stress
    syndrome), 134–136
Muscle, tendon, and ligament tears,
    147–149
Myostatin function modifiers, **127**

NA (Narcotics Anonymous), 109
Nandrolone, **126**
Narcotics Anonymous (NA), 109
Narrow external focus, 39
Narrow internal focus, 38
Nasal hyperventilation, 35
National Athletic Trainers'
    Association, 244
National Basketball Association
    (NBA), **88–90,** 149, **236**

National Center for Catastrophic Sports Injury Research, 141

National Collegiate Athletic Association (NCAA), **88–90,** 141, 239, 249

National Football League (NFL), 86, 87, **88–90,** 131, 142, 149, **236**

National Hockey League (NHL), **88–90**

National Institute on Drug Abuse, 86

NBA. *See* National Basketball Association

NCAA. *See* National Collegiate Athletic Association

Neck injuries, 144–146

Negative emotions
injury recovery and, 153
mood disorders and, 182, **183**

Neuralgia, and case study, 17

Neurocognitive testing, 33

Neuroendocrinological system, and anabolic steroids, 108

Neurological symptoms, of concussion, **143**

Neurophysiological program, for mental preparation, 33

Neuropsychiatric effects, of anabolic steroids, 108

Neuroticism/subliminal reactivity, and personality profile, 33

NFL. *See* National Football League

NHL (National Hockey League), **88–90**

Nicotine, 64, 80, 81, 102–104, **121, 123**. *See also* Tobacco

Non–rapid eye movement (NREM) sleep, 74

Nonsteroidal anti-inflammatory drugs (NSAIDs), 149, 150

Norandrosterone, **126**

Norepinephrine, 81. *See* Selective norepinephrine reuptake inhibitors

NREM (non–rapid eye movement sleep), 74

NSAIDs (nonsteroidal anti-inflammatory drugs), 149, 150

Nutrition, and energy management, 11, 70–73. *See also* Eating disorders

Nutritional supplement contamination, and banned substances, **89**

Obesity, increase in childhood, 220, 221

Obsessive-compulsive personality disorder, 20–21

Olympics, and drug testing programs, 87

On-site services, for mental health care, 196

Opiates, 13

Osteoarthritis, 149

Over-the-counter (OTC) amphetamine analogs, 104–105, **121**

Owners, of sports teams, 209

Oxcarbazepine, 184

Pain control. *See also* Injury recovery
common mental disorders and, 186–189
emotions and, 154
key clinical points, 161
substance use and, 86
symptom screening form and, 217
working with medical staff and, 208–209

Paralysis, and catastrophic injury, 141–146

Patellar tendonitis, 137–139

Patellofemoral syndrome, 138

Patterned relaxation breathing, 34

PCL (posterior cruciate ligament), 150–152

PCS (postconcussive syndrome), 244–245

Peptide hormones, 108, **127**
Performance anxiety, 165, 169–170, 191
Performance enhancers, and substance use, 86–87, 91, **126–128**
Persistence, and mental preparation, 43–44
Personality conflicts, and working with teams, 202–203
Personality profile, 33
Personalization, of goals, 45
Phenylpropanolamine, **121**
Phobic anxiety, 170
Phosphate system, and energy, 69
Physical cues, and precompetition routine, 48
Physical stressors, **54**
Physicians, and medical staff, 204, 206
Playing in the zone, 38, 39
Plyometric training, 45, 148, 239
POMS (Profile of Mood States), 235, 238
Positive self-talk
  basic mental skills and, 4, 36–38
  high athletic achievement and, 31, 32
Postconcussion Symptom Scale, 245
Postconcussive syndrome (PCS), 244–245
Posterior cruciate ligament (PCL), 150–152
Precompetition anxiety, and case study, 4–5
Precompetition routines
  attention-deficit disorders and, 177
  complex mental skills and, 6, 47–49
Pregabalin, 17
Premature death, and anabolic steroids, 108
Prevention programs, and injury, 238–239

Probenecid, **128**
Proficiency, and youth sports development, 221, 222
Profile of Mood States (POMS), 235, 238
Propranolol, 170, 191
Protein, and energy regulation, 71
Psychiatric services, 196
Psychosis, and marijuana use, 98–100
Psychosomatic disorders, and stress, 55
Psychotherapy, 189–190

Questionnaire for Eating Disorder Diagnoses, 241
Quetiapine, 19, 20–21, 76, 99, 171, 184, 207, 247

Ramelteon, 19, 76, 247
Rapid eye movement (REM) sleep, 74
React, and shifting of attention or focus, 39
Reactive emotions, and injury recovery, **132,** 154
Realism, and goal setting, 45
Reflect, and shifting of attention or focus, 40
Rehabilitation, and injury recovery, 16, 130, 137, 151, 156–157
Relaxation
  attention shifting and focus, 39
  basic mental skills and, 4, 33–36
  stress and reflex system for, 53–54, 58–59
  sustained attention and, 177
Religion, and stress control, 63–64
REM (rapid eye movement) sleep, 74
Repressive/subliminal coping, and personality profile, 33
Rest, ice, compression, and elevation (RICE), 133

Return-to-play phase, of injury recovery, 16, 130, 157–158, 235, **236–237**
RICE (rest, ice, compression, and elevation), 133
Risk factors, for hamstring strains, 136
Risperidone, 100
Road trips, and clinicians, 199
Rotator cuff injuries, 139, 147–148
Running. *See* Track and field

Salbutamol, **127**
Salt, and fluid replacement, 72
Sedatives, 13
Selective androgen receptor modulators, **126**
Selective estrogen receptor modulators, **127**
Selective serotonin reuptake inhibitors (SSRIs), 19, 167, 171, 183, 191
Self-awareness, and emotional competencies, 30
Self-confidence, and pyramid of mental skills, **3, 30, 199.** *See also* Confidence
Self-evaluation, and complex mental skills, 6, 32, 45–47. *See also* Evaluation
Serotonin-norepinephrine reuptake inhibitors (SNRIs), 19, 167, 183, 191
Sertraline, 191, 209
Sexual behavior, and alcohol use, 95
Shin splints, 134–136
Shoulder injuries, 139–140, 147–148, 152–153
Side effects
    of medications for attention-deficit disorders, 177
    of stimulants, 81, 106
Simple concussions, 142
Sleep and sleep disorders. *See also* Insomnia
    alcohol use and, 14, 95

anxiety disorders and, 170–171
circadian rhythm of, 74
common mental disorders and, 18–19
energy regulation and, 73, 74, 75
evidence base for, 246–248
future directions in, 248
medication management for, 19, 246
pain control and, 154
scope of practice in sports psychiatry and, 10–12
sleep apnea and, 75
sleep debt and, 74
stress and, 56–57
symptom screening form and, 216
Smokeless tobacco, 102
SNRIs. *See* Serotonin-norepinephrine reuptake inhibitors
Snuff, 103–104
Soccer
    coaches of, 246
    common mental disorders and, 20–21, 168–169, 185–186
    development and, 223
    energy management and, 70–71
    examples of goals, **46**
    injury recovery and, 133–134, 139, 144
    mental preparation and, 37, 42, 44, 47, 49–50
    narrow external focus and, 39
    stress control and, 9–10, 59, 62–63
    substance use and, 249
    team cohesion and confidence in, 6–8
    team goals and, 203–204, **205**
    training programs and burnout prevention, 77
    working with medical staff and, 206–208
Socialization, and emotional competencies, 31

Social networks, and stress control, 8.
See also Support networks
Softball, 6, 39, 41, 145–146, 180–181,
225–226
Somatic symptoms, and stress
reaction patterns, 8
Somatoform disorders, 19, 186–189
Spice (marijuana substitute), 98
Spine injuries, 144–146
Spirituality, and stress control, 63–64
Spironolactone, **128**
Sports mental health programs, 22
Sports psychiatry. *See also* Coaches;
Culture; Development; Energy
management; Gender; Injury
recovery; Mental disorders;
Mental preparation; Pain
management; Sleep and sleep
disorders; Stress; Substance use
and misuse; Teams, medical
staff, and sports leadership
core competencies in, 2, **3**
development of as practice area, 1
evidence base for practice of, 223
future directions in, 234
key clinical points, 26–27
scope of practice for, 1–26
SSRIs. *See* Selective serotonin
reuptake inhibitors
Stanozolol, **126**
Steroids. *See* Anabolic steroids
Stimulants. *See also* Amphetamines;
Caffeine; Methylphenidate
common mental disorders and,
167–168
effects of on athletic performance,
121–125
energy regulation and, 80–83
stacking of, 13, 15, 104–105
stress control and, 64
substance misuse and, 86, **90**, 100–
106
Stress
basic principles in recognition and
control of, 53–54

breathing patterns and, 34
characteristic response to, 67
definition of, 54
early recognition of symptoms of,
57–58
facts about, 56–57
key clinical points, 67–68
methods for coping with, 59–67
relaxation reflex and, 58–59
scope of sports psychiatry and, 8–
10
sleep disorders and, 75
substance use and, 64–65
support networks and, 60–61
symptoms of common reactions
to, 55, **56**
time management skills and, 62–
63
types of physical and mental
stressors, **54, 57**
Stress control therapy, 189
Substance use and misuse. *See also*
Alcohol use; Anabolic steroids;
Cocaine; Marijuana; Nicotine;
Performance enhancers;
Stimulants
athletes and reasons for, **13, 87**
evidence base for, 248–250
future directions in, 250
key clinical points, 110–111
overview of issues in, 85–92
prescription forms of, 105–106
scope of practice in sports
psychiatry and, 12–15
stress control and, 58, 64–65
symptom screening form and,
217
Sugars, and aerobic metabolic system,
69
Suicide, and steroid use, 86
Support networks. *See also* Social
networks
depression and, 183, 184
injury recovery and, 155
stress control and, 60–61

Surgery, return to play following, 235, **236–237**
Swimming, 246. *See also* Diving
Symptom screening form, 215–217
Synephrine, **121, 124**

Team assistance programs, 195
Teams, medical staff, and sports leadership
  case study on team cohesion and, 6–8
  characteristics of successful teams, 200
  evidence base for, 245–246
  future directions in, 246
  key clinical points, 213
  issues in working with medical staff and athletic trainers, 204–209
  overview of issues in working with, 195–196
  provision of mental health services for teams and, 197–204, **205**
  scope of sports psychiatry and, 22–23
Tennis, 24–25, 37, 40, 65–66, 71–72, 79–80, 109–111, 148–149
Tennis elbow, 140
Testosterone, 107, **126**
Tetrahydrogestrinone, **126**
THC (delta-9-tetrahydrocannabinol), 97, 98
Therapeutic alliance, and mood disorders, 184
Therapeutic use exemptions, for substance use, **90,** 206
Therapeutic writing, 238
Thiazides, **128**
Thinking and thoughts, and stress control, 59–60
Tibolone, **126**
Time management, and stress control, 62–63

Timetable, for completion of goals, 45
Tobacco, 13, 15, 80. *See also* Nicotine; Smokeless tobacco; Snuff
"Tommy John procedure," 148
Topiramate, 152, 207
Track and field, 4–5, 70, 72, 135–136, 170, 171–172, 181–182
Training programs
  burnout prevention and, 77
  stage models of youth sports development and sports-specific, 222–223
Training-to-train stage, of youth sports development, 222
Transition out of sports, after injury, 158–160
Travel
  energy management and, 74
  sleep and, 247
Trazodone, 12, 19, 20, 76, 171, 190, 247, 248
Triamterene, **128**
Trust, and mental health care, 197

Unwinding routine, and sleep, 10
Urine testing programs, for substance use, 87, 248
Utilization rates, for mental health services, 240–241, **242–243**

Varenicline, 102, 103
Venlafaxine, 19, 21, 189, 191
Verbal communication, and learning styles, 178
Verbal cues, and precompetition routine, 48
Videotape self-modeling, 32
Visual cues, and precompetition routine, 48
Visualization, and basic mental skills, 4, 31–32, 41–43
Volleyball, **132, 133**

WADA (World Anti-Doping Agency),
        87, **88–90,** 91
Wakefulness, and energy regulation,
        74, 247–248
Weight gain, and alcohol use, 95
Women's National Basketball
        Association, **236**
World Anti-Doping Agency (WADA),
        87, **88–90,** 91

Youth sports, and developmental
        issues, 220–223

Zeranol, **126**
Zilpaterol, **126**
Zolpidem, 17, 19, 76, 110, 154, 171,
        190, 191, 247, 248
Zopiclone, 247